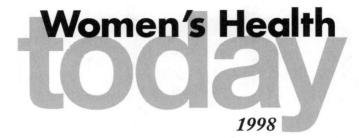

Women's Health today

1998

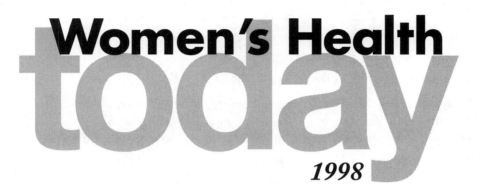

Women's Health today

1998

Over 500 Essential New Tips to Help You:

- Lose Weight
- Fight Fatigue
- Slow Aging
- Outsmart Disease

Featuring "The Hormone Connection"

Edited by Sarí Harrar

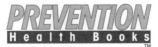

Rodale Press, Inc.
Emmaus, Pennsylvania

Copyright © 1998 by Rodale Press, Inc.
Illustrations copyright © 1997 by Narda Lebo

All rights reserved. No part of this publication may be reproduced or transmitted in any form or by any means, electronic or mechanical, including photocopying, recording, or any other information storage and retrieval system, without the written permission of the publisher.

Prevention Health Books is a trademark of Rodale Press, Inc.

Printed in the United States of America on acid-free ∞, recycled paper ♻

The credits for this book are on page 295.

ISBN 0–87596–511–3 hardcover
ISBN 0–87596–512–1 paperback

Distributed in the book trade by St. Martin's Press

2 4 6 8 10 9 7 5 3   hardcover
2 4 6 8 10 9 7 5 3 1 paperback

──── OUR PURPOSE ────

*"We inspire and enable people to improve
their lives and the world around them."*

Women's Health Today 1998 Editorial Staff

EDITOR: Sarí Harrar

MANAGING EDITOR: Sharon Faelten

CONTRIBUTING WRITERS: Betsy Bates; Lisa Bennett; Pamela Boyer; Marisa Fox; Laura Goldstein; Toby Hanlon; Sarí Harrar; Chantey Jamison; Janis Jibrin, R.D.; Sid Kirchheimer; Yun Lee; Barbara Loecher; Eils Lotozo; Gale Maleskey; Holly McCord, R.D.; Peggy Morgan; Marty Munson; Kristine Napier; Sara Altshul O'Donnell; Cathy Perlmutter; Linda Rao; Maureen SanGiorgio; Caroline Saucer; Steve Schwade; Ed Slaughter; Susan C. Smith; Carol Spiciarich; Maggie Spilner; Laurence Roy Stains; Michele Stanten; Sharon Stocker; Susan Telingator; Margo Trott; Densie Webb, Ph.D.; Teresa A. Yeykal

BOOK RESEARCHER AND PERMISSIONS COORDINATOR: Susan E. Burdick

COPY EDITORS: Kathryn A. Cressman, Karen Neely

ART DIRECTOR: Darlene Schneck

COVER DESIGNER: Lynn N. Gano

BOOK DESIGNERS: Christopher R. Neyen, Christopher Stengel

LAYOUT DESIGNER: Karen Lomax

MANUFACTURING COORDINATOR: Melinda B. Rizzo

OFFICE MANAGER: Roberta Mulliner

OFFICE STAFF: Julie Kehs, Mary Lou Stephen

RODALE HEALTH AND FITNESS BOOKS

VICE-PRESIDENT AND EDITORIAL DIRECTOR: Debora T. Yost

EXECUTIVE EDITOR: Neil Wertheimer

DESIGN AND PRODUCTION DIRECTOR: Michael Ward

RESEARCH MANAGER: Ann Gossy Yermish

COPY MANAGER: Lisa D. Andruscavage

BOOK MANUFACTURING DIRECTOR: Helen Clogston

Board of Advisors for Rodale Women's Health Books

JEAN L. FOURCROY, M.D., PH.D.

Past president of the American Medical Women's Association (AMWA) and past president of the National Council of Women's Health in New York City

CLARITA E. HERRERA, M.D.

Clinical instructor in primary care at the New York Medical College in Valhalla and associate attending physician at Lenox Hill Hospital in New York City

DEBRA RUTH JUDELSON, M.D.

Senior partner with the Cardiovascular Medical Group of Southern California in Beverly Hills, Fellow of the American College of Cardiology, and past president of the American Medical Women's Association (AMWA)

JOANN E. MANSON, M.D.

Associate professor of medicine at Harvard Medical School and co-director of women's health at Brigham and Women's Hospital in Boston

MARY LAKE POLAN, M.D., PH.D.

Professor and chairman of the department of gynecology and obstetrics at Stanford University School of Medicine

ELIZABETH LEE VLIET, M.D.

Founder and medical director of HER Place: Health Enhancement and Renewal for Women and clinical associate professor in the department of family and community medicine at the University of Arizona College of Medicine in Tucson

LILA AMDURSKA WALLIS, M.D.

Clinical professor of medicine at Cornell University Medical College in New York City, past president of the American Medical Women's Association, founding president of the National Council on Women's Health, and director of continuing medical education programs for physicians

CARLA WOLPER, R.D.

Nutritionist and clinical coordinator at the Obesity Research Center at St. Luke's/Roosevelt Hospital Center in New York City

Contents

For the best interactive guide to weight loss, fitness, nutrition, and living a more fulfilling life, visit our Web site at http://www.healthyideas.com.

Introduction

If you've ever endured the teeth-on-edge tension of premenstrual syndrome (PMS) or sweated through a menopausal hot flash, then you've experienced the undeniable influence of female hormones on your body and your emotions. If you've ever taken birth control pills or used hormone-replacement therapy (HRT), then you know that these powerful little substances can be harnessed to do your bidding, but often at a price: uncomfortable or even dangerous side effects.

Yet PMS, birth control, and menopause are not the whole hormone story. Researchers are finding out that a woman's hormones also affect her health in subtle and surprising ways. Dozens of conditions have hormonal links—from heart disease to brittle bones, arthritis to asthma, depression to headaches, and beyond. And what's more exciting, medical science is finally beginning to use those links to improve women's well-being.

That's why this book focuses on hormones. Inside, you'll find expert-endorsed self-care tips to ease hormone-related health conditions. You'll read the latest information on HRT and the Pill—with frank advice about when taking hormones is the best decision, and when it's not. You'll discover new ways to cope with PMS and menopausal discomfort, including natural, hormone-free remedies for menstrual cramps and hot flashes. There's a peek at new hormones that you'll be hearing more about in the future, and an honest look at links between estrogen and cancer.

You'll also find the latest discoveries for outsmarting disease, eating healthy, shedding extra pounds, overcoming fatigue, and looking youthful. As always, we've taken the biggest breakthroughs in women's health research and turned them into empowering hints that you can use, safely and with confidence, to feel wonderful and look great. Gathered from the top researchers and best medical writers in the nation, this is information your doctor may not even know about yet. Now, it's in your hands. Use it in good health!

Sarí Harrar

Sarí Harrar
Editor

part one

Hormones and Your Health

1

the Hormone Connection

Every day, it seems there's another story in the news about the amazing effects of estrogen on the female body. Whether it's maintenance of bone tissue, prevention of heart disease, or even healthier teeth and gums, estrogen is able to work its potent magic on nearly every part of our bodies. Indeed, women have long suspected that changes in our moods and overall health weren't "all in our heads" but were actually caused by shifting hormones.

Thanks to research devoted to women's health, we now know much more about how and why estrogen affects us so profoundly. According to Elizabeth Lee Vliet, M.D., medical director and founder of HER Place women's health centers in Tucson and Dallas and author of the book *Screaming to Be Heard: Hormonal Connections Women Suspect and Doctors Ignore*, among the new understandings about estrogen are these.

❖ **Estrogen is potent.** It normally only takes extremely minute quantities—as little as a billionth of a gram—to affect your body's organs.

❖ **Estrogen does many jobs.** Estrogen receptors are located throughout your body, not just in reproductive organs. From your joints to your hair follicles, from your digestive system to your blood vessels and beyond, there are estrogen receptors ready to grab hold of estrogen as it circulates in your bloodstream. As a result, this hormonal gadabout performs 400 different functions in your body beyond its primary duties of regulating menstruation and supporting pregnancy.

❖ **Estrogen goes to your head.** Estrogen receptors are located in many areas of your brain, including the hypothalamus, which directs your body's many rhythms, such as sexual desire, appetite, and sleep; the limbic system, which controls certain aspects of emotion and behavior; and the cortex, the center of thinking and reasoning.

❖ **Not all estrogens are created equal.** The estrogen receptors are very specific for the primary estrogen (17-beta estradiol) made by the ovaries before menopause. Dr. Vliet points out that if you are experiencing problems while taking estrogen supplements, check with your doctor to make sure that you're taking the type that's right for you.

So why has it taken so long for doctors to acknowledge the importance of hormones? Physicians tend to ignore the intuitive wisdom that women might have about their bodies, says Dr. Vliet. "Once, many health problems were wrongly attributed to women being neurotic. Now, we can conclusively show with science the role hormones play in our bodies."

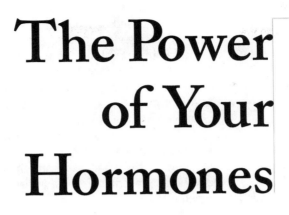

The Power of Your Hormones

W hat does the word *hormones* make you think of? Puberty, pregnancy, and menopause—the three major, hormone-powered transitions in a woman's life?

How about asthma. Varicose veins. Depression. Truth is, a woman's hormones strongly influence physical and emotional health on a daily basis, and have a pronounced effect on many common health conditions, from heart disease to brittle bones, phlebitis to acne.

Here are a dozen conditions affected by a woman's hormones, with self-care advice from women doctors—experts who know about the hormone connection not only from their medical school training and work with women patients but also from personal experience. It's advice you can trust.

Acne: Clear Up Cyclical Blemishes

Some women get occasional pimples or blackheads. Others experience frequent or ongoing bouts of pimples, blackheads, and whiteheads beginning in puberty. Some women notice that acne tends to flare up at their times of ovulation and fade after their menstrual periods begin.

The woman who is most likely to get acne will generally have both overproducing oil glands and a tendency for cells lining the pores to clog. These two

Don't Let Hormones Keep You Awake

Having trouble sleeping? For many women insomnia may be caused by fluctuating levels of two important hormones: estrogen and progesterone.

How? Estrogen influences the production of brain chemicals that keep you alert. Progesterone can make you sleepy. When levels of both are at a low ebb toward the end of your cycle, transient insomnia can be one result, says Suzanne Trupin, M.D., head of the department of obstetrics and gynecology at the University of Illinois College of Medicine at Urbana–Champaign and an expert on the effects of hormones on a woman's body. In fact, insomnia is the number one complaint of women who experience premenstrual syndrome, and it is a common nuisance for postmenopausal women as well.

Insomnia can become a problem for women beginning in their late thirties, when hormone levels begin to drop. If you experience insomnia that seems hormone related on a regular basis, consider getting your levels of follicle-stimulating hormone (FSH) checked. This hormone is one of the first indicators to change as your body begins preparing for menopause.

If FSH levels indicate that you're approaching menopause, you can nudge your hormonal chemistry a little, in a way that may make sleep easier, says Dr. Trupin. She suggests eating fruits and vegetables rich in plant estrogens, such as apples, carrots, cherries, green beans, oats, peas, potatoes, soybeans, and bean sprouts.

HEALTH FLASH

---

problems work together to trap and incubate bacteria on the skin. The result is a chronic formation of whiteheads (called closed comedones), blackheads (open comedones), pimples, and even cysts.

Self-care tip: Wash with benzoyl peroxide liquid. To reduce the number of bacteria that cause acne, gently wash your face with a benzoyl peroxide cleanser or a mild salicylic acid liquid every morning, says Susan C. Taylor, M.D., assistant clinical professor of medicine in the department of dermatology at the University of Pennsylvania School of Medicine in Philadelphia.

If you also break out on your back and chest, use the liquid to wash these areas as well, says D'Anne Kleinsmith, M.D., a staff dermatologist at William Beaumont Hospital in Royal Oak, Michigan.

Then, stick with oil-free moisturizers and cosmetics. Although many women who have acne will never need moisturizers, says Dr. Kleinsmith, there is a small group of women who have oily skin only on their foreheads and noses, while their cheeks and jaws are actually dry. These women should apply moisturizers that are oil-free and noncomedogenic—meaning they won't clog pores—to the dry areas of their faces.

Also, wear only oil-free cosmetics that are labeled "noncomedogenic" or "non-acne-forming" so that they won't clog your pores, says Dr. Kleinsmith.

Asthma: Anticipate Estrogen-Related Attacks

Some women describe asthma as feeling as though they're trying to breathe through a straw. The description fits perfectly because, during an attack, airways in the lungs squeeze shut, making it difficult to draw in air. At the same time, the narrowed airways become inflamed and filled with mucus, stifling the airways still further.

A family history of asthma and exposure to viruses or allergens set the stage for asthma. Women make up about 60 percent of adult asthmatics, but a disproportionate number of them suffer severe attacks and account for 75 percent of hospitalizations for the disease. Research shows a strong link between asthma attacks and the ebb and flow of hormones during the menstrual cycle.

Researchers working in an emergency department—where women suffering severe asthma flare-ups often wind up—divided a 28-day menstrual cycle into four weeklong intervals based on typical fluctuations in estrogen levels, and noted each patient's status upon arrival. A rather dramatic pattern emerged: Nearly half of the 182 women in the study were in one particular 7-day span in their cycles, the perimenstrual stage (the 3 days preceding their periods and the first to fourth days of bleeding).

"What we were seeing was the lungs' response to estrogen withdrawal," says Emil M. Skobeloff, M.D., lead author of the study and clinical assistant professor of emergency medicine at Allegheny University of the Health Sciences in Philadelphia. Estrogen appears to benefit asthmatic lungs in two ways, says Dr. Skobeloff. It calms the destructive overreaction of the immune system to triggers and makes the lungs less twitchy. This protective effect is particularly evident after ovulation, during cycle days 19 to 25, when the levels of the hormone are very high. The lowest number of emergency department visits (only 10 percent) occurred during this interval. It seems that the flare-ups don't stem simply from a difference between high and low estrogen levels but are provoked by the abrupt drop (the steepest plunge on that roller coaster) that occurs in the perimenstrual stage. This hormonal free fall provokes a powerful reaction in the lungs, increasing their sensitivity and reactivity to such an extent that they may not respond as well to normal asthma medications.

Does this mean that doctors will begin prescribing estrogen supplements for asthmatics? That would require much more research, says Dr. Skobeloff. "We'd have to examine the implications for women in their childbearing years and balance those concerns against the threat of out-of-control asthma."

For now, a woman's best bet is to keep a diary of her asthma symptoms according to her menstrual cycle. It should include her medications, activities, twice-a-day peak-flow meter results, and any emergency room visits or hospitalizations. Doing this for a couple of months is likely to highlight any patterns, which can then be brought to the attention of her physician and become part of her monthly plan. For instance, it might be possible for a patient to cut down on medication during good times of the month and increase it when trouble is expected, says Dr. Skobeloff. "We've had women tell us for years that they've had flare-ups connected to their cycles, but we haven't taken it seriously enough. Perhaps now that will change."

Self-care tip: Since estrogen therapy for asthma is not yet available, be prepared in advance for attacks by marking your quick-action inhalers "rescue medicine." Most people being treated for asthma use two different kinds of prescription inhalant drugs: long-acting and short-acting. If you're having an attack, you should use only a short-acting drug such as albuterol (Proventil), metaproterenol (Metaprel), or pirbuterol (Maxair). These drugs kick in almost immediately.

Depression: Understand a Woman's Unique Risks

If you're depressed to the point that you can't sleep, can't concentrate, and don't want to get out of bed, you're not alone. Women are more likely than men to experience mild depression. And more than twice as many women as men have severe depression that can linger for several months, even years, if not treated.

Research suggests that our genes and biochemistry, our circumstances, and our personal history can all, independently or in combination, contribute to depression. Depression is an illness, not a character flaw, and experts say that it runs in families. People with severe depression seem to have a brain chemistry that predisposes them to the condition. Hormonal changes that precede menstruation and follow pregnancy also appear to play some role. Losses, disappointments, difficult relationships, stress, and past traumas can all contribute. So can other illnesses or certain prescription drugs, including oral contraceptives.

Self-care tip: For mild depression, try confiding in friends. When you're depressed, bed may seem like the safest place to be. It isn't. Social isolation contributes to depression, says Carol Landau, Ph.D., clinical professor of psychiatry and human behavior at Brown University School of Medicine in Providence, Rhode Island. If you're down, make a particular point of seeking out and confiding in supportive friends, even if only by phone.

But steer clear of whiners and complainers. Try to avoid relationships that are all work and no gain. While it's important to get out there and be with people, avoid taking on too many responsibilities, since stress feeds depression. By all means, don't let guilt or a sense of obligation keep you in a relationship that you don't enjoy. They'll make you feel worse, not better.

Gum Disease: Scrub It Away before, during, and after Pregnancy

Gum disease—dentists call it gingivitis—moves into your mouth when a sticky film of bacteria, food, and saliva (called plaque) takes up residence at and below your gum line. Left alone, it hardens into tartar, triggering inflammation and infection. If plaque and tartar collect on your teeth, you get cavities. If they sneak into your gums, you get gingivitis.

If you don't take action, you may end up with full-blown periodontitis, where bacteria from the dental plaque actually undermines the bone and structures that hold your teeth in their sockets.

Women are at increased risk of developing gingivitis during pregnancy, says Rita D. Zachariasen, Ph.D., professor of physiology at the University of Texas Health Science Center at Houston. Estrogen and progesterone (female hormones produced by your ovaries) seem to enhance conditions for the growth of certain types of plaque-forming bacteria, while reducing the ability of your gums to heal once gingivitis occurs, according to Dr. Zachariasen. Therefore, you should pay special attention to cleaning your teeth during pregnancy and whenever you are taking oral contraceptives since ovarian hormones are elevated at these times.

Pregnancy's flood of hormones can be especially hard on the gums. Scientists estimate that 60 to 75 percent of pregnant women will have gingivitis, says Dr. Zachariasen. Prevention is the key. Studies show that women who are plaque-free when they enter pregnancy or who start taking oral contraceptives can avoid swollen, bleeding gums, or at least minimize the problem.

*Self-care tip:*Brush and floss. You probably already own the two simplest tools for fighting gingivitis: a toothbrush and dental floss. "Used properly and regularly at least once a day, they can thoroughly remove the plaque and bacteria from your teeth and gums," says Caren Barnes, professor of clinical dentistry at the University of Alabama School of Dentistry in Birmingham.

If you're pregnant, brush and floss thoroughly and carefully after each meal, says Mahvash Navazesh, D.M.D., associate professor and vice-chairman in the department of dental medicine and public health at the University of Southern California School of Dentistry in Los Angeles.

But don't scrub too hard. Plaque is sticky like jelly, not sticky like glue. Attack it with a soft-bristled toothbrush, held at a 45-degree angle to the gum line.

Migraines and More: Avoid Menstrual Cycle Head Pain

What women have suspected for years has been confirmed: Headaches really are worse for women than for men.

Why? The reason may be estrogen. Changes in estrogen levels that govern women's menstrual cycles can cause headaches. Headache-prone women have more head pain during menstruation and ovulation. And those cycle-related throbbers last longer, and are more intense, and, worse yet, are harder to treat, harder to prevent, and harder to eradicate once they've begun.

In addition to hormonal changes, headaches can be caused by triggers that are as individual as women are. Joan Miller, Ph.D., a clinical psychologist in Marietta, Georgia, and author of *Headaches: The Answer Book*, cites several common provokers. They include tension, certain foods (such as lunchmeats or aged cheeses), caffeine withdrawal, skipping meals, environmental factors (pollen or pollution, for example), and certain physical causes, like problems associated with sinuses, vision, teeth, fevers, or head traumas.

Self-care tip: For occasional headaches, Sandra McLanahan, M.D., executive medical director of the Integral Health Center in Buckingham, Virginia, recommends taking the herb feverfew. "Research on feverfew suggests that it can be effective as a headache remedy. I've used it with success for patients with headaches," she says. "I recommend taking two feverfew capsules (available at health food stores) three times a day until your headache is gone." Studies indicate that feverfew has anti-inflammatory properties, which is why it might be particularly effective for migraine headaches. (For more ways to stop a migraine or tension headache before it starts, see chapter 20.)

Osteoporosis: Outwit Hormonal Bone Robbers

The earlier you take action against osteoporosis, the better. This disease could easily become yesterday's news if, starting now, you eat calcium-rich foods and engage in regular weight-bearing exercise.

"Osteoporosis is 100 percent preventable," says Susan Ward, M.D., clinical assistant professor of medicine at Jefferson Medical College of Thomas Jefferson University and associate director of the Jefferson Osteoporosis Center at Thomas Jefferson University Hospital, both in Philadelphia. Women's bodies were originally designed to not last much past menopause, when estrogen production slows and finally ceases, according to Dr. Ward. The lack of estrogen triggers an increase in bone resorption, or bone loss.

Self-care tip: Bone up on calcium. Premenopausal women need at least 1,000 milligrams of calcium a day, says Doris Gorka Bartuska, M.D., director of endocrinology, diabetes, and metabolism clinical services at Allegheny University of the Health Sciences. Once past menopause, women should be getting 1,200 to 1,500 milligrams a day, she says.

The best sources of calcium? Low-fat dairy products. Topping the list are nonfat yogurt (1 cup has 452 milligrams), skim milk (1 cup has 302 milligrams), and part-skim mozzarella cheese (1 ounce has 181 milligrams). Of course, taking calcium carbonate, calcium gluconate, or other forms of calcium supplements is the easist way to ensure that you get what you need each and every day of the week. (For more ways to prevent osteoporosis, see chapter 14.)

Panic Attacks: Outsmart Progesterone

As debilitating as they are unpredictable, panic attacks are relatively common. They happen to perfectly reasonable people, like you. And for some women they're more likely to strike during the last week of the menstrual cycle, when levels of the hormone progesterone fluctuate.

"A large number of adults have had panic attacks at some time in their lives," says Irene S. Vogel, Ph.D., a psychologist and director of Vogel Psychology Associates in the Washington, D.C., metropolitan area. "Some people never have more than one or two and don't even know that they've had one." They may blame their symptoms on something else, such as drinking too much coffee.

We're all more likely to have panic attacks during periods of stress. But some of us seem to inherit a vulnerability to attacks, say researchers, since the attacks appear to run in families. For reasons that scientists don't completely understand, panic attacks are more common in women than men.

Self-care tip: Talk yourself out of it. "Tell yourself, 'Okay, I'm having a panic attack. I know that I'm not having a heart attack or dying or going crazy. This won't last long. It will pass. I'll get through it,'" says Dr. Vogel. This self-talk, part of an approach called cognitive behavioral therapy, should take the edge off your anxiety, and your symptoms should start to fade.

While you're reminding yourself that you're going to be fine, try deep breathing or some other relaxation technique, like progressive relaxation, adds

Dr. Vogel. Relaxation helps diminish symptoms, end attacks, and lower the odds of future attacks.

Phlebitis: Relief When Pregnancy and the Pill Raise Risks

Simply translated, phlebitis means that the veins in your legs—those closest to the surface—are inflamed. A variation called deep-vein phlebitis is more serious, says Lenise Banse, M.D., a dermatologist and vein expert at the Northeast Family Dermatology Center in Clinton Township, Michigan. Deep-vein phlebitis affects veins buried deeper and is usually caused by a clot in the affected veins.

Genetics, smoking, and varicose veins put women at risk for phlebitis, be it mild or serious, says Toby Shaw, M.D., associate professor of dermatology at Allegheny University of the Health Sciences. "Also, if phlebitis runs in your family, birth control pills add to your risk since they can promote blood coagulation, and a clot is coagulated blood."

The hormone connection? Since 80 to 90 percent of people with phlebitis are women—and since phlebitis risk rises during pregnancy, when a woman's body unleashes a torrent of hormones—experts think that female hormones are somehow involved. As yet, they haven't uncovered the precise link.

Serious, deep-vein phlebitis is usually treated in a hospital with clot-busting medication. Women with superficial phlebitis, however, can try using self-care techniques to alleviate the redness, itching, pain, and swelling that results from inflammation.

Self-care tip: For immediate relief, Dr. Shaw recommends cool compresses made with Domeboro astringent solution, sold at drugstores. Empty one packet of powder into a basin filled with cool water, mix, then wet a clean washcloth in the solution. Wring out the washcloth and apply it to the inflamed area, she says.

Snoring: Silence Night Noises Caused by Low Estrogen

There once was a woman in Davis, California, who snored so loudly that a neighbor had her arrested in the middle of the night under the city's new anti-noise statute.

"We think of snoring as being normal and sometimes even cute," says Kristyna M. Hartse, Ph.D., associate professor of psychiatry, human behavior, and otolaryngology at St. Louis University School of Medicine and director of the Sleep Disorders Center at St. Louis University Health Sciences Center. "But there's nothing normal or cute about it."

And while men are more frequently dragged by their wives to doctors' offices for snoring treatments, women may snore just as often, experts say. Among the reasons women snore are low estrogen, having had a hysterectomy, or being postmenopausal. Why? Experts suspect that a lack of estrogen makes muscles more relaxed—including the muscles in the airway running from the nose to the voice box. Flabby muscles and tissue vibrate, creating the snorts that keep sleep at bay.

Self-care tip: Sleep on your side. "Snoring is usually worse when you sleep on your back," says Laurel Wiegand, M.D., associate professor of medicine in the division of pulmonary and critical-care medicine at Pennsylvania State University College of Medicine in Hershey. So try to sleep on your side or stomach.

To aid these antisnoring positions, sew a tennis ball into the back of your pajama top or nightgown. That way sleeping on your back will be too uncomfortable, and you'll automatically roll to your side or stomach.

Stress: Calm Female Stress Hormones

"Women are probably under more stress than ever before," says Camille Lloyd, Ph.D., professor in the department of psychiatry and behavioral sciences at the University of Texas Medical School at Houston. At work we have more responsibility but less job security. We're juggling demands made by our bosses, our kids, and our spouses. Our relationships are less secure—consider the divorce rate. And we're less likely to have extended family and lifelong friends to lean on, since everyone relocates so often, says Dr. Lloyd.

Add it up, and too much responsibility, too little control, and too few resources amount to too much stress, says Dr. Lloyd. Plus, women tend to absorb the stress felt by those who are close to them, compounding the problem.

"Research shows that women are more sensitive to the stress of people close to them," continues Dr. Lloyd. "If their husbands are under stress or their kids are under stress, they experience more stress themselves."

In addition, women's unique hormonal makeup enhances our reactions to stress. We have naturally higher levels of the hormone cortisol, which maintains the turbo-charged, fight-or-flight mode we enter when stress strikes. And high levels of progesterone in the days before our menstrual periods begin have a similar effect. This sensitivity to stress once gave women a survival advantage. But our stress-response system can't tell the difference between a deadline-intense project at work, an injured child at home, and a marauding mammoth.

That's not healthy. Studies suggest that your body's physiological reaction to high levels of sustained stress—increased blood pressure, an outpouring of adrenaline, and other changes—makes you more susceptible to serious disorders like heart disease. You may also find yourself depressed, irritable, despairing, or edgy, says Sharon Greenburg, Ph.D., a clinical psychologist in private practice in Chicago. Or you may find that you can't sleep, concentrate, or remember things.

Self-care tip: Take a moment to relax. Stress is most damaging if it's unrelenting. Even a few moments of relaxation can help considerably, says Susan Heitler, Ph.D., a clinical psychologist in Denver and creator of the audiotape *Anxiety: Friend or Foe?*

"Take mini-breaks," she says. "If you're at work and you start feeling stressed, get up and stretch or talk to a co-worker for a couple of minutes." If you're at home, take a break in a quiet room. Then give yourself a longer break at least once every day. Read a magazine, go for a walk, or simply luxuriate in doing nothing at all.

Varicose Veins: Soothe the Ache after Pregnancy or Anytime

If you're tired of the throbbing ache of varicose veins, take heart. You can ease the agony.

"Varicose veins are like a pair of stretched-out panty hose," says Dr. Banse. They're stretched and baggy—the veins, not the hose—because the valves in your legs just aren't doing their job. Blood, which should flow toward the heart, ends up flowing back toward your feet, putting pressure on veins.

What puts you at risk? "Genetics, mostly," says Dr. Shaw. If your mother had varicose veins, you probably have them, too. But estrogen production, pregnancy, being constantly on your feet, and aging play a part as well.

Self-care tip: Pull on a pair of support panty hose, says Dr. Banse. This will keep your veins tight so they can't stretch out. Tights are even better, she adds, especially the Lycra exercise tights that go so well with long tunics and sweaters.

Or enlist the support of compression hose. "If you're on your feet all day, buy stockings that provide 20 to 30 millimeters of pressure," says Dr. Shaw. The numbers are on the package. Look for them at your local drugstore.

And pull those panty hose on while you're still in bed. Whether you use regular support hose or compression support hose, "keep the stockings by your bed at night and put them on before you get out of bed in the morning, before gravity pulls blood through the valves to pool," says Dr. Shaw.

Yeast Infections: Cut the Birth Control Link

Sooner or later, most women get yeast infections, says Janet McCombs, Pharm.D., clinical assistant professor at the University of Georgia College of Pharmacy in Athens. And it's easy to see why, say other women doctors.

The vagina is a delicate ecosystem that is easily unbalanced, says May M. Wakamatsu, M.D., instructor of obstetrics and gynecology and reproductive biology at Harvard Medical School. A variety of microscopic organisms normally reside as peaceful neighbors in the vagina, among them the yeastlike fungus *Candida albicans*. But taking antibiotics for other conditions can kill off certain flora and leave Candida to go on a rampage. This results in Candida vaginitis, or a yeast infection, the second most common form of vaginitis experienced by women.

Yeast cells seem to have their own estrogen receptors, and that stimulation of those receptors by hormones in the Pill may cause yeast to grow. Yeast infections may be 20 percent more likely in women taking birth control pills.

Self-care tip: Start with a nonprescription remedy. "For the average yeast infection, over-the-counter antiyeast suppositories and creams (such as Gyne-Lotrimin or Monistat 7) are very effective," says Kathleen McIntyre-Seltman, M.D., professor of medicine in the department of obstetrics and gynecology at the University of Pittsburgh School of Medicine. And use suppositories and creams at bedtime, according to the package directions.

2 Love, Lust, and Your Hormones

If you've ever seen a female cat in heat, rolling around lasciviously, you know how powerfully hormones affect animals' sexual behavior. But do hormones affect the sex drive in humans? "Like other animals, we come under the spell of our hormones—but what sets us apart is that we're not slaves to them," says Theresa L. Crenshaw, M.D., a specialist in sexual medicine from San Diego and author of *The Alchemy of Love and Lust*. Our emotions, maturity, and family and social influences also have a big effect on our sexual and romantic urges.

Still, she emphasizes, "There is no question that hormones distinctly affect the intensity of the sexuality and emotions that women and men experience. And the fluctuations in those hormones during our lives influence the way we relate to lovers at different ages." Dr. Crenshaw shared with us her theories on how hormones affect love and lust in heterosexual relationships throughout our lives.

Your Teen Years: "Hormonal Madness"

This is a time of hormonal madness, says Dr. Crenshaw. Estrogen, the female hormone, surges in girls. How does it affect our sex drives? Estrogen gives us a "receptive" sexuality—a desire for foreplay, penetration, touching, love, and approval, though not a strong desire toward orgasm. Oxytocin, a hormonelike

For Natural Lubrication, Say "Open Sesame"

Here's a simple kitchen-cabinet remedy for beating the vaginal dryness that often comes with hormonal changes in your forties, fifties, sixties, or beyond. This at-home technique could make sexual intimacy—and daily living—more comfortable and enjoyable during this time of your life.

"Some women report having great success using sesame oil to relieve vaginal dryness," says Adriane Fugh-Berman, M.D., former head of field investigations for the Office of Alternative Medicine at the National Institutes of Health in Bethesda, Maryland. Before you go to bed, soak a quilted cotton cosmetic square in sesame oil, squeeze out the excess oil, insert it into the vagina, and leave it in overnight. Remove the square the next morning.

Repeat every day for a week, then once a week for as long as necessary. "The sesame oil is supposed to induce an estrogen-like effect," says Dr. Fugh-Berman.

---

chemical that increases sensitivity to and desire for touch, also plays an important role in adolescent girls.

What about those girls who love intercourse and climax easily? All females possess low levels of testosterone, while all males have small quantities of estrogen. Dr. Crenshaw theorizes that sexually aggressive girls probably have higher-than-average testosterone levels or lower-than-average social constraints.

In teenage boys, testosterone, the "macho hormone," is at its height. It's responsible for the wet dreams and obsessions with sexual encounters that are typical of many young men. Although boys have oxytocin just like girls, the influence of testosterone tends to overwhelm their desire for touching.

The differences in the needs of the sexes are so great at this time that most teen romances are tempestuous and short-lived. Occasionally, however, "love comes to the rescue, bridging differences," points out Dr. Crenshaw. Love, she continues, is the "great equalizer" between couples of all ages.

Your Twenties: Estrogen at Its Peak

At this age, most women and men continue to be emotionally and sexually incompatible—although, as with teenagers, there are always exceptions. The one thing twentysomething males and females do have in common: They're at the apex of their physical desirability. One of the reasons for this is that the level of dehydroepiandrosterone (DHEA), a sex hormone that both women and men possess in equal amounts, peaks in both sexes between the ages of 25 and 30. This hormone increases sex drive and produces pheromones, our unique scent-prints that are important in erotic attraction. (DHEA has also garnered a great deal of attention in the media recently because some scientists believe that supplements have an "anti-aging effect." But so far, the research is inconclusive.)

Men at this age are "somewhat less focused on orgasm than in adolescence, but not by much." Due to experience, twentysomething males are usually much more concerned with pleasing their lovers; in fact, "some become so preoccupied with satisfying women that they become emotionally disconnected from the sex act." But, due to testosterone's tyranny, men are still attracted to "uncomplicated couplings such as one-night stands and casual affairs."

Estrogen is at its height in women now; we're more fertile and sexually oriented. Women still tend to be more concerned, however, with getting male love and approval than with satisfying their own sensual needs, says Dr. Crenshaw, who believes that estrogen contributes to an increased desire for permanent relationships and children as well.

Your Thirties: Better Orgasms

Subtle changes occur in women's hormonal balances during this decade. Our estrogen levels decline slightly, making testosterone's influence more noticeable. As a result, a thirtysomething woman is usually able to reach orgasm more quickly and may become multiorgasmic (if she wasn't before). Our greater levels of experience and maturity team with these chemical changes to make us more sexually assertive and concerned with our own pleasure.

Ironically, most men start to become more relationship-oriented in their thirties, although scientists don't know whether this is due to hormonal shifts or to social and psychological forces. At any rate, monogamy usually becomes more appealing to men during this time.

Your Forties: Secure and Self-Reliant

This is the first time that biological forces are no longer so dramatically dividing men and women. Men at this age are less obsessed with reaching orgasm and value communication and touching more, due to continuing declines in testosterone and increases in emotional maturity. They last longer before climaxing, too, thanks to hormonal influences and experience.

Women's estrogen levels drop farther, leaving relatively higher testosterone levels that help us shift our focus to orgasm. We have probably overcome sexual inhibitions by this time and are more secure and self-reliant.

Your Fifties: The Compatibility Decade

By this point, says Dr. Crenshaw, "men and women are more perfectly matched, biologically and psychologically, than they ever have been (assuming that they are healthy)." A fiftysomething man who is emotionally mature can be a terrific lover because of his experience, his enjoyment of foreplay and cuddling, and further declines in testosterone. Likewise, because of confidence and maturity, women are more likely to initiate sex and to be innovative sex partners.

The one potential drawback: Some women undergoing menopause without hormone-replacement therapy (HRT) have such severe symptoms, such as depression and lack of vaginal lubrication, that their sex lives suffer. This can usually be remedied, but you should always consult a physician before attempting to treat any menopausal symptoms.

Many men experience a "viropause" that is similar to (but usually not as dramatic as) menopause. Caused by declines in testosterone levels, the side effects include depression and anxiety, loss of energy and competitiveness, and lack of desire and sexual stamina. These symptoms—which can cause great distress—can usually be alleviated with testosterone therapy, although many physicians ignore this problem.

Your Sixties and Beyond: The Importance of Touch

The positive relationship trends of the fifties continue. DHEA is still decreasing in both sexes. Estrogen drops even farther in women (unless they're on HRT), and testosterone becomes more influential now, sometimes even resulting in a deeper voice and faint mustache. Testosterone diminishes in men, bringing estrogen's influence to the forefront (some men even develop breasts). Because of this decline in testosterone, fantasy stimulation is less effective, and men may need more mechanical stimulation in order to get an erection. Women may lubricate a bit less (because of lower estrogen levels) but continue to be as responsive as before.

Barring debilitating disease, there is no reason that men and women can't enjoy sex for the rest of their lives. They may not be able to have intercourse as frequently if medical or pharmacological problems intervene, but they can enjoy oral sex and cuddling as well as true communication and sharing.

③ Triumph over Hell Week

I t's not all in your head. You really do want to hang a "Do Not Disturb" sign around your neck the week before your period. You really do get cramps that make you want to crawl pitifully into bed. Your cravings for chocolate are utterly overwhelming. And just where did that bag of potato chips go, anyway?

But you've resolved not to give in to menstrual or premenstrual discomfort. Your job, your kids, and your life itself are just too demanding. Besides, you're not the type to hide under the covers for days on end. So what's a real woman, beset with the very real symptoms of premenstrual syndrome (PMS), cramps, and other menstrual challenges to do? For the best advice that advocates of natural healing have to offer, read on.

PMS and the Progesterone Connection

PMS is so ubiquitous among women that one British doctor calls it the world's most common disease. "Sixty to 80 percent of all women have premenstrual changes that are mildly annoying," says Kathleen Ulman, Ph.D., staff psychologist at Women's Health Associates at Massachusetts General Hospital in Boston and instructor in the department of psychiatry at Harvard Medical School. "About 3 to 5 percent of women have severely disruptive symptoms like

Relieve Cramps with Fish Oil

A daily dose of fish oil may dramatically ease menstrual distress, according to the first-ever study of fish oil's effect on women's monthly cramps.

When 37 young women took fish oil capsules twice a day for two months, they had a marked improvement in cramps and other menstrual symptoms, including nausea and headaches, according to researchers at Children's Hospital in Cincinnati, Ohio.

The women were also able to cut their usual doses of cramp-relieving ibuprofen in half. This was not the case when they spent two months taking a placebo capsule—women saw little change in symptoms or ibuprofen use. The results are thought to apply to older women as well.

Researchers suspect that the body uses the fatty acids in fish oil, called omega-3 fatty acids, in place of omega-6 fatty acids found naturally in the body. When the body tries to build prostaglandins, the prime substances believed to cause cramps, from the omega-3 fatty acids, cramps are much weaker.

Women in the study took 1.8 grams of omega-3 fatty acids a day in capsule form. Could you get that amount of fish oil—and the benefits—in fillet form?

Maybe, says Frank M. Biro, M.D., study author and associate professor of clinical pediatrics at Children's Hospital. But every day, you'd have to eat 4 to 6 ounces of some kind of fish, such as salmon or sardines, that is high in omega-3 fatty acids.

profound depression, flashes of rage, and unremitting exhaustion."

What causes PMS? No one, not even British physician Katharina Dalton, who coined the phrase "premenstrual syndrome" back in 1953, is entirely certain. What scientists do know, though, is that female reproductive hormones, specifically progesterone, probably play a significant role.

Dr. Dalton notes that there are more than 150 recognized symptoms of PMS that affect teenage girls, menopausal women, and everyone in between. The good news, she says, is that nearly 100 different treatment options exist to help relieve PMS.

Medical options include daily doses of synthetic hormones or drugs such as the antidepressant fluoxetine hydrochloride (Prozac) and the anti-anxiety drug alprazolam (Xanax). For women looking for a natural, nondrug route, alternative practitioners offer the following advice.

Drug-Free Relief

"We know that stress-management techniques can alleviate many PMS symptoms," says Dr. Ulman, who runs PMS stress-management groups. Here are the strategies that she has found to be the most successful.

Keep a menstrual journal. In a small notebook note your mood and physical symptoms for each day of your cycle. Many women with PMS find that stresses that they would otherwise tolerate well (or ignore) at other times of the month seem to make PMS worse.

"When you learn what triggers your symptoms and what your bad days may be, you'll know when you have to take it easy, go home a little early, and save the hard stuff for next week," says Dr. Ulman.

Test-drive a calming discipline. It doesn't matter which relaxation technique you choose, as long as it works for you, says Dr. Ulman. "Deep breathing, yoga, and meditation are all excellent for PMS," she says.

Take a walk. "I have some very exciting news for women with PMS," reports Mary Jane DeSouza, Ph.D., an exercise physiologist with the Center for Fertility and Reproductive Endocrinology at New Britain General Hospital in Connecticut. Dr. DeSouza conducted a study of 45 sedentary women. She found that women who took easy to moderately brisk ½-hour walks three or four times a week experienced significant improvements in PMS symptoms.

Food, Vitamin, and Herbal Therapies That Work

Making a few dietary changes could ease or even end your premenstrual syndrome and other menstrual problems, says Loretta Mears, D.C., a chiropractor and certified clinical nutritionist in private practice in New York City. "For many of the women that I work with, PMS problems are usually related, in one way or another, to nutritional problems." Here's what she and other nutritional experts recommend.

Eat small meals—frequently. "I find that eating five small meals a day, with a good balance of complex carbohydrates and a moderate amount of protein, helps many women," says Dr. Ulman. (Half of a turkey sandwich on wholewheat bread is a good example of such a meal.)

The combination of carbohydrates and protein helps buffer mood swings, says Diana Taylor, R.N., Ph.D., director of the Perimenstrual Symptom Management Research Program at the University of California School of Nursing in San Francisco. "What doesn't help is going for hours without eating and then grabbing a candy bar," she says. Simple sugars, like candy, soft drinks, juice drinks, cookies, and ice cream, cause your body to release additional insulin, which can cause a low-blood-sugar rebound effect, sometimes resulting in fatigue and irritability, according to Dr. Taylor.

Hydrotherapy: Soak Away Menstrual Distress

Therapeutic use of water is a simple, time-tested treatment that works especially well for menstrual cramps. "The soothing effect of lying in a tub of very warm water helps relax tense uterine muscles, so that's why it helps your cramps," says Irene von Estorff, M.D., assistant professor of rehabilitation medicine at New York Hospital–Cornell University Medical College in New York City.

"Instead of a nice hot bath, however, you could use another, more portable variation on hydrotherapy when you have cramps—a moist hot pack," Dr. von Estorff suggests. Making your own moist heating pad is simple, she says. Dampen a terry cloth towel in hot (not boiling) water, wring it out so that it's not dripping, and place it over your crampy lower abdomen. Lie still, relax, and let it cool naturally. Repeat as necessary.

Skip the java. Studies have shown that as little as one cup of coffee a day can increase the tension and anxiety symptoms of PMS. Even decaffeinated beverages can contain enough caffeine to stimulate symptoms in sensitive women.

To avoid withdrawal headaches (not unusual in coffee drinkers who try to quit), gradually replace caffeine by substituting decaffeinated versions of your favorite beverages, whether coffee, tea, or cola, over a couple of weeks, recommends Dr. Taylor.

Pump some iron. Inadequate iron intake may cause excessive menstrual bleeding, according to Linda Ojeda, Ph.D., author of *Menopause without Medicine*. Excessive bleeding, in turn, can lead to iron-deficiency anemia, which can cause fatigue. Dr. Ojeda and others recommend that women with heavy periods eat iron-rich foods to prevent iron deficiency.

The most efficiently absorbed iron, called heme iron, is supplied by foods such as red meat, liver, egg yolks, and fish. If you're watching your intake of fat and cholesterol, a multivitamin/mineral supplement with iron is a sound alternative, Dr. Ojeda says. Vegetarians who get nonheme iron from grains, beans, and dried fruit must also take vitamin C to enhance absorption, she says.

Get raspberry for relief. "Raspberry leaves (the botanical name is *Rubus idaeus*) contain fragrine, a specific constituent that tones the uterus and helps ease cramping," says Kathleen Maier, a physician's assistant and herbalist who founded the Dreamtime Center for Herbal Studies in Flint Hill, Virginia, and who is a former advisor on botanical medicine to the National Institutes of Health in Bethesda, Maryland. Maier recommends brewing a strong cup or two of raspberry-leaf tea, available at most health food stores, for cramp relief.

Try the "mothering" herb. "When you want a good mother herb, motherwort's wonderful," says Maier. "I use 10 to 15 drops of motherwort (*Leonurus* *cardiaca*) tincture (a concentrated herb extract that you can add to water, juice, or tea) for menstrual cramps at midcycle, or ovulation time, daily until bleeding starts. Most women see a noticeable improvement in their cramps after one month, but I'd say that, generally, it takes three to four cycles to establish a difference."

Quell cramps with black cohosh. "Black cohosh is an antispasmodic—it quells muscle spasms, especially in the uterus," says Maier. "It relaxes the uterus and decreases cramps. But I use it in general relaxation formulas when there's also shoulder tension." The botanical name for black cohosh is *Cimicifuga racemosa*.

Get regular with Vitex tincture. Vitex (*Vitex agnus-castus*) has long been used in European herbal medicine. It is believed to inhibit the secretion of the peptide hormone prolactin by the pituitary gland. For irregular menstrual periods, take a dropperful in a small glass of water two or three times a day for six to eight weeks after every irregular period, suggests Susun S. Weed, herbalist and teacher from Woodstock, New York, and author of the *Wise Woman* book series on herbs. For heavy bleeding or flooding, take 25 drops two to three times daily for several months.

Control heavy bleeding with lady's-mantle. In tincture form, lady's-mantle (*Alchemilla vulgaris*) controlled heavy menstrual bleeding or episodes of menstrual flooding in virtually all of the approximately 300 women who participated in a clinical test, says Weed. When taken after heavy bleeding began, lady's-mantle took three to five days to be effective. When taken one to two weeks before menstruation, lady's-mantle prevented heavy bleeding. Weed recommends taking 5 to 10 drops of the fresh plant tincture in a beverage three times daily for up to two weeks out of the month.

More pain control with crampbark and valerian. "Heavy bleeding accompanied by nasty cramps responds well to a blend of 2 parts crampbark tincture mixed with 1 part valerian tincture," says Rosemary Gladstar, author of *Herbal Healing for Women*. The botanical name for crampbark is *Viburnum trilobum*, and for valerian, *Valeriana officinalis*.

Prelude to the Change

Julie is an investment consultant; Elaine is a fashion designer with her own boutique; Deanna works with learning-disabled children. (All asked that we not use their last names.) These three women, all in their forties, also have in common an array of puzzling symptoms and a series of frustrating visits to their gynecologists.

For Julie the problem began as a sudden, heavy period. "I bled off and on for almost two weeks. It seemed like I had to change tampons every hour. I was really frightened," she recalls.

Elaine experienced a decided drop in libido. "That lusty feeling I had in my thirties and early forties just died. I didn't have the same erotic feelings and intense orgasms," she says.

Deanna's symptoms were more extreme. "I thought I was losing my mind," she says. "I was anxious; I couldn't concentrate. The memory loss was most frightening, though. I had to be constantly talking to myself to keep myself on track."

All were told by their respective doctors that their symptoms were probably hormonal (not one physician said the word "premenopausal"). Julie is putting up with heavier periods for now. Elaine is taking the Pill to help regulate her cycle. Deanna insisted on having her estrogen level tested; it turned out to be almost nil. After starting hormone-replacement therapy (HRT), she reports that her mental fog has lifted. The experience left each wondering, "What's

Checking women's estrogen levels—with blood tests or newer, more accurate saliva tests—may help pinpoint where they are in the slow, hormonal shift that leads up to and through menopause. Such tests can also show how their bodies are adapting to hormone-replacement therapy (HRT). But do you need regular hormone tests? Gynecologists and health insurance companies debate the merits of testing a woman's estrogen levels regularly during menopause.

Women who have irregular periods, who experience hot flashes yet still have menstrual periods, who have very heavy bleeding that may require a hysterectomy, or who have postmenopausal bleeding and aren't taking HRT are all good candidates for estrogen testing, says Loren Greene, M.D., an endocrinologist and clinical associate professor of medicine at New York University School of Medicine in New York City. A screening will show whether premenopausal changes, called perimenopause, are the cause, and can help a doctor decide how to treat the problem, she says. Sometimes a biopsy of the lining of the uterus or an ultrasound to determine the thickness of the uterine wall is helpful to see the effects of estrogen, says Dr. Greene. Pap smears can be used to check estrogen levels, although they provide only a rough indication.

Repeated testing for women who are taking hormone-replacement therapy is not usually necessary, Dr. Greene notes. These tests don't provide the kind of information that helps tailor a hormone-replacement regimen to your particular needs, she says. Deciding on the right dose and form of hormone therapy requires something more basic: straightforward talk between a woman and her doctor about her unique symptoms, her health history, and her lifestyle—things a blood or saliva test won't reveal.

happening to me?" Little did these women know that their agonies could be summed up in one word: perimenopause.

All in Your Hormones, Not in Your Head

The term *perimenopause* (literally "around menopause") is fairly new, and its definition hinges largely on how scientists define menopause. "We can say for sure that a woman is in menopause after she's had no periods for 12 months," says Sherry S. Sherman, Ph.D., director of the endocrine and musculoskeletal branch of the geriatrics program at the National Institute on Aging in Bethesda, Maryland. "But right now, we can't tell women exactly when perimenopause starts or how long it lasts." Given that over the next two decades an estimated 40 million American women will go through menopause, more research is clearly needed. "Women are getting hot flashes even though they are having periods. It's disturbing to them," says Dr. Sherman. Many of the symptoms once labeled menopausal may turn out to be perimenopausal.

Just as puberty is a gradual process leading up to a girl's first period, perimenopause begins a few years before menopause, around age 47. Some women may have symptoms even earlier. The average age at menopause is 51, although it can occur earlier in women who've had chemotherapy or hysterectomies.

"You can pick up the first hormonal signs of perimenopause from around age 35, when fertility starts to decline," says Wulf H. Utian, M.D., chairman of reproductive biology at Case Western Reserve University in Cleveland and executive director of the North American Menopause Society. Even though a woman may still ovulate, her eggs die off at a faster rate.

During a woman's forties, the egg-producing follicles in her ovaries become resistant to follicle-stimulating hormone (FSH), which normally sparks ovulation. In a desperate bid to stimulate the follicles to release eggs, the pituitary gland churns out extra FSH, causing spikes in estrogen levels. At the same time, progesterone, one hormone that triggers menstruation, is produced sporadically. So instead of a progressive decline in hormones, there's a rollercoaster effect, which is what causes perimenopausal symptoms.

Coping with Unexpected Bleeding

The most common symptom of perimenopause is irregular bleeding, experienced by as many as 70 percent of women in their forties. "Estrogen keeps building up the endometrial lining of the uterus, but if a woman doesn't ovulate, there's no progesterone to trigger menstruation," says Nanette F. Santoro, M.D., assistant professor and director of reproductive endocrinology in the department of obstetrics and gynecology at the University of Medicine and Dentistry of New Jersey–New Jersey Medical School in Newark. The endometrium may build up to such an extent that when a woman finally does get her period, the flow is quite heavy (as in Julie's case). Midcycle spotting may also occur, or periods may stop and start again.

Because overgrowth of the endometrium can set the stage for uterine cancer, any irregular bleeding must be checked out. Like Julie, many women undergo an endometrial biopsy or a dilation and curettage (a D and C, the surgical scraping of the uterine lining). "The biopsy was painful, and I had to wait for the results, which was very anxiety provoking," Julie says. "And I still have the bleeding. But I'll have to live with it because I have a family history of breast cancer, so I don't want to take hormones." (Taking estrogen may slightly increase a woman's risk of breast cancer.)

Others can bypass the biopsy and D and C by using a type of ultrasound procedure called saline infusion sonohysterography, or SIS. With it, doctors can confirm that the uterine lining is normal.

Loss of sex drive and sexual pleasure, such as the decreased libido that Elaine experienced, are other chief symptoms of perimenopause. Lower estrogen levels may reduce blood flow to the pelvis, causing less engorgement and lubrication during sex. While thinning of vaginal walls and painful intercourse are more common after menopause, women in their forties can also experience vaginal dryness.

But I'm Too Young for Hot Flashes

In addition to irregular bleeding, perimenopausal women may be surprised by an array of unexpected symptoms, including hot flashes. "For me, having hot flashes was like being hit by lightning," says Deanna. "I certainly wasn't expecting it. I was barely 49, and I was still having what I thought were regular periods."

Some experts believe that hot flashes tend to strike during months when a woman skips a period, while others note that women with an earlier, longer perimenopause are more prone to hot flashes than those with a later, shorter perimenopause. There's some evidence that the severity of a woman's hot flashes corresponds to the intensity of her menstrual cramps and that the tendency to have them may be inherited. Only 10 to 20 percent of women in their forties experience hot flashes, but many others have what are sometimes called hot flash equivalents, including insomnia, headaches, heart palpitations, dizziness, and tingling sensations in the skin.

"Insomnia can be one of the first signs that you're heading toward menopause," says Mary Jane Minkin, M.D., clinical professor of obstetrics and gynecology at Yale University School of Medicine and co-author of *What Every Woman Needs to Know about Menopause*. Fluctuations in estrogen and progesterone can affect the sleep/wake cycle, and hot flashes are more common at night. "Some women wake up in the middle of the night and don't know why. The sweats may not be severe, just enough to disrupt sleep," says Dr. Minkin.

Headaches and heart palpitations may also occur right before menstruation, and women may experience fatigue, irritability, mood swings, anxiety, poor concentration, and memory loss—symptoms often associated with premenstrual syndrome (PMS). In fact, many women first develop PMS or see their usual symptoms worsen during perimenopause.

"It's often hard to differentiate between PMS and perimenopause," says

Investigating Abnormal Bleeding

Perimenopausal women who experience abnormal bleeding are usually sent for an endometrial biopsy or a dilation and curettage (D and C, the surgical scraping of the uterine lining) to make sure that there is no precancerous growth in the uterus. But saline infusion sonohysterography (SIS) could make D and C's unnecessary 75 percent of the time.

SIS, a painless office procedure now done in many major medical centers, involves putting sterile saline into the uterus, then placing an ultrasound probe in the vagina to inspect the uterine lining. Even small abnormalities can become apparent, allowing doctors to separate women who may need hormone therapy to control abnormal bleeding from those with growths, such as fibroids or polyps, which may need to be removed. "With SIS the only time women will need to go to the operating room for D and C's will be for treatment, not diagnosis," says Steven R. Goldstein, M.D., director of the gynecological ultrasound unit at New York University Medical Center in New York City.

Studies show not only that SIS is better at finding problems (including cancer) than endometrial biopsy plus D and C but also that it's considerably cheaper. A biopsy followed by a D and C might run $4,000 in a city medical center, compared with around $850 for SIS.

Sally K. Severino, M.D., executive vice-chairman at the University of New Mexico Medical Center in Albuquerque. "The majority of women who seek treatment for PMS are in their thirties and forties. They seem to have the worst symptoms and the most difficult time managing them." The shortened menstrual cycle also means the symptoms come more frequently.

While birth control pills may lessen PMS in some women, antidepressants can help if symptoms are primarily anxiety or depression, says Dr. Severino. Studies show that depression rates spike during perimenopause. Experts believe that the women at greatest risk are those who have had major depression or depressive symptoms while taking birth control pills.

Is It Time for Estrogen?

The question of whether a woman should take hormones during perimenopause is almost as thorny as whether she should take them after menopause. Oral contraceptives can help control irregular bleeding and diminish perimenopausal symptoms by smoothing out fluctuating levels of hormones, and because perimenopausal women still need contraception, the Pill may be a good option for many. "Birth control pills are not really hormone-replacement therapy," says Dr. Santoro. "They contain a higher dose of estrogen than we use in HRT, but they do take perimenopausal women off the hormonal roller coaster."

There is another possible drawback to the Pill for perimenopausal women, however. Taking oral contraceptives may make it harder to determine when a woman has gone through menopause, since Pill-users' periods often stop altogether. It can also interfere with the blood tests that doctors use to measure hormone levels once a woman is believed to be in menopause.

Traditionally, physicians have not prescribed HRT until a woman has not had a period for at least a year, feeling it's dangerous to add extra hormones to those being produced naturally. But since the estrogen dose in HRT is much lower than in the Pill, some practitioners now give estrogen (in pill or patch form) if a woman appears to be fairly close to menopause. Most agree that women need not wait until their periods stop for 12 months to seek treatment for troublesome symptoms. "You don't treat diabetes only after someone has an insulin level of zero, so why withhold estrogen replacement until the estrogen level is zero?" asks Harriette Mogul, Ph.D., director of the menopausal health program at New York Medical College in Valhalla.

Not all physicians prescribe hormones before menopause. "I still take the position of waiting until a year after a woman has stopped menstruating before giving HRT because I can't be 100 percent positive that she's not going to get pregnant," says Dr. Santoro. (Extra estrogen can harm a developing fetus.)

Dr. Utian agrees, noting that hormone therapy during perimenopause is difficult to manage since natural estrogen levels fluctuate.

Stepping off the Roller Coaster

Whether a woman eventually decides to take the Pill or estrogen—or do nothing—for perimenopausal symptoms, she shouldn't wait to take steps to prevent heart disease and osteoporosis, which can strike with force after menopause. Experts suggest you take these steps first.

If you smoke, stop. Smoking decreases estrogen production, which may aggravate hot flashes and bring on menopause an average of two years earlier.

Get calcium. Make sure your calcium intake tops 1,500 milligrams a day, with 400 international units of vitamin D to aid absorption.

Focus on fruits and veggies. Cut back on fat and sugary carbohydrates, and eat a minimum of five servings of fruits and vegetables a day. This will help you fight midlife weight gain and control cholesterol levels, and it will afford some added protection against heart disease, diabetes, and some forms of cancer.

Add weight-bearing exercise. Walk, jog, jump rope, or engage in some other form of weight-bearing activity for 30 minutes at least three times a week. These measures should help you fight midlife weight gain and maintain healthy bone mass and cholesterol levels while still in your perimenopausal years.

The Pill's Surprising Health Benefits

5

What if you could take a drug that not only prevented pregnancy but also strengthened your bones, made your periods lighter, and dramatically reduced the risk of ectopic pregnancy, endometriosis, pelvic inflammatory disease, and certain gynecological cancers? That drug is available—and has been for 36 years. It's the birth control pill.

If you're surprised, you're in good company. A recent survey of 247 women receiving care at Yale University Health Services found that very few could identify any benefits from the Pill other than contraception and convenience. "That the Pill offers women major health benefits is one of the best-kept secrets in America," says David Grimes, M.D., an obstetrician and gynecologist with the University of California at San Francisco/San Francisco General Hospital. When it comes to oral contraceptives, he adds, "there is gross misinformation and gross confusion."

Fear and outdated attitudes about the Pill, the most effective form of contraception short of sterilization, are keeping it out of the hands of women over the age of 35. As a result, their rate of unintended pregnancy is nearly as high as that of teenagers: Fully 77 percent of women in their forties who become pregnant did not intend to do so.

The Pill certainly isn't the best choice for everyone, but it's an option for most women. In deciding whether to use it, a woman should consider the total possible impact on her health—benefits as well as risks. Over the past few decades, researchers have identified those risks. And during that time the Pill itself has been greatly modified to minimize them.

Doctors Say the Pill Is Safe— For Most

Research on the safety of oral contraceptives shows that birth control pills do not greatly increase a woman's risk of breast cancer or stroke, as previously thought.

"The Pill was introduced in 1960. If it really did make a difference in cancer rates, we should be up to our ears in breast cancer by now, but we are not seeing any kind of epidemic related to the use of the Pill," says Anita Nelson, M.D., associate professor of obstetrics and gynecology at Harbor–University of California, Los Angeles, Medical Center in Torrance.

In a major research project based in Oxford, England, researchers analyzed 90 percent of studies about oral contraceptives and cancer risk done around the world. They found a small increase in breast cancer risk among current Pill users, but they also discovered that, among women who had stopped taking the Pill, there was virtually no associated breast cancer risk after 10 years. The project did not find major differences in risk among women in different age groups.

The findings from the Oxford study tell women and physicians once again that taking the Pill does not cause breast cancer. Rather, scientists say that the Pill may enhance the growth of undetectable cancers that already exist in a woman's breast.

"Taking the Pill is about as small a risk as you can measure," says Eugenia E. Calle, Ph.D., director of analytic epidemiology for the American Cancer Society in Atlanta and one of the Oxford project collaborators. Study results are reassuring not only because the risks were found to be small but also because cancers diagnosed in Pill users were less advanced than cancers found in nonusers, says Dr. Calle.

In another study researchers from Kaiser Permanente Medical Care Program, Southern California, in Pasadena interviewed 295 women (or the close relatives of women who had died) who had suffered strokes and found that low-estrogen oral contraceptives do not appear to increase the risk of stroke.

HEALTH FLASH

Inside Today's Birth Control Pills

The Pill has generally consisted of estrogen and progestin (the synthetic form of the female hormone progesterone), with some pills offering just progestin. But today's versions have much lower hormone doses than their predecessors. These "second-generation" pills contain one-fifth the estrogen and progestin of earlier versions. (So-called third-generation pills, offering low-dose estrogen along with newer forms of progestin, were introduced in the United States in 1993). By offering the minimum hormone levels that effectively suppress ovulation, today's Pill is less likely to cause the adverse effects—some of them life-threatening—that frightened women in the 1970s.

In another major change, doctors are now more careful in prescribing the Pill. Years of research have shown that the most serious effect of birth control pill use—the development of a blood clot that could lead to a heart attack or stroke—is limited mainly to smokers, particularly those over 35. The combination of lower hormone doses and more careful prescribing has virtually eliminated the danger of blood clots once associated with the Pill. Users now face a negligible increase in their risks of blood clots, from 1.6 in 10,000 when not on the Pill to 3.2 in 10,000 for Pill users.

The big news is that although the Pill still has side effects, most of them actually improve a woman's health. Nevertheless, a recent national survey found that women seem overly sensitive to the Pill's perils, with only 25 percent of the 1,000 women in the survey judging birth control pills as "very safe" and 29 percent considering them unsafe. Here are some of the benefits that the Pill offers women. Keep in mind that all these benefits involve the standard pills containing both estrogen and progestin but probably don't apply to progestin-only formulations such as the mini-pill, Depo-Provera injections, or Norplant implants.

Reduced risk of ovarian cancer. This is one of the most deadly of all female cancers since it's rarely diagnosed at an early, curable stage. Pregnancy, breast-feeding, and other events in a woman's life that stop ovulation reduce her risk of getting ovarian cancer. Since the Pill prevents pregnancy largely by suppressing ovulation, researchers had long suspected that it could help prevent ovarian cancer.

Proof came in the late 1980s, when the federally sponsored Cancer and Steroid Hormone study (CASH), involving more than 9,000 women, was published. The CASH study as well as several smaller, more recent studies confirm that, on average, Pill users have a 40 percent lower risk of ovarian cancer than other women. "Keep in mind that this is just an average number," says Leon Speroff, M.D., an obstetrician and gynecologist with Oregon Health Sciences University in Portland. "The longer you take the Pill, the greater the benefit. Taking it for more than 10 years yields an 80 percent reduction in ovarian cancer risk." And this protection seems to persist for at least 15 years after women stop taking the Pill.

Reduced risk of endometrial cancer. Taking estrogen alone increases a woman's risk of cancer of the endometrium (the lining of the uterus). But combining progesterone with estrogen effectively eliminates this risk. That's why postmenopausal women who still have uteruses must take estrogen and progesterone as hormone-replacement therapy (HRT), while those who've had hysterectomies can safely take estrogen alone.

The Pill also contains progesterone (in the form of progestin), in amounts that actually protect against endometrial cancer. The CASH study found that women who took the Pill for at least a year halved their risk of the disease. As with ovarian cancer, this protective effect persists for at least 15 years after women stop taking the Pill. In addition, international studies have shown a decrease in rates of endometrial cancer in several countries after the Pill was introduced.

"If you ask most women whether taking the Pill will reduce their risk of cancer, they will say, 'Absolutely not,'" remarks Gilbert Haas, M.D., an obstetrician and gynecologist with the University of Oklahoma Health Sciences Center in Oklahoma City. "But that's a perception that clearly doesn't reflect medical reality."

Reduced risk of ectopic pregnancy. The rate of ectopic, or tubal, pregnancies in the United States has tripled in the last few years to reach what Dr. Grimes terms epidemic proportions. Ectopic pregnancy occurs when a fertilized egg implants in a fallopian tube rather than in the uterus, and it is now the leading cause of maternal death in early pregnancy. By suppressing ovulation, the Pill cuts a woman's risk of ectopic pregnancy by 90 percent.

Reduced risk of pelvic inflammatory disease (PID). PID results from untreated infections of the female reproductive organs. Two-thirds of cases are due to sexually transmitted infections, such as gonorrhea and chlamydia. PID is a major cause of infertility since the infections can eventually scar and block the fallopian tubes. Although many PID cases are "silent," the classic symptoms are lower abdominal pain, vaginal discharge, fever, nausea, and vomiting.

Women on the Pill have half the PID rate of nonusers, perhaps because the Pill thickens cervical mucus, making it harder for infection-causing bacteria to spread to reproductive organs. But the Pill should never be relied on for protection against sexually transmitted infections.

Help against endometriosis. In up to 10 percent of women, patches of endometrial tissue escape the uterus during menstruation and turn up elsewhere in the body, often on the ovaries but also on the uterus's outer surface and on the fallopian tubes. Scar tissue may form wherever these endometrial lesions are present. This condition—endometriosis—is a major cause of infertility, detectable in up to 60 percent of infertile women.

Ovulation fuels endometriosis by causing menstrual periods, which can trigger new lesions. Since the Pill suppresses ovulation and causes lighter periods, it can help prevent endometriosis and ward off recurrences in women who have been treated for it surgically or with drugs.

Increased bone density. Although the evidence is mixed, Pill users seem to have slightly greater bone mass than nonusers. Greater mass helps ward off the bone-thinning disorder osteoporosis, which affects many postmenopausal women. "It makes sense that the estrogen in the Pill would help increase bone density since estrogen-replacement therapy is the most effective treatment we have to stop bone loss after menopause," says Dr. Speroff.

Unanswered Questions

Despite the Pill's long history of use, a few uncertainties remain. The most important one concerns the possibility that estrogen may increase a woman's risk of breast cancer. The controversy over estrogen and breast cancer centers mainly on estrogen as part of HRT, used primarily by older women to relieve the acute symptoms of menopause and to prevent osteoporosis. Studies of women who've been on HRT have yielded contradictory results, some suggesting that users face a higher risk of breast cancer and others finding no increased risk.

Although the list is not long, some women are not good candidates for the Pill, mainly those with an increased risk of blood clots: smokers, women who've had blood-clotting disorders, and those with risk factors for heart disease or stroke, including hypertension, elevated cholesterol, diabetes, or a strong family history of heart disease. In addition, women who've had breast cancer should avoid the Pill.

While the Pill offers significant benefits and minimal risks, it does not guard against sexually transmitted diseases (STDs). No matter what contraceptives they use, women of any age with multiple sex partners—or even just one partner whose sexual history is questionable—should use condoms. To optimize their protection against both pregnancy and STDs, some women may want to use both the Pill and a condom.

The Pill and Older Women

For years, the Pill was reserved primarily for younger women. The Food and Drug Administration (FDA), in fact, recommended that women over 40 avoid the Pill, out of concern that it could increase their risk of potentially fatal blood clots. But more recently, studies have shown that second-generation, low-dose pills pose no greater risk to women in their forties than to younger women. The FDA reached that conclusion in 1989, proclaiming the Pill safe and effective for all premenopausal women. Nevertheless, many women in their thirties and forties aren't aware that the Pill is an option for them.

News that most women of reproductive age can use the Pill—and that it can have important positive effects on women's health—has gotten too little publicity, contends Dr. Grimes. He blames the media for ignoring good news about products and focusing instead on their hazards. "Bad news sells," he says.

6

Picking the Right Estrogen- Replacement Therapy

I f you could take all the estrogen products that are available and line them up on one shelf, you might think you were in the cereal aisle of your supermarket. The sheer variety is overwhelming.

First, there are all the different types of estrogen. You practically need a degree in pharmacology to pronounce their names, let alone understand the chemical differences between them—estradiol, conjugated estrogens, estropipate, esterified estrogen, and estrone. What's more, estrogens come in a variety of delivery systems: pills, transdermal patches, creams, and even a vaginal ring. And most of these products come in different dosages.

How do you know what's right for you? True, all forms of estrogen-replacement therapy are intended to ease menopause in one way or another. They may stop what are called vasomotor symptoms—symptoms like hot flashes and night sweats. Or quench symptoms of urogenital atrophy: vaginal dryness, painful intercourse, and urinary tract discomfort. Or halt bone loss that can lead to crippling osteoporosis. And there's even the tantalizing—albeit preliminary—evidence that estrogen supplementation may halve a woman's risk of heart disease.

Thinking that there's one perfect estrogen for everyone is like suggesting to every cereal lover in the supermarket that they only buy a big white box marked "Breakfast Flakes." The point is that there is no single perfect estrogen and not every estrogen does it all. The woman who switches to the patch because a pill has made her queasy also has to say goodbye to the rise in heart-healthy high-density lipoproteins (HDLs—the so-called good cholesterol) that can come with the pill. And she may find that she has skin irritation from the patch. A switch in any direction has its trade-offs—and some trades are more serious than others.

Customizing Your Therapy

What to do? Prioritize, says Howard Zacur, M.D., Ph.D., director of the estrogen consultation service at Johns Hopkins University in Baltimore. "List your goals in order of importance to you—whether it's relief of vasomotor symptoms or something bigger, like bone protection."

If you're not sure of what your needs are, a complete physical examination and a cholesterol test can determine whether cardiovascular protection is an urgent need for you. A bone-density test can help you figure out whether bone protection should be a top concern or—if you're already on estrogen—whether it is helping your bones enough.

Look below for your number one priority, and we'll tell you which form of estrogen can give it to you.

Relief from Dryness

Without adequate amounts of estrogen, the tissues in the vagina and urinary tract become dry, atrophied, and easily traumatized. Vaginal dryness can cause painful intercourse as well as uncomfortable itching. Many women also experience an increase in urinary tract infections and irritation of the urethra, which can cause painful urination.

If these annoying and persistent complaints are your only reasons to take estrogen-replacement therapy, a localized form of estrogen, supplied by prescription vaginal estrogen creams or the vaginal ring, may be all you need. The downside is that localized estrogen doesn't prevent hot flashes or help your heart or bones. "If someone came to me saying, 'I want to prevent heart disease,' I wouldn't advise her to use a vaginal cream," says Valerie L. Baker, M.D., a gynecologist and reproductive endocrinologist at the University of California, San Francisco. Nor would the vaginal ring be the way to go.

If you're looking to get the added benefits of relief from hot flashes and night sweats and protection against bone loss and/or heart disease (an effect that looks promising but has not yet been proven), you'll need the pill or patch form of estrogen.

Vaginal creams are applied directly within the vagina. Depending on whom you ask, that's either a blessing or a mess. Creams, however, may be a quick way to combat vaginal dryness, which is the only thing that they are intended to do. While it can take a month to get relief from dryness by using a pill or patch, creams may bring relief slightly faster (the vaginal tissues absorb them very well). When used as prescribed, creams also don't elevate blood levels of estrogen significantly or consistently because the estrogen stays mostly in the vagina, says Brian Walsh, M.D., director of the menopause clinic at Brigham and Women's Hospital in Boston.

If you use the cream sporadically or find success with smaller amounts than recommended on the package, you may have even smaller amounts of estrogen circulating in your body.

Vaginal rings were first designed for contraception. But Estring, manufactured by Pharmacia and Upjohn, has become available in the United States for estrogen-replacement therapy. About the size of a diaphragm, it is inserted by either the woman or her physician and kept for up to three months in the vagina, where it releases a steady, low dose of estrogen. Clinical studies show that it works well to relieve both vaginal dryness and urinary tract complaints. It may be more convenient and certainly less messy than creams. And unlike creams, you don't have to think about when to apply it.

"The ring is specifically designed to deliver estrogen locally and in doses too low to provide blood levels of estrogen comparable to those caused by the patch or pill. Very minimal levels get into the blood," says Dr. Zacur. Like the creams, the ring won't provide relief from hot flashes or a benefit to your bones or heart.

Relief from Hot Flashes

When the body lacks adequate levels of estrogen, it tricks the brain into thinking that your body's temperature is too high. As a result, blood flow to the skin increases, and you become overheated and flushed, and you begin to per-spire. If taming hot flashes or night sweats is your number one goal, your only choices are estrogen pills or the transdermal patch because nothing else gets enough estrogen to the temperature regulation center in your brain.

If doctors tend to prescribe the pill called Premarin more frequently, it's most likely because of all the studies on it. "Because it's the most widely tested estro-gen, I think it's worth considering if a woman chooses oral estrogen," says Nanette F. Santoro, M.D., associate professor and director of reproductive en-docrinology in the department of obstetrics and gynecology at the University of Medicine and Dentistry of New Jersey–New Jersey Medical School in Newark.

Nonetheless, the patch can also relieve hot flashes and night sweats. The patch is self-adhesive and releases estrogen through the skin into the blood-stream. It is applied to the buttocks or abdomen, according to the manufac-turer's instructions, and changed once or twice a week (depending on the brand you choose).

If you haven't chosen between the pill or the patch, turn to your next prior-ity—heart or bone protection, perhaps—to give you a hand. And keep in mind that if you're set on relieving hot flashes and night sweats, there may be some ways to do that without using estrogen supplements, such as by eating foods containing soy.

Bone Protection

If one of your priorities when choosing a type of estrogen therapy is to pro-tect your bones, know that certain doses of several oral estrogens and one trans-dermal patch are indicated by the Food and Drug Administration (FDA) for preventing bone loss. Other pills and patches are likely to follow as the manufacturers do the necessary studies to convince the FDA of the products' bone-protecting abilities.

When using estrogen for bone protection, the most important factor seems to be dosage. Go too low, and your bones get no benefit. The challenge is that there is no magic cutoff point (yet) under which bones are not being helped. Each product has to show efficacy on its own.

So far, a few products have been shown to benefit bones with dosages approved by the FDA.

Type	Minimum Bone-Protecting Dose (mg.)
Estraderm patch	0.05
Estrace	0.50
Premarin	0.625
Ogen	0.75
Ortho-Est	0.75

Even though a product may be FDA approved for osteoporosis prevention at only one particular dose, that doesn't mean a physician can't prescribe a higher dose. In fact, a few of the experts we spoke to felt that some of the approved doses were too low for maximum bone protection. If the table suggests that the dose you're currently taking might not be high enough for bone benefits, you have a couple of choices. One, of course, is to ask your doctor about taking more estrogen. But remember: There are risks and benefits to be balanced.

Heart Protection

If heart disease protection tops your list of reasons to take estrogen, both the pill and the patch have benefits to offer. But the benefits of each are slightly different.

If lowering your cholesterol numbers is what the doctor ordered, then oral estrogens may offer the most powerful heart protection. Because the pill requires digestion, it passes through the liver. This so-called first-pass effect is responsible for increasing the good HDL cholesterol and decreasing the bad low-density lipoprotein (LDL) cholesterol.

"If you're looking for major cholesterol changes, you need to take your estrogen orally," says Dr. Walsh. "The changes can be significant. We're talking about a 15 percent increase in HDL. From that alone, you could expect to reduce your risk of heart disease by something on the order of 40 percent." (Keep in mind that while population studies link estrogen to heart disease prevention, well-controlled trials to prove the point are still under way. So at this point, no estrogen has FDA approval for heart protection.)

As far as dose goes, "the level of estrogen needed for the heart is probably comparable to the level needed to protect bones," says Bruce Carr, M.D., director of the division of reproductive endocrinology at the University of Texas Southwestern Medical Center at Dallas. "But there isn't enough research to be specific yet."

Now the downside. Oral estrogens can raise triglyceride levels, which can help promote the buildup of plaque in arteries (again, the first-pass effect at work). Women who have had blood clots or are at risk for them and who have had gallbladder disease should discuss with their doctors the decision to take oral estrogens. If you're looking for less of an effect on your cholesterol, the patch could help you out.

Overall, the patch may come in second place (after pills) for cardiovascular benefits—but that's still pretty good. Although oral estrogens have the most beneficial effect on cholesterol levels, research shows that estrogen from patches as well as pills provides a direct benefit to blood vessels—improving blood flow, for example. "In the long run, the benefits via direct action on the blood vessels may be as helpful in preventing heart disease as estrogen's effect on cholesterol," says Dr. Baker.

Unlike oral estrogens, the patch doesn't increase triglycerides. Even though studies aren't conclusive, it is likely to have minimal or no effect on blood clotting. So it's considered safe for women who can't take pills for those reasons, though any decision like this should be discussed with your doctor.

Of course, when it comes to protecting the heart, there are ways to do it in addition to estrogen therapy: Eat a low-fat diet, exercise, reduce stress, and of course, don't smoke.

Estrogen and Cancer: What Every Woman Needs to Know

For a woman with debilitating hot flashes, the relief provided by hormone-replacement therapy (HRT) may be a blessing. A woman with a personal or family history of crippling osteoporosis may be relieved to find that HRT can protect against bone loss. A woman at risk for heart disease may feel reassured that HRT can help protect against heart problems.

In these situations, HRT's short-term side effects—including water retention, bloating, breast tenderness, irritability, abdominal cramps, and irregular, menstrual-like bleeding may be worth tolerating.

But long-term risks are less clear. Although HRT has been around in some form for more than 50 years, the possibility of long-term hazards is a matter of intense medical debate. Here, we look at what is currently known and unknown about the connection between long-term use of HRT and cancer.

Endometrial Cancer:
When Hormones Raise the Risk

According to the National Cancer Institute, approximately 35,000 new cases of endometrial (uterine) cancer develop each year; about 2,900 women die from

Factor Mammogram Effects into Your HRT Decision

Thought you had heard about all the side effects of hormone-replacement therapy (HRT)? Now, theoretical concerns have been raised that HRT might make early breast cancer detection with mammograms more difficult. A study from the University of Washington in Seattle showed that about 25 percent of women using HRT have denser-than-normal breast tissue, which might mask cancerous growth, according to Anita Nelson, M.D., associate professor of obstetrics and gynecology at Harbor–University of California, Los Angeles, Medical Center in Torrance, California.

Does the news mean that you should forgo HRT? No way. While some experts have raised these concerns about detection troubles, others point out that there are no studies to show that this delays a woman's diagnosis of breast cancer, notes Dr. Nelson.

"Until the risks outweigh the benefits of HRT, I feel my patients are better off using it," Dr. Nelson says. Benefits include protection from heart disease and brittle bones. But it's not for everyone. For a woman with a strong family history of breast cancer and no risk factors for heart disease or osteoporosis, the risks from HRT may be too high, she says. However, Dr. Nelson says she would favor HRT if that woman also smokes cigarettes, because smoking can increase heart disease risk. "Every woman should balance the risks and benefits based on her own health needs."

HEALTH FLASH

endometrial cancer annually. It is the third most common form of cancer in women.

A woman with a uterus who takes unopposed estrogen (estrogen alone) for 10 or more years has a 4- to 10-fold greater risk of developing endometrial cancer than a woman who doesn't take it. And that increased risk persists for 5 to 15 years after she has stopped HRT. Endometrial cancer, however, is usually caught early and thus generally has an excellent survival rate. But you wouldn't want to be the exception—nor would you want to develop cancer at all. Here are answers to common questions about HRT and endometrial cancer.

How does estrogen cause cancer? To be precise, estrogen itself does not cause cancer. Estrogen promotes a dangerous, precancerous condition called endometrial hyperplasia—an excessive buildup or proliferation of the cells that line the uterus.

Does all hyperplasia develop into cancer? No. Hyperplasia can develop into cancer if it is neglected and if you are predisposed toward uterine cancer. A family history of endometrial cancer is a warning flag, as is obesity. Other risk factors may include conditions such as diabetes, high cholesterol levels, and high blood pressure.

The greatest risk factors, however, appear to be the dose of estrogen you take and the duration of hormone therapy. The more unopposed estrogen you take, and the longer you take it, the greater your likelihood of developing hyperplasia.

What are the symptoms of hyperplasia? Hyperplasia often causes unexpected (breakthrough) bleeding or unusually heavy or long-lasting bleeding. Be aware that hyperplasia can develop in the years before menopause, when your body's menstrual cycles become irregular and unpredictable.

Every woman on estrogen must be alert to unusual bleeding, such as heavy bleeding or spotting between scheduled periods, and inform her doctor. Tests such as an endometrial biopsy or a dilatation and curettage (D and C, a procedure in which the uterus is scraped clean of its lining) can determine if you have hyperplasia.

What can I do to protect myself against endometrial cancer? To combat the dangers of unopposed estrogen, health care practitioners now prescribe progestin (a synthetic progesterone) in tandem with estrogen for women with a uterus.

Called combination therapy, the estrogen-and-progestin regimen has slowly gained a foothold as the HRT standard. Progestin suppresses hyperplasia by preventing the thick uterine buildup. In rare cases hyperplasia can develop even if a woman is taking progestin—possibly because the woman is supersensitive to the effects of estrogen. Larger progestin doses may be needed. The key thing to remember is that women on combination therapy still need to pay attention to unusual bleeding.

How often do I need to take progestin to guard against hyperplasia and cancer? Although no one yet knows the precise minimum number of days you need to take progestin to reduce the risk of endometrial cancer, studies suggest that most women are protected if they take progestin for at least 12 days of each month.

How much progestin do I need? If your HRT regimen calls for taking progestin for 12 to 14 days of the month, then the usual daily dose is 10 milligrams of medroxyprogesterone acetate. If you take progestin every day, the usual dose is 2.5 to 5 milligrams of medroxyprogesterone a day. But you may need a larger dose if you show signs of hyperplasia.

Is it ever possible to take unopposed estrogen? If you have a uterus and take progestin and find that you cannot tolerate its side effects (which can include bleeding, chronic headaches, nausea, cramps, irritability, and depression), you can continue to take unopposed estrogen, but most doctors won't recommend that you take that risk. If you do opt for unopposed estrogen, you must commit to annual tests (usually endometrial biopsies) to monitor the health of your endometrium.

As you would expect, you should not take estrogen at all if you have endometrial cancer.

How effective is progestin? Several studies suggest that women who take a combined therapy of both estrogen and progestin have a lower incidence of hyperplasia or endometrial cancer than women who do not take HRT at all. That said, however, it must be noted that the long-term effects of progestin on the endometrium won't really be known for many years.

Breast Cancer and HRT: The Debate Goes On

The possibility of a link between estrogen and breast cancer is an explosively controversial subject. On one side of the debate are physicians who say that the vast body of scientific research—somewhere in the neighborhood of 30 studies—has found no conclusive connection between breast cancer and estrogen replacement.

On the other side of the estrogen/breast cancer argument are those scientists and physicians who are uncomfortable with any increased cancer risk. They suspect a link between estrogen and breast cancer for many reasons. Breast cancer is much more common in women than men. Estrogen is known to affect breast tissue, occasionally encouraging abnormal cell growth and harmless, benign cysts in the breasts (a condition known as fibrocystic breast disease). Some forms of breast cancer are estrogen dependent, meaning they grow in the presence of estrogen. Then, too, extensive tests have shown that estrogen is associated with the development of breast tumors in animals.

Breast cancer is a major concern for women. Approximately 10 percent of women will develop breast cancer at some time in their lives. Some 175,000 to 180,000 cases of breast cancer are diagnosed in the United States each year, and 46,000 women die from this cancer annually. About three-quarters of all breast cancers occur in women over age 44, during the perimenopausal and postmenopausal years.

While the association between estrogen use and breast cancer is hotly debated, there is evidence that long-term HRT use can increase the risk to a statistically significant degree. A Harvard University study found that women who took estrogen for five or more years after menopause had a 32 percent higher risk of breast cancer than women who had never taken the hormone. In those women who also took progestin, the risk rose to 41 percent. At greatest risk were women ages 60 to 64 who had used hormones for five years or longer. They had a 71 percent higher risk of breast cancer than women who never took estrogen. The researchers also found that the risk of dying from breast cancer was 45 percent higher among estrogen-users.

This Harvard study is significant in the number of participants—69,000 postmenopausal nurses took part in the Nurses' Health Study from 1976 to 1992—and in the fact that the study examined all forms of HRT. The researchers found no difference in the effect of different forms or doses of estrogen.

Please remember, however, that these higher risks do not predict that most women on HRT will develop cancer. In fact, the study predicts that the actual percentage of women who will develop breast cancer in the next five years is still low. About 3 percent of 60-year-old women who have been taking estrogen for five years will develop breast cancer, compared to 1.8 percent of 60-year-old women not using hormones. Nonetheless, this greater percentage is enough to cause many women to reevaluate hormone-replacement therapy.

Are other risk factors associated with breast cancer? Many experts assert that estrogen in and of itself doesn't cause breast cancer. Other risk factors must be present. A family history of breast cancer, early onset of menstruation, late menopause, first childbirth after age 30, obesity, inactive lifestyle, and smoking are among the factors linked to breast cancer. Age is also a risk factor—the older you are, the more likely you are to develop this cancer.

Can I take HRT if I had breast cancer years ago? For some women this question is a very real concern. Everyone agrees that HRT is inappropriate for someone who is currently being treated for cancer. Medical experts disagree, however, about what is appropriate if you had cancer in the past. Many doctors are uncomfortable recommending HRT when its safety and benefit for successfully treated breast cancer patients have not been tested in controlled clinical trials.

8

Cool Off Those Hot Flashes, Naturally

Menopause doesn't bother everyone. In fact, only about 15 out of 100 women will experience severe symptoms while going through the change of life, says Margery Gass, M.D., director of the University Hospital Menopause and Osteoporosis Center at the University of Cincinnati. "We estimate that 25 percent of women will sail through menopause with no trouble whatsoever," she says, "while some 60 percent will experience varying degrees of hot flashes, mood swings, vaginal dryness, and other discomforts associated with menopause." The remainder experience occasional but not significant discomfort.

For women with severe or bothersome concerns associated with menopause, medical science offers hormone-replacement therapy (HRT). But it's not the perfect solution for every woman.

And so more women are turning to natural solutions, such as herbs, vitamins, and other alternative approaches to menopause—with promising results. In fact, many natural options are so effective that mainstream doctors have begun to incorporate them into treatment programs for menopausal patients. Here's what practitioners say are the best alternative options for treating menopausal problems.

Soy Makes Sense

Diets abundant in soy products contain a group of natural chemical compounds called phytoestrogens that possess estrogen-like qualities, says Wulf H.

Dong Quai: Hype or Herbal Healer?

Suddenly, the Chinese herb dong quai is everywhere. The root of a Chinese plant that botanists call *Angelica sinensis*, this herb is purported to ease hot flashes at menopause—and to contain estrogen-like substances. But according to Varro E. Tyler, Ph.D., professor emeritus of pharmacognosy at Purdue University in West Lafayette, Indiana, and author of *Herbs of Choice*, research so far has not backed these claims.

Dong quai hasn't been evaluated clinically by standard Western medical methodologies, Dr. Tyler says. In China most herbs are used in combination with a dozen or so other botanicals. Several formulas containing dong quai with other herbs have been examined in China and Japan, but it has never been studied adequately by itself. Although many people testify to its effectiveness in treating menopausal symptoms, scientific evidence of its utility is lacking. So at present, it's tough to say if the herb is effective or not.

As for the idea that dong quai contains estrogen-like compounds, the truth is that no chemical has ever been identified in this plant.

Dong quai is usually administered in doses totaling 2 grams per day for menopausal symptoms. At that dosage level, it appears reasonably safe, Dr. Tyler says. But consumers of dong quai should shun the sun as much as possible or wear sunscreen because substances in the herb may cause the user to develop a skin rash following sun exposure.

Utian, M.D., Ph.D., chairman of reproductive biology at Case Western Reserve University in Cleveland and executive director of the North American Menopause Society.

Phytoestrogens come in two general forms: isoflavones and lignans. Isoflavones are found in soy foods like tofu and soy milk; lignans are found in whole grains, flaxseed, and to a lesser extent, fruits and vegetables.

What's their benefit to menopausal women? "If a woman wants to relieve her menopausal symptoms and doesn't want to go on hormone-replacement therapy, certainly one or two daily servings of soy products is a reasonable approach," says Mark Messina, Ph.D., a nutritionist in Port Townsend, Washington, a participant in the Asian food conference, and author of *The Simple Soybean and Your Health*. One small six-month study showed that soy did increase bone strength, adds Dr. Messina. But until phytoestrogens are studied further, he says that women at risk for osteoporosis shouldn't assume that phytoestrogens have the same bone-protecting benefits as HRT.

"Soy foods, the richest food source of phytoestrogens, may be the reason why Asian women have fewer menopausal symptoms than American women do. I recommend adding two servings of soy foods four or five days a week," says Jane Guiltinan, a doctor of naturopathy, clinical professor, and medical director of the teaching clinic at Bastyr University of Naturopathic Medicine in Seattle. Dr. Guiltinan also suggests that you add flaxseed, walnuts, and oats to your diet for rich sources of plant estrogen.

"We already know about a lot of benefits to eating less animal protein," says Gregory L. Burke, M.D., vice-chairman and professor in the department of public-health sciences at Bowman Gray School of Medicine of Wake Forest University in Winston-Salem, North Carolina. "I say, 'Go ahead,' to women who ask if they should replace animal protein with soy protein as they near menopause."

Experts offer these easy, tasty ways to add soy to your diet.

Add soy milk to your cereal. Admittedly, soy milk doesn't taste like cow's milk. But when chilled, it's perfect for pouring over your cereal. Look for calcium-added nonfat or low-fat soy milk in health food stores.

When cooking, substitute soy milk for cow's milk. Replace cow's milk with equal amounts of soy milk in practically any recipe, including cream sauces, shakes, baked goods, and puddings, suggests Dr. Messina.

Whip up a breakfast smoothie. For a delicious, satisfying breakfast treat, combine 1/2 cup unsweetened orange or apple juice, 1 medium banana, and 3 ounces tofu in a blender. Blend until smooth. If you like, add frozen strawberries or substitute them for the banana.

Use soy cheese. An excellent substitute for cow's-milk cheese, soy cheese is lower in fat and salt. It is available in some grocery stores and health food stores in an ever-growing variety of flavors, including mozzarella (try it in lasagna or on pizza), Cheddar, American, and Monterey Jack.

Try soy protein. Textured vegetable protein is made from defatted soy flour and found in health food stores and some grocery stores. Its meaty texture makes it a ringer for ground beef when used in spicy tacos, chili, or sloppy joes.

Taming the Wild Hot Flash

Of all the changes heralding menopause, most women agree that the hot flash is the most notorious. Most research or experimentation with natural remedies for menopause has focused on this symptom.

Hot flashes arise when estrogen levels fall, says Nancy Lee Teaff, M.D., in her book *Perimenopause—Preparing for the Change*. Estrogen affects the hypothalamus, your brain's "thermostat." When estrogen levels begin to ebb, your body's ability to regulate your temperature goes haywire. As a result, blood vessels may dilate inappropriately.

Starting as a sudden warmth in your face, head, or chest, a hot flash can spread like wildfire in just seconds, and as your body tries cooling itself off, you start sweating. The kicker to a reddening, drenching, hot flash can be a bout of shivering chills, as your body reacts to your wide-open pores and dampened skin.

If you're among the estimated 75 to 85 percent of women who experience hot flashes, alternative practitioners offer these time-tested herbal soothers for relief. You can find these remedies at herb stores.

Cool off with black cohosh. Black cohosh (the botanical name is *Cimicifuga racemosa*) has been proven to be as effective as estrogen for the relief of hot flashes, according to Varro E. Tyler, Ph.D., professor emeritus of pharmacognosy at Purdue University in West Lafayette, Indiana, and author of *Herbs of Choice*. (You may need to use it for up to four weeks before you feel better, however.)

To find the best dosage, start with 10 drops in a beverage twice a day and increase the dose by 5 drops every other day until you are satisfied with the results, suggests herbalist and teacher Susun S. Weed of Woodstock, New York, in her book *Menopausal Years: The Wise Woman Way*. Some women take black cohosh daily, others take it simply when needed, and some take it for any two consecutive weeks each month.

Ease with motherwort. Motherwort (*Leonurus cardiaca*) is a magnificent herbal ally for moderating menopausal symptoms such as hot flashes and night sweats, according to Weed. She dilutes 5 to 15 drops motherwort tincture, a concentrated herb extract made from fresh, flowering tops, in a little water or tea. Take it as needed to cool hot flashes—or several times a day to prevent them.

Don't overlook common chickweed. Chickweed (*Stellaria media*) has provided hot flash relief for many women, says Weed. She uses 25 to 40 drops of fresh plant tincture in a beverage once or twice a day to reduce the severity and frequency of hot flashes. Most women experience results within a week or two of regular use, she says.

Reset your thermostat with elder flower. This herb (*Sambucus canadensis*) specifically resets the body's thermostat, says Weed. For women who have frequent hot flashes or night sweats, 25 to 50 drops of fresh elder blossom tincture in a beverage several times a day should bring rapid results.

Chill out with violet. Violet (*Viola odorata*) can also cool hot flashes, says Weed. Eat the fresh leaves in your salad (violets grow in many lawns) or brew a strong tea by steeping 1 ounce of dried violet leaves in a quart of boiling water overnight. Strain, refrigerate, and drink within 48 hours. Weed suggests drinking at least a cup a day.

Easing Vaginal Dryness

During menopause, the lining of your vagina may become drier, thinner, and less flexible, due to lessening amounts of estrogen. You notice it most during sex—you may find that you don't become as lubricated when you're aroused, so sex is uncomfortable (or impossible). Here's what healers say you can do to remedy the situation.

Have sex regularly. Regular sexual activity promotes better circulation to the vagina and can increase lubrication, says Adriane Fugh-Berman, M.D., former head of field investigations for the Office of Alternative Medicine at the National Institutes of Health in Bethesda, Maryland. So a good way to protect yourself against menopausal vaginal dryness is to have sex regularly—and it doesn't have to be with a partner.

Apply vitamin E. Some women find that vitamin E oils, when used regularly, ease vaginal dryness.

Use an herbal salve. Herbal salves or ointments that contain both St.-John's-wort and calendula will ease a dry, irritated vagina, says Rosemary Gladstar, author of *Herbal Healing for Women*. In her book, Gladstar also offers this simple recipe for a soothing medicinal paste: Mix enough slippery elm powder with aloe vera gel to form a thick paste; apply inside the vaginal lips and vagina.

Try a water-based lubricant. If you aren't lubricated, drugstore remedies such as Astroglide, K-Y Jelly, and Replens (which lasts for up to three days per application) can also reduce the friction and discomfort of intercourse.

Beyond Estrogen: New Hormones on the Horizon

These days, hormones are making news. In bookstores and pharmacies, at the newsstand, and on the Internet, we read or hear about substances that promise to make us feel better, help us look younger, and free us from disease. But are they safe? Do they live up to their claims? Here's the lowdown on the hottest hormones.

Melatonin: Too Good to Be True

Melatonin has catapulted to fame in a blizzard of news reports and several books about its purported benefits. Proponents claim that melatonin supplements can cure or prevent cancer, heart disease, Alzheimer's disease, depression, schizophrenia, sudden infant death syndrome, epilepsy, autism, Parkinson's disease, sleep disturbances, sexual problems, and the flu.

If this list of benefits sounds too good to be true, your instincts are correct. At this juncture, there is only one credible claim: Melatonin is a promising medication for some sleep disturbances. But using melatonin even for this purpose is premature. Optimal doses, when to take them, long-term side effects, and potential drug interactions are unknown. In addition, the concentrations of over-the-counter products that contain melatonin vary widely, making it difficult for consumers to know exactly what they're taking.

Think Twice about the Male Hormone

New evidence suggests that adding testosterone to your hormone-replacement therapy (HRT) regimen may raise your breast cancer risk.

Testosterone isn't just a male hormone—women's bodies also produce it. And when levels fall during menopause, a woman may feel fatigued, lose her sex drive, or have hot flashes, even when on HRT. Taking testosterone can correct those problems—but may cause another. In a study of more than 4,000 post-menopausal women, researchers found that women who developed breast cancer had higher levels of testosterone and estradiol (a type of estrogen).

"Testosterone can be converted to estrogen in a woman's body, and the presence of high estrogen levels is a suspected risk factor for breast cancer," explains Mary K. Beard, M.D., associate clinical professor of obstetrics and gynecology at the University of Utah School of Medicine in Salt Lake City, spokesperson for the American College of Obstetricians and Gynecologists, and author of the book *Menopause and the Years Ahead*.

Still, more research must be done to determine the real risk from testosterone, according to Dr. Beard. "The number of women in this study who developed breast cancer was very small," she says. "The study needs to be repeated by several large centers to confirm its findings."

Meanwhile, if your HRT regimen includes testosterone, Dr. Beard suggests talking with your doctor to be sure your HRT takes into account your personal and family history of breast cancer. In addition, consider trying a lower dose of testosterone to see if it is just as effective.

What is it? Melatonin, a hormone found in nearly all plants and animals, helps to coordinate many cyclical life processes. In some animals it's involved in seasonal behaviors such as molting, hibernation, and mating. In humans it appears to help regulate daily sleep patterns. It also plays a role in physical growth and development, reproduction, and the immune response to infection.

Melatonin production drops as we age. Researchers speculate that this natural age-related decline may be one reason that older adults sometimes have difficulty falling asleep and staying asleep.

The bottom line: A great deal more research is needed before recommendations concerning proper sleep-aid dosages and treatment schedules can be made. Accurate guidelines are important because taking melatonin at the wrong time and in the wrong amounts can backfire, inducing sleep when alertness is required and vice versa. Furthermore, overdoses can produce grogginess, vivid dreams, depression, and headaches. Possible long-term side effects, especially on the cardiovascular system, are unknown.

Women with severe allergies, rheumatoid arthritis, and cancers such as lymphoma and leukemia should be particularly cautious because of melatonin's apparent role in immune response. Those taking corticosteroids, such as prednisone, should not take melatonin because of possible drug interactions. The ways in which supplemental amounts of melatonin interact with other drugs are unknown.

Estrogens of the Future

The words *raloxifene*, *droloxifene*, *idoxifene*, and *toremifene* are meaningless today, but tomorrow they may be as familiar as estrogen and progesterone. Their developers believe that they may duplicate most of estrogen's positive effects while eliminating many of its undesirable effects.

What are they? These drugs, called estrogen analogs, could become the new generation of hormones not only for treating breast cancer but also for use in postmenopausal hormone-replacement therapy (HRT).

The bottom line: Stay tuned. These hormones are still being developed in pharmaceutical labs. So far, raloxifene and droloxifene haven't triggered endometrial proliferation (an overgrowth of the lining of the uterus that can lead to endometrial cancer) as regular estrogen can. If they prove to lower the risk of osteoporosis and heart disease without raising the likelihood of breast and endometrial cancers, they may have a future role in HRT.

DHEA: Not Ready for Prime Time

DHEA (dehydroepiandrosterone) is everywhere, from pharmacies to books to the World Wide Web. But if you're trying to stave off a debilitating disease or if you long to recapture the energy of your youth, there is little evidence—at least in human studies—that DHEA will do anything except lighten your wallet...and perhaps raise your risk of endometrial cancer or make existing cancer grow faster.

What is it? Each morning, the adrenal glands (which sit atop the kidneys) release a form of DHEA into the bloodstream. From there DHEA works its way to the body's tissues and is converted into small amounts of the sex hormones testosterone and estrogen. DHEA levels decline steadily as we age, leading some researchers to speculate that this hormone causes us to age, get sick, and die. But scientific evidence for this is scant so far.

The bottom line: Claims that DHEA can prolong life are unfounded—in fact, the opposite has been found in experiments with laboratory mice. Claims that DHEA can prevent heart disease and cancer, melt away excess body fat, rev up sex drive, or boost immunity are also without basis, according to researchers who study this hormone. In fact, DHEA could raise your risk of endometrial cancer, according to researchers at the National Institute on Aging.

Prometrium: Not (Yet) Available in the United States

Prometrium emerged as one of the happy surprises of the Postmenopausal Estrogen/Progestin Intervention (PEPI) Trial, the first major controlled study to evaluate the effects of HRT in women.

What is it? Prometrium is a natural form of progestin, a hormone added to estrogen in HRT regimens to reduce the risk of endometrial cancer. In the PEPI study, compared to the standard progestin used in HRT in the United States, prometrium did as good a job of preventing endometrial cancer and a better job of preserving estrogen's beneficial influence on levels of lipids, blood fats that can raise or lower the risk of heart disease.

Forms of prometrium are available in Europe and Canada. Experts speculate that prometrium may be approved soon as a component of HRT in the United States.

The bottom line: A few doctors are prescribing micronized progesterone, which can be dispensed in its "raw" state without Food and Drug Administration (FDA) approval, from special pharmacies. By following a "recipe" from the October 1989 issue of the journal *Obstetrics and Gynecology*, pharmacists can produce capsules that are similar to prometrium. This approach is neither standardized nor well-studied, but if you want to try it and your doctor is willing to write a prescription and monitor you, you can contact the National Association of Compounding Pharmacists at (281) 933-8400.

Testosterone: The "Male" Hormone That Women Need, Too

Increasingly, HRT formulas for postmenopausal women include testosterone. But do you need it? What are the risks, if any?

What is it? Contrary to popular belief, testosterone isn't exclusively a male hormone. Although it is an androgen—a hormone responsible for masculinizing physical characteristics—in females it is produced by the ovaries, adrenal glands, and fat cells.

In women testosterone depletion at menopause has been associated with thinning pubic hair, diminished muscle mass, flagging energy, memory loss, and declining libido.

The bottom line: Most women who take testosterone do so to improve their sex drives. Several studies have indicated that estrogen/testosterone combinations are more effective than estrogen alone in enhancing libido. The object of such therapy is to achieve a balance of the two hormones—testosterone to increase desire and estrogen to prevent vaginal dryness and thereby reduce pain associated with intercourse.

The two preparations that have been approved by the FDA combine estrogen and methyltestosterone, a synthetic form of testosterone, in a single pill. The testosterone dose of one pill, Estratest, is only one-fourth that of the other, Premarin with methyltestosterone. Testosterone is also available alone.

If you're considering taking testosterone supplements, keep the following in mind: The effects attributed to testosterone were demonstrated only in women with levels below the normal range. And it may take some experimenting to get the desired effect. Finally, the long-term effects of testosterone supplementation are not well-understood. There is evidence that testosterone may prevent osteoporosis, but there is also concern that it will reduce the beneficial effects of estrogen on lipid levels, and that it may raise the risk of breast cancer.

part two

Outsmarting Disease

2

the Hormone Connection

Call it menstrual cycle medicine: By paying attention to the ebb and flow of hormones during the monthly cycle, women and their doctors are beginning to care for some of our biggest health problems more effectively. And more of these specially timed treatments may be on the horizon.

Chronobiologists—those who study biological rhythms—have long suspected that the body's rhythms can directly influence health problems as well as their treatment. Not only do researchers know that a woman's shifting hormones can affect many health conditions but they're also discovering that well-timed treatments can better ease discomfort and may even save lives. Here are some examples.

❖ **Greater breast cancer survival.** When researchers at the Milan Cancer Institute in Italy looked at the survival rates of 1,175 women after breast cancer surgery, they found that women whose surgeries were performed during the luteal phase of their menstrual cycles—the phase after ovulation—had a greater chance of survival than women whose surgeries were performed during the first, or follicular, phase.

❖ **Fewer migraines.** Among women who get migraine headaches, a majority report that some, if not all, of their headaches are related to their menstrual cycles. The most common times for head pain are during menstruation or at ovulation—two times during the month when there are decreases in the blood levels of a form of estrogen called estradiol. Women who receive estradiol during these low times can successfully counter menstrual-cycle-related migraines, says Philip Sarrel, M.D., professor of obstetrics, gynecology, and psychiatry at Yale University School of Medicine.

❖ **Less depression.** Since estrogen is known to have some positive effects in combating depression and anxiety in women, some doctors try to work with a woman's cycle by prescribing antidepressants and anxiety-lowering medications during the luteal half of the menstrual cycle, when estrogen levels—and moods—are lowest.

❖ **Simpler surgery.** Doctors have learned to reduce complications during many kinds of surgery by scheduling operations around a woman's menstrual cycle if she is prone to cyclical, hormone-sensitive conditions such as asthma, abnormally fast heart rate, or severe chest pain, says Dr. Sarrel.

Are You Turning Into Your Mother?

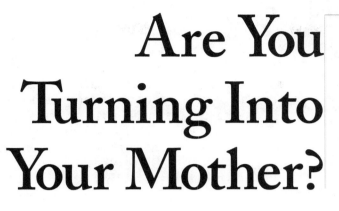

As a child, Kathi Marangos always found her birthday cake a bit hard to swallow. Each sugary bite reminded her of a birth mother who gave her up for adoption and of a biological family she didn't know. But she recalls her 18th birthday as especially bittersweet. "That's when my mother found me," she says. "She hired a private detective so she could give me information about my family."

Marangos at once felt transformed into the proud daughter of a ski lodge manager and a Harvard graduate. But at the same instant, she felt the chill from her biological family's dark side, with its frightening predisposition toward depression, heart disease, and colon cancer.

Today, 35-year-old Marangos and her doctor keep an eye out for any sign of cancer, while she makes sure her family sticks to a low-fat diet. "I'm so glad to know my medical history," she says. "I can use it to protect myself and my kids from our genetic shortcomings."

Sleuthing for Inherited Risks

If only more Americans would see the light, says Michael Crouch, M.D., director of the Baylor Family Practice Residency Program in Houston and a leading expert on inherited health risks. Tracing your roots to learn your fam-

Consider All the Consequences of Genetic Test Results

Thanks to genetic tests for everything from some breast cancers to cystic fibrosis, from muscular dystrophy to Huntington's disease and beyond, women can now glimpse their future health. But before you sign up for any of the hundreds of genetic tests now available, carefully weigh the medical benefits against the social and economic consequences that could arise, advises E. Virginia Lapham, Ph.D., a social scientist and associate professor of pediatrics at Georgetown University in Washington, D.C., who has studied the consequences of genetic testing.

In a study of 332 people who had genetic disorders in their families, Dr. Lapham and other researchers found that in many cases genetic information had been used against them by insurers or employers. One in 4 people in the study thought the information was used to refuse her family life insurance, more than 1 in 5 thought it was used to deny her health insurance, and more than 1 in 10 thought the information led to job discrimination. "Information about one person in the family can even result in the termination or denial of insurance coverage for the whole family," says Dr. Lapham, whose work was funded by Office of Ethical, Legal, and Social Implications Branch of the Human Genome Research Institute, which is part of the National Institutes of Health based in Bethesda, Maryland.

Before you agree to any genetic testing, Dr. Lapham suggests that you gather information to help you weigh your own options. Read the fine print in your insurance policies and employee records to see if you are obligated to disclose test results. With your doctor's help, assess the likelihood that you carry the genes for a life-threatening or debilitating condition. Ask yourself if the results of the testing would radically change your health care decisions. (For example, would you undergo a mastectomy if you tested positive for the breast cancer susceptibility gene?) If you decide to proceed, you'll have a clearer sense of what the future holds—not just for your health, but for your financial and social well-being as well.

HEALTH FLASH

ily's health history may be the single most important thing you ever do to bolster your well-being, according to Dr. Crouch.

Why? Because any disease that runs in your family puts you at risk. And regardless of whether the risks stem from you genetic code or from habits nurtured in your childhood, many family-linked ills can be kept at bay if you know the right steps to take.

Children of alcoholics, for example, are between two and four times more likely to become alcoholics than other people. "People who recognize patterns of alcoholism in their families tend to note the red flags in their own lives and are more likely to seek help or avoid problems in the first place," says Dr. Crouch.

What's more, doctors alerted by family histories can aggressively look for and treat specific health problems. "Consider breast cancer, for example," says Steven Esrick, M.D., a family physician in Northampton, Massachusetts, who is physician in charge at Kaiser Permanente Northampton Health Center and who also helps direct preventive-care programs in the northeastern United States for Kaiser Permanente, the largest nonprofit health maintenance organization (HMO) in the country. "It's reasonable for most women with a family history of the disease to start having mammograms at the age of 40."

"I know one woman who lost her mother and one sister to ovarian cancer at a young age," says Dr. Esrick. Because this cancer tends to be fatal and is difficult to detect early, even with frequent screening, the woman chose to have her ovaries removed. Not the decision for everyone, to be sure. "But because this woman knew her risks," says Dr. Esrick, "she was better able to weigh the options and to make the right decision for herself."

The New Family Tree

People in this country are hardly strangers to unearthing family history. Nearly half say they've at least dabbled in genealogy, and tens of millions have compiled some kind of family tree. Still, Dr. Esrick says he is amazed by how few people know even the barest of details of their relatives' medical histories. Only now, thanks to health maintenance organizations and other managed-care groups, is this trend starting to change. Under Dr. Esrick, for example, Kaiser-Permanente recently began an ambitious effort to gather family health information from all 114,000 of its patients in New York, Connecticut, and Massachusetts.

"What you're really looking for are patterns," says Dr. Crouch. Most crucial, he explains, are cases of cancer, high blood pressure, heart disease, diabetes, depression, and alcoholism—all common, life-threatening hereditary diseases that you can do something about.

"Another important pattern," Dr. Crouch says, "is the ages at which your relatives developed diseases." For example, women whose mothers had breast cancer prior to menopause run a much higher risk themselves. "It's hardly worrisome if several relatives died in their eighties due to heart disease," says Dr. Crouch. "But it's a different kettle of fish if they died at 35 or even 55."

Dr. Crouch constructs a health history for every patient but tells people not to worry just because a couple of relatives have suffered from heart disease or struggled with addiction. "My guess is that there's a genetic component to almost every disease," he says. "But few of them are caused entirely by genetics." In other words, having a diabetic grandfather raises your risk—it doesn't necessarily doom you to the disease.

Neither does a clean record mean that you can quit taking good care of yourself, says Bruce Bagley, M.D., a member of the board of directors of the American Academy of Family Physicians. "Just because you don't have a history of hypertension or heart disease doesn't mean a doctor won't still urge you to have your blood pressure checked, to eat a healthy diet, and to exercise." But when doctors can tie in family history, he says, blanket health warnings are made personal.

"Sure, no one should smoke," Dr. Bagley says. "But if someone looks at her family history and sees low cholesterol coupled with a two-pack-a-day cigarette habit, she may come to realize that it was really Dad's smoking that caused his heart attack. That's a pretty strong impetus for a person to quit."

This type of nudge can be crucial for people with silent conditions like high blood pressure and elevated cholesterol, says Dr. Esrick. Why change your habits if the disorder doesn't make you feel bad? "What feels bad," he points out, "is what happened to your parents."

No wonder Dr. Esrick often finds that his patients aren't ready to discuss their family's medical past until they're about the same age as a mother or brother was when she or he became ill or died. "I had one patient who finally came in because he's 47 and his father had a heart attack at 50," says Dr. Esrick. "Now he's taken up walking two days a week, he's reduced his weight, and, because he lost someone he cared about, he's agreed to take cholesterol-lowering medication."

Dr. Esrick's gospel is steadily sinking in. "A lot more people are being counseled and screened," he says. "And it's not just that more people are getting mammograms, Pap smears, and cholesterol tests. It's that the right people are being given the right tests."

Solving the Mystery: Detective Work

Investigating your family's health history doesn't have to be difficult, Dr. Esrick says, but it does take a little time. An ideal family health tree includes details about all your close relatives, both living and dead. What's the best way to

Preventable Perils: Are You at Risk?

Here's one rule of thumb: The more close relatives you have who suffered one of the conditions listed below, and the younger they were at the time, the likelier you are to have inherited a predisposition to the illness. Here's how to size up your risk and improve your odds.

Breast cancer. Only 5 to 10 percent of all breast cancers are inherited. Scientists have pinpointed a mutated gene, BRCA1, linked to both breast and ovarian cancer, and 1 percent of Jewish women carry it.

If it runs in your family: You may want to start yearly mammograms at the age of 40 instead of 50. If many members of your family developed the disease at a young age, you might ask your doctor about being tested for the mutated form of BRCA1.

Colon cancer. Between 10 and 15 percent of all colon cancers are inherited; family genes lead to about 20,000 new cases each year.

If it runs in your family: Ask your doctor about a sigmoidoscopy, which examines the interior of the lower colon. Regular, low doses of aspirin may offer protection, as does a low-fat, high-fiber diet.

Depression. Some types of depression run in families and occur in generation after generation. Not everyone with a vulnerable genetic makeup will develop depression, but stress is believed to trigger its onset.

If it runs in your family: Your doctor is more likely to suggest early intervention if you become depressed and your family history includes suicide attempts or major depressions requiring hospitalization.

Diabetes. If you have one parent with Type I (insulin-dependent) diabetes, you typically have a 4 to 6 percent chance of getting it yourself. If one parent has Type II (non-insulin-dependent), your risk is 7 to 14 percent. African-Americans, Mexican-Americans, and Pima Indians are at especially high risk.

If it runs in your family: Exercise regularly, lose weight if you're obese, and eat a low-fat, high-fiber diet.

Heart disease. If your mother or grandmother had a heart attack or bypass surgery before age 65, or your father or grandfather did before age 55, it raises your risk significantly, especially if you're African-American.

If it runs in your family: Swear off smoking and have your cholesterol level tested. If it's over 240, you need to have your blood analyzed for low-density lipoprotein (LDL), or "bad," cholesterol. An LDL level higher than 160 will likely prompt your doctor to prescribe cholesterol-lowering drugs and to advise you to exercise and cut back on fatty foods.

High blood pressure. A family history of high blood pressure increases your risk of developing the condition, which in turn boosts your odds of having a stroke sixfold.

If it runs in your family: Have your pressure checked regularly, watch your weight, exercise, and eat a diet low in fat and high in calcium, potassium, and magnesium.

Family Facts: Where to Find Them

The following agencies can help you track down your relatives, research your heritage, and, after you've compiled a health history, gauge your risks or those facing your children.

If You're Building Your Family Tree

National Genealogical Society offers two publications ($6 each) that explain ways to track down family health records. Send a written request to 4527 17th Street N, Arlington, VA 22207.

Family History Library of the Church of Jesus Christ of Latter-Day Saints houses the world's largest collection of genealogical records (church members are only a fraction of the database). The staff can answer brief questions and refer you to sources. You can also check the databases at more than 1,800 Family Search Centers in the United States and Canada. For information, write to 35 Northwest Temple, Salt Lake City, UT 84150; or call (801) 240-2331.

National Society of Genetic Counselors will refer you to professional genetic counselors, who flag hereditary illnesses and determine your risks. Once you've compiled your family health history, send a written request to the society at 233 Canterbury Drive, Wallingford, PA 19086. For more information, call (610) 872-7608.

If You're Seeking Your Birth Parents

Few Americans know less about their family health histories than the five million people who were adopted. Confidentiality has been the watchword for adoption agencies since the 1930s. These agencies can help you learn more.

International Soundex Reunion Registry provides a free service that matches data on adopted children with data on biological parents who have given up a child for adoption. Call or write for a registration form at P.O. Box 2312, Carson City, NV 89702; (702) 882-7755.

American Adoption Congress has local support groups across the country for adoptees, birth parents, and adoptive parents. Write to 1000 Connecticut Avenue, NW, Suite 9, Washington, DC 20036; or call (202) 483-3399.

Concerned United Birthparents provides support and some search help through a monthly newsletter and 14 local branches around the country. Write to 2000 Walker Street, Des Moines, IA 50317; or call (800) 822-2777.

Adoptee Liberty Movement Association holds search workshops at 62 chapters worldwide. The organization also provides a registry for people adopted from foreign countries who are seeking their biological relatives. Write to P.O. Box 727, Radio City Station, New York, NY 10101; or call (212) 581-1568.

get started? Before you call Aunt Edna, read this advice from Dr. Crouch and Dr. Esrick on assembling your own family health history.

Focus first on old-timers. Start with older family members since they're more likely to have suffered whatever ailments run in your bloodline. After tracking down information on your parents, grandparents, aunts, uncles, and siblings, you can compile the data for your spouse and children. If you're ambitious, you can fill in facts on cousins, nieces, and nephews.

Be tenacious. Placing a few phone calls is all it takes for some people. Others send out questionnaires or plan a big reunion so family members can swap medical details. Of course, close-knit families have a distinct edge over those separated by geography or personal disputes. But even deep gaps can be bridged. One method is to send any estranged relatives a note describing how a comprehensive health tree will benefit the whole family.

Be sensitive. Locating relatives is the easy part, says Dr. Crouch. Often tougher, he says, is convincing them to open up about their maladies and provide details. Health topics are highly sensitive; some are taboo to older people. Remember that not long ago it was the norm in this country to keep mum on miscarriages, mental illnesses, and even cancer.

Ethnicity, too, remains a delicate topic, albeit an important one. "For example, we worry about hypertension in blacks because they suffer more damage from the disease earlier in life. But in the South, especially," Dr. Crouch says, "if a mother was Creole, it's often not talked about because some people don't want to know what the racial background really is."

If one relative is tight-lipped, see if your chatty aunt might be more forthcoming. But in the end, says Dr. Crouch, don't sweat a few unknown details about an unreachable uncle or long-lost grandparent. Your goal is simply to gather as much information as you can.

Get all the facts. For each of your close relatives, try to find out:

- ❖ Full name and dates of birth, marriage, divorce, and remarriage
- ❖ Ethnic background
- ❖ Height and weight
- ❖ Average amount that she drank or smoked
- ❖ Any health problems, from recurring headaches and frequent colds to allergies and even limps. Pay special attention to heart attacks, strokes, cancers, diabetes, high blood pressure, high cholesterol, miscarriages, and major surgeries. List the age at which an event occurred or a condition was diagnosed.
- ❖ Any depression or substance abuse and all suicide attempts
- ❖ Date and cause of death

Tease out as much information as you can. If a grandmother died of stroke, was it caused by a blood clot or by bleeding in the brain? Did she also have high blood pressure? If she died of cancer, what kind?

Controlling Your Health

Organize your tree so that you and your physician can easily compare the health histories of two or more family members. The more close relatives you see who developed a hereditary illness and the younger they were at the time they got sick, the more significant your own risk. Some illness patterns—if all your aunts had osteoporosis, for instance—will be obvious. But your doctor might notice threats that you miss and possibly refer you for tests or even suggest that you see a genetic counselor, who can help gauge your risk of certain hereditary diseases.

"Some people will always be worried about finding an incurable disease in their bloodlines—though I'm of the school of thinking that knowledge is a good thing even if the news is bad," says Dr. Crouch. Not everyone agrees. Both patients and doctors worry that insurance companies might use this information to deny coverage to high-risk individuals, such as women who carry the gene mutation that raises the odds of breast cancer. Still, more than 10 states already have laws on the books banning this type of discrimination.

And though there's no immediate advantage to finding out that a relative had an incurable illness such as Lou Gehrig's disease, the day will come when doctors can actually repair defective genes. Until then, Dr. Crouch says, there's a lot we can do about the big things people die from, such as heart disease, hypertension, and cancer—especially if a family tree leads to an early diagnosis.

"In the balance of things," Dr. Crouch says, "learning more about your family history is about as close as you can get to controlling your destiny."

Too Young for a Mammogram?

Enduring the brief discomfort and inconvenience of a yearly mammogram pays off, says Daniel B. Kopans, M.D., associate professor of radiology at Harvard Medical School and director of breast imaging at Massachusetts General Hospital in Boston. This test can save breasts and lives. "Scientific research overwhelmingly supports annual mammography screening beginning at age 40," states Dr. Kopans.

And in cases of high risk, even women under 40 may potentially benefit from regular mammograms. "Annual mammography screenings for women in their forties as well as for older women could reduce their chances of dying from breast cancer by as much as 40 percent," says Stephen Feig, M.D., professor of radiology at Jefferson Medical College of Thomas Jefferson University and director of breast imaging at Thomas Jefferson University Hospital, both in Philadelphia.

Of course, mammograms aren't infallible. They have been criticized for being less reliable in younger women. But together with monthly breast self-exams and annual physicians' exams, they're the best protection we have. "The good news about breast cancer," says Dr. Kopans, "is that it's treatable—and for most women, it's curable." So don't wait any longer to start taking care of your breasts.

Why You Shouldn't Wait

Women under the age of 50 are not immune to breast cancer. Granted, the breast cancer rate for women under 50 is lower than for women over 50 (about 15 in 1,000 for women during their forties, 24 in 1,000 for women during their fifties, and 34 in 1,000 for women during their sixties). "But simply because there are so many more women between 40 and 49 in the population, the number of women in that age group with breast cancer is greater than the number of women in their fifties with breast cancer," says Dr. Kopans.

Yearly Mammograms Make Sense for Many

Should women over 40 receive regular mammogram screenings? When the National Cancer Advisory Board (NCAB) recently suggested that a woman and her doctor should decide the issue for themselves, it stirred up a loud controversy. And it's no wonder—in the United States breast cancer is the single leading cause of death for women ages 40 to 49.

In response to these recommendations, the National Cancer Institute and the American Cancer Society recommended regular screenings every one to two years for women who are of average risk for developing breast cancer. What is the best for women in their forties who are concerned about the risk of breast cancer? The best answer combines both suggestions, says Barbara Rimer, Ph.D., chairman of the NCAB and director of cancer prevention, detection, and control research at Duke University Medical Center in Durham, North Carolina.

"Women need to make the decision of how often to have mammograms based on their own personal history as well as on their own preferences and values," Dr. Rimer says. "Those who have had a family history of breast cancer, previous biopsies with a diagnosis of atypical hyperplasia (precancerous cell growth), and other risk factors might lean toward having a mammogram every year." Otherwise, says Dr. Rimer, every two years is certainly within range. If you're still undecided, talk with your physician, Dr. Rimer advises, and together you can decide what makes you feel safest—and what makes sense for you.

HEALTH FLASH

Mammography is your earliest warning system. "Think of breast cancer as an air bubble rising from the ocean bed," Dr. Kopans explains. "As it rises, it gets bigger and bigger. The doctor examining your breasts in the office is like a snorkeler—she can dive just below the surface and pick up cancer that has expanded to a certain size. But give a doctor scuba gear—a mammogram—and she can go even deeper, catching cancer at a much earlier stage." In fact, for a woman in her forties, mammograms make it possible to spot a small tumor about two years before she or her doctor could detect it with a manual exam.

Catching breast cancer early is especially important to young women. That's because breast cancer has a tendency to grow more rapidly in women under age 50. The reason this happens isn't exactly clear. It is thought that women who are genetically predisposed to breast cancer are likely to develop the disease at younger ages. Plus, higher levels of circulating hormones like estrogen may be factors. Whatever the reason, the point is, says Dr. Kopans, that younger women have smaller windows of opportunity in which to catch cancer in its earliest, most curable stage.

And studies have shown that, especially in women under the age of 50, having annual screenings is much better than a screening every two years. An early catch can be breast-saving. Early detection increases the likelihood that cancer will be limited to one small well-defined lump that can be successfully treated without removing the breast. A doctor can simply excise the lump with a bit of surrounding tissue and the underarm lymph nodes. With a follow-up course of radiation, lumpectomy is as effective as mastectomy in curing small localized cancers.

Catching breast cancer early can also be life-saving. Experts say annual mammograms beginning at age 40 can save lives just as well as mammograms beginning at age 50. In fact, according to Dr. Feig, for every 100,000 women ages 40 to 49 who are screened with annual mammograms, anywhere from 180 to 300 lives can be saved over a 10-year period.

The Under-50 Challenge

One drawback to screening all women beginning at age 40 is the additional number of surgical biopsies that result. Mammograms can't definitively differentiate between cancerous and noncancerous lumps; they only warn that something is there that shouldn't be. That "something" is often nothing more than benign fibrocystic change. Yet every spot that's still suspicious-looking after additional imaging (such as ultrasound) must be diagnosed with a biopsy—performed either as a needle biopsy or an open surgical biopsy. Because breast cancer becomes more common as women age, only 22 percent of the biopsies on women in their forties reveal cancer, compared with 36 percent for women in their fifties and 45 percent for women in their sixties.

Ultimately, that's good news for younger women. But there's no discounting the fact that biopsies provoke anxiety. Still, it's better to err on the side of caution. And biopsies needn't be a big deal. Skilled breast surgeons typically perform them in hospital outpatient facilities, using local anesthesia. Many biopsies can be performed accurately by taking out slivers of tissue with special needles. Occasionally, you may find out the results before you leave the hospital, but most often, you'll need to wait several days.

The biggest challenge in screening younger women, however, is missing lumps that are of concern. Younger women may have an extra hoop to jump through on the way to a good mammogram because they tend to have "dense breasts." (Density is a term used in mammography; it has no relationship to how breasts feel upon examination.) Breasts are made up of glandular (milk-producing) tissue, connective tissue, and fat. Younger women usually have a higher proportion of dense glandular tissue to fat, which is less dense. Child-

How to Get the Best Mammogram

Dense breasts shouldn't be a barrier to a good mammogram. Here's how you can ensure the best picture.

Go to a breast-imaging center. That way you're assured the equipment, technologists, and radiologists are dedicated to mammography. "A radiologist who interprets at least 15 mammograms a day is more likely to be better at it," says Stephen Feig, M.D., professor of radiology at Jefferson Medical College of Thomas Jefferson University and director of breast imaging at Thomas Jefferson University Hospital, both in Philadelphia.

Look for the seal of approval. Make sure the Food and Drug Administration (FDA) seal of approval is prominently displayed in the breast-imaging center. Besides setting radiation limits, the Mammography Quality Standards Act sets standards for mammogram equipment and record keeping. Every health professional involved, including the technologist who takes the pictures and the radiologist who reads them, has to be well-trained and practiced. Even if it's a mobile van, the mammogram facility must be certified.

Don't go with tender breasts. The most comfortable time to have a mammogram is right after your period, says Rachel F. Brem, M.D., acting director of breast imaging at Johns Hopkins Medical Institutions in Baltimore. If you can't schedule your screening for that time, dull discomfort by taking an over-the-counter pain medication (Dr. Brem suggests Extra-Strength Tylenol) about an hour before you have the x-ray.

Skip the talcum powder and antiperspirant. Ingredients in these products can show up as little speckles on the x-ray film, which could be misinterpreted as calcifications, tiny deposits of calcium salts in breast tissue that could be early signs of breast disease, says Dr. Brem.

Get a second reading. Go to a facility that does double readings on all mammograms. That means that two radiologists routinely read each mammogram.

Your insurance company probably won't pay for a second reading. But get it anyway. The cost of a second reading varies and could be about one-third to two-thirds the cost of the mammogram. What your insurance company may pay for is a second opinion, meaning you take your films to another radiologist to be interpreted. You may want to get a second opinion if an abnormality shows up and your doctor suggests a biopsy.

bearing and breastfeeding—as well as gradual changes that occur with normal aging—may shift that proportion toward fat.

The advantage for women with fatty breasts is that fat shows up black on a mammogram, whereas a tumor shows up white. But dense tissue shows up white, too. So like a snowman in a snowstorm, breast cancer in a woman with dense breasts can be difficult to distinguish.

Dense breasts may be harder to read, but no breasts are inscrutable. "No woman has breasts that can't be evaluated on mammograms," says Dr. Kopans. Merely increasing the amount of radiation is one way to produce a clearer x-ray.

And you don't need to worry about excessive radiation dosages anymore. Four years ago, the federal Mammography Quality Standards Act limited mammograms for the "average" breast to 0.3 rad per film—that's 10 times less radiation than was used in the early 1970s. Even if you start annual mammograms when you're 35, by the time you're 75, "the benefit to you will still be 25 times greater than the cumulative risk from radiation," says Fred Mettler, M.D., chairman of the department of radiology at University of New Mexico Health Sciences Center in Albuquerque.

Life-Saving Screening Guidelines

Everyone agrees that mammograms are the best breast-health test we have. They correctly identify tumors 75 to 90 percent of the time. The most recent review of data from Swedish screening programs shows that breast-cancer deaths for women in their forties can be reduced by at least 24 percent and perhaps by as much as 40 percent by screening annually.

The best advice? Follow these breast-saving guidelines developed by *Prevention* magazine after extensive interviews with breast-cancer experts.

Make it an annual event. If you're age 40 or older, begin scheduling annual mammograms for all the reasons already mentioned.

Start sooner if breast cancer runs in the family. If your mother or sister had breast cancer before menopause, begin scheduling annual mammograms at age 35 or 5 to 10 years before the age at which your relative's cancer was diagnosed. A family history of premenopausal breast cancer is an important risk factor, says Curtis Mettlin, Ph.D., director of cancer control and epidemiology and chief of epidemiologic research at Roswell Park Cancer Institute in Buffalo, New York. "Close surveillance is called for," he says.

Take care if you've had Hodgkin's disease or a problem biopsy. If you had Hodgkin's disease as a teen or have had a precancerous breast biopsy, take special precautions. A teenage case of Hodgkin's disease that was treated with radiation subjected you to large doses of radiation, most likely in the chest area, just as your breasts were developing. And that's when breast cells are most vulnerable. Compare: Radiation doses used for Hodgkin's disease are about 4,000 rads, says Dr. Kopans; mammogram doses are an average of no more than 0.3 rad per film—and the risk, if any, is negligible at this low dose, he says. So a woman who had Hodgkin's as a teenager has a 35 percent chance of developing breast cancer by the time she's 40.

Another situation in which you need to take special precautions is if you've

Lumps: When Not to Worry

For three out of four women, lumpy breasts are simply a normal fact of life. Every month, your body has a dress rehearsal for what would happen if you became pregnant, according to C. H. Baick, M.D., founding director of and breast surgical oncologist at the Breast Health Center in Santa Ana, California. Your body brings in extra fluids that you might need. As you get older, the cleanup after menstruation isn't as effective. Fluids are left in your breasts, forming lumps.

In premenopausal women, only 1 lump in 12 is malignant. But it's still important to have any suspicious lumps checked out by a doctor before you write them off as harmless, says Lydia Komarnicky, M.D., radiation oncologist at Thomas Jefferson Hospital in Philadelphia and co-author of *What to Do If You Get Breast Cancer.*

Although most lumpiness can be blamed on hormonal changes in your body, you can try some strategies to help smooth things out.

Dry your whistle. Cut back on alcohol, advises Susan Lark, M.D., a physician in private practice in Los Altos, California, and author of *The Woman's Health Companion.* "Alcohol elevates levels of estrogen in your system, which makes breast lumpiness worse."

Defat your diet. A low-fat, high-fiber diet can help rid your system of excess estrogen, notes Dr. Lark. A high-fat diet impairs estrogen excretion and raises estrogen levels by promoting the growth of bacteria. That growth increases the absorption of estrogen back into your body. "Vegetable-eaters excrete estrogen more effectively," she says. Significant sources of fat include salad dressing, cheese, margarine, and many meats.

Drink an un-cola. Avoiding caffeine could help cut back on lumpiness, notes Dr. Komarnicky. "Some people do seem to be very sensitive to caffeine. When they stop drinking cola or eating chocolate, their lumps decrease in size or go away, and breast tenderness decreases also."

had a breast biopsy with the diagnosis of lobular carcinoma in situ or atypical hyperplasia. "These are not diagnoses of cancer. They're just changes in cell patterns that you see under the microscope," says Dr. Kopans. But they do appear to be risk factors for breast cancer. So if you've been treated for Hodgkin's as a teenager or had a problem biopsy, discuss mammography screening with your doctor. Both situations require close monitoring.

Postpone, if you're not yet thirtysomething. If you're age 30 or younger, it's best to postpone mammograms. "Although the level of radiation used in mammography is very low, breasts are more sensitive to radiation at a younger age," says Dr. Feig.

Help and Hope for the Female Heart

Ask your women friends how they protect themselves, and they'll tell you about locking their doors, driving defensively, and what kinds of airplanes are the safest. They'll tell you about regular mammograms, and they'll tell you about not using products with broken safety seals.

Even so, most women are still leaving their most vulnerable spots unguarded: their hearts. When *Prevention* magazine undertook two nationwide surveys—one of female readers and one of women across the country—the publication found that women aren't even aware that their heart health is an area that's begging for protection. And the surveys revealed that doctors aren't doing nearly enough to educate us about how vulnerable our hearts are and about the essential steps we should be taking to protect them.

The good news: There's plenty that women can do.

Bridging a Dangerous Information Gap

Heart disease is the number one threat to women's lives—yet most women aren't even aware that they should be concerned about this matter of the heart. Women worry about breast cancer. But for every woman who dies of breast cancer, five die of heart disease. In the *Prevention* surveys, only one-third of the public and 37 percent of the magazine's readers were aware that their risk of dying from heart attacks is greater than their risk of dying from breast cancer.

A Heart-Saving Action Plan for Women

If there's one word women need to know when it comes to heart health, it's "action." In a *Prevention* magazine survey of American women, one in four who had heart attack symptoms didn't seek immediate medical attention. "I was particularly concerned about these results," comments Bernadine Healy, M.D., a cardiologist, former director of the National Institutes of Health in Bethesda, Maryland, and renowned women's health advocate. "Women still minimize symptoms, even the most compelling ones."

The classic symptom of heart disease for both men and women is heaviness, tightness, or discomfort in the chest. That may be accompanied by shortness of breath or sweating. The discomfort may radiate into the neck, shoulders, or stomach. For women any of the following may also signal a heart attack.

❖ Chest discomfort that occurs during mental stress or when resting (in men chest discomfort is most likely to occur during physical exertion).

❖ Nausea and pain, often just under the breastbone, can be aside from or along with chest discomfort; the nausea is not relieved by antacids or burping, and there may even be vomiting.

❖ Any of these symptoms accompanied by weakness in the chest, arms, or shoulders or unusual fatigue that may worsen with activity.

If you feel any of those important signals, take these steps immediately.

❖ Go directly to the emergency room if you're short of breath or have an excruciating chest pain that you've never felt before.

❖ Call your physician if you have other symptoms. Be as specific as possible about what you're feeling and where the feeling is. Don't dismiss what you're feeling just because you are not having chest pains.

Your doctor can tell you what the next step should be. "If you can't reach a physician on the telephone within a few minutes, go to an emergency room," says Dr. Healy. If it's not serious, you might be embarrassed. But if it is a heart attack, you just might save your life.

HEALTH FLASH

Beyond that, many women think that heart disease is like *Monday Night Football* or Steven Seagal movies—sort of a guy thing. But beginning at menopause, women's rate of heart disease slowly rises. By age 75, it's the same as that of men. Yet of survey respondents ages 75 and older, only one in three recognized the risk of heart disease. The danger is that women who mistakenly think they're immune to heart disease may not go out of their way to prevent it.

For years, scientists didn't suspect that women were prone to heart disease either. This gave doctors, and even women themselves, an excuse to ignore heart disease symptoms, notes Bernadine Healy, M.D., a cardiologist, former director of the National Institutes of Health in Bethesda, Maryland, and renowned women's health advocate. But now the truth is out and women need to know it. Women do indeed get heart disease and they do die of heart attacks—but usually about 10 years later in life than men do. Exception: Throughout their lives, women with diabetes can have heart disease risks higher than those of nondiabetic men. Other women whose risks may shoot up more quickly than their peers' are women who've experienced early menopause or have had surgical removal of their ovaries.

Take Control

A surprising number of American women—nearly three out of five—say that their physicians have not talked to them about heart disease. That number includes a substantial number of women over age 60, whose risk is the highest.

"This is not acceptable," says Marianne J. Legato, M.D., associate professor of clinical medicine and co-founder of the Partnership for Women's Health at Columbia University College of Physicians and Surgeons in New York City and co-author of *The Female Heart*. Women who are at high risk need to hear about it. And younger women shouldn't wait until they're at risk to start thinking about heart disease. The earlier women begin healthy lifestyles, the better, says Dr. Legato. That means the agenda for your next doctor's appointment is clear: If your doctor doesn't raise the heart disease subject, take the initiative and ask for a review of your risk factors. Here are the most powerful ways you can predict your risk.

Know your cholesterol ratio. To know your risk, you need to know the cholesterol number that matters most. American doctors deserve kudos for being scrupulous about two basic measures of heart disease risk. Nine out of 10 women say that during routine examinations their doctors are checking their blood pressures and weights.

The bad news is that many women and doctors are overlooking cholesterol checks, an essential measure of heart disease risk. One-quarter of *Prevention* readers said their doctors have not recommended that they get their cholesterol checked at all.

Even worse: When women do get their cholesterol checked and find out they have total cholesterol levels higher than 150, they don't come away with the number they most need to know—their total cholesterol/high-density lipoproteins (HDLs) ratio. "You can't beat that ratio for predicting heart disease risk—it's better than total cholesterol, HDL, low-density lipoproteins (LDLs), or even triglycerides," says William Castelli, M.D., medical director of the Framingham Cardiovascular Institute in Massachusetts.

To find your ratio, you divide your total cholesterol number by your HDL number. Your ratio should be 4.0 or lower. Laboratories often calculate this ratio for you and include it on your blood test results.

Looking at your total cholesterol and HDL numbers together, in the form of the ratio, is essential because, in women, high HDL can make up for high total cholesterol, says Dr. Healy. Remember that HDL is the "good" cholesterol, admired for its ability to herd "bad" LDL out of the body. Especially before menopause, women tend to have much higher HDL than men (testosterone may suppress HDL). That can make a woman's total cholesterol *look* really awful. Dr. Healy offers the example of a woman with total cholesterol of 240, which is risky for a man and could also be dangerous for a woman. "But if her HDL is 85, then her cholesterol level is actually good," Dr. Healy says. If doctors and women don't pay attention to HDL, women might end up taking cholesterol-lowering medication that they don't really need.

Conversely, "low" total cholesterol doesn't guarantee women immunity from heart disease. A woman with total cholesterol lower than 200 might assume she's safe if she doesn't know that she has low HDL—and she may not do enough to improve her heart disease profile.

Wondering where you stand? Ask your doctor for specifics. "Don't get into a situation in which you're told, 'Your numbers are okay; I looked at them,'" says Dr. Castelli.

If your total/HDL ratio is higher than 4.0, ask your doctor to check your triglyceride level. (This may mean returning to your doctor's office for another blood test, though sometimes the first test will also measure triglycerides.) If a woman's total/HDL ratio is bad and her triglyceride level is high (over 150), it might help the doctor diagnose a newly recognized pattern of symptoms called syndrome X, or polymetabolic syndrome.

"To put it bluntly, women with these symptoms are galloping toward heart attacks," says Dr. Castelli. "A particularly dangerous type of fat particle called the small dense beta VLDL particle tends to clog up their arteries. They need to know that they're susceptible, because they must be especially careful about staying on a prudent diet." The good news about high triglycerides—and syndrome X in general—is that lifestyle changes can eliminate the risk. "Most of these women would be cured by losing 15 pounds around the waist," says Dr. Castelli.

If you've reached menopause or have family or personal risk factors for heart disease—especially new risk factors (like recent weight gain)—get your cholesterol numbers retested every year if your readings are less than optimal. If you're healthy, under age 50, have no risk factors for heart disease, and have a good total/HDL cholesterol ratio, some experts say that a cholesterol recheck every four to five years is sufficient. But still others say annual tests are best for all women.

Measure your waist and hips. Virtually no physicians measure women's waist/hip ratio (WHR). WHR has been shown to be a better way to judge who's at risk for heart disease than weight alone. Even people who aren't overweight can have an increased heart disease risk if too much of their weight is located around their middles.

Among the women surveyed, only 8 percent have doctors who measure their waists and hips. Some doctors say that they don't need to wrap a tape measure around each patient to clarify whether that particular person has a dangerous pattern of central obesity or not. In the most obvious cases, "eyeballing it" may be enough. But just as your doctor puts you on a scale to get a precise reading of your weight, a precise reading of your WHR is important, too.

If your doctor doesn't check your WHR at all, grab a tape measure and record the following measurements: your waist in inches, then the widest part of your hips in inches. Next, divide your waist measurement by your hip measurement. This is your WHR. Your target is a ratio of 0.8 or less. Except for very slender women, the risks of heart disease rise steeply in women whose ratios are higher than 0.8. The good news, says Dr. Castelli, is that it's not so hard to change your WHR. "I've seen people's waist/hip ratios reverse even after they've lost just 5 pounds," he notes.

Heart-Healthy Hormones

After menopause, we need to consider hormone-replacement therapy (HRT) for heart health. Very few of the women surveyed by *Prevention* knew that HRT reduces women's risks of heart disease.

The fact is, the incidence of heart disease and death in postmenopausal women who take estrogen supplements is almost half that of women who have never used it. Research shows that estrogen can reduce blood pressure, keep blood vessel walls from collecting plaque, and prevent blood vessels from constricting. Some scientists speculate that these benefits may prove to be even more important than estrogen's well-documented effect on cholesterol levels: It can raise HDL and lower LDL by as much as 15 percent.

The experts also acknowledge that HRT is not right for every woman. The decision about whether to begin the therapy must be based on a careful evaluation of each individual's risk factors for heart disease and other health considerations. Even when women do decide to use HRT, they must be closely supervised by a knowledgeable physician. Dosages and the forms of therapy—which hormones are included and whether they are in the form of a pill or a patch, for

Emotional Rescue: Why Your Heart Needs It Now

Anger, depression, and social support all play roles in heart health for women. Here's how to assess and improve your emotional profile.

Learn to defuse anger. "Anger is probably as much of a risk factor for coronary disease (in women and in men) as cholesterol, smoking, high blood pressure, and a sedentary lifestyle," says Redford Williams, M.D., professor of psychiatry and director of the Behavioral Medicine Research Center at Duke University Medical Center in Durham, North Carolina.

It's not the occasional moment of rage that ruins your heart, it's when you regularly explode outward or hold anger inside and stew. Both of those tactics can send levels of stress hormones like cortisone and adrenaline, as well as blood pressure, into the stratosphere.

Dr. Williams suggests that you learn to disarm that anger by asking yourself three questions.

1. "Is the situation that's causing my anger important to me?" A no answer can knock out a lot of anger right from the start. If the answer is yes, go on to the next question.
2. "Is my anger appropriate to the objective facts of the situation?" Again, a no may remove a lot of anger right away. But maybe it is appropriate: "If blizzard conditions mean you're going to spend the next three nights at the Newark airport and miss Christmas with your family, any jury would rule that you have a right to be angry," says Dr. Williams. If the answer is yes, go on to the next question.
3. "Is there anything I can do to modify the situation that's causing my anger?" Confront the situation in an assertive way. Don't blow up at the ticket clerk—that won't eliminate the blizzard. But if the ticket clerk won't let you call to tell your family, you can insist on seeing his manager. "Don't explode," says Dr. Williams. "Ask for what you want."

example—often need individualized adjustments in order for women to maximize benefits and minimize side effects.

Align Mars and Venus

Women need to ask their partners for heartening support. The survey found that women may be a little too considerate for their own good—by being more concerned about their male partners' hearts than those partners are about the women's health. Why? Woman may be more "other oriented" than men are, says Redford Williams, M.D., professor of psychiatry and director of the Behavioral Medicine Research Center at Duke University Medical Center in Durham, North Carolina.

Recognize and ease depression. Depression is dangerous to the heart in both men and women, according to research. But research has shown that women are more likely to suffer depression than are men.

If depression persists, it's vital to get help. "It's as treatable as a broken leg, but first the illness must be recognized," says Dr. Williams. "Depression is a persistent sadness, lack of energy, or feeling of guilt. These emotions are often accompanied by changes in biological functions such as a lack of interest in sex or changes in sleeping and eating patterns," he says. If such symptoms interfere with your daily activities for a period of two weeks or more, your depression is serious enough to warrant medical attention.

Treatment doesn't necessarily mean medication. Studies show that cognitive/behavioral therapy ("talk therapy" that helps you learn new, positive, and realistic ways to think) can work just as well as pharmacological therapy, says Dr. Williams.

Spend time with friends and confidants. You've heard of cocooning. You've heard how concerns about safety are keeping people tucked away in their homes, isolated from others. Some research has turned up a link between loneliness and increased heart disease risk. Having a confidant not only reduces heart disease risk, it even improves the prognosis for people who already have heart disease, says Dr. Williams. The confidant could be your spouse, a family member, or a friend.

If you don't already have a confidant, you can win one over by becoming a good one yourself. "Be a good listener," suggests Dr. Williams. "When someone tells you that her back hurts, don't immediately respond by saying, 'Let me tell you about my ankle!'" Instead, he says, "Acknowledge their feelings. Say, 'Back pain really can be awful. Tell me more.' If you're a good confidant, that will make her more likely to be a confidant for you."

Or perhaps both men and women incorrectly assume that women aren't vulnerable to heart disease, suggests psychotherapist Mary Nakata, lifestyle counselor at the Pritikin Longevity Center in Santa Monica, California.

Either way, the point is that a significant other's loving support can improve heart health, says Dr. Castelli. Partnering up is especially important when you already have heart disease, he says. "We've learned that when the patient talks to a doctor alone, without her partner, treatment won't be as successful as when the whole family hears the information and realizes that lifestyle changes are something they have to do together."

Where to start? "Make an appointment to talk with your partner about your heart health," suggests Dr. Williams. "Sometimes it's hard to engage a man in dialogue about this sort of thing. A woman can say, 'I want to set a time for us to talk about this health problem. When is good for you?'"

Then ask specifically for what you need. If your partner is always bringing ice cream into the house, Dr. Legato suggests saying something like, "My cholesterol is terrible, and I have a real problem resisting ice cream. Can you help me out with this?" Engage him in collaboration.

The outcome? It may work. Or it may not. Ultimately, Dr. Legato says, women can't afford to wait for someone else to save them. "We have to take care of ourselves. If we wait for our partners or someone else to rescue us, it won't happen," she says. "Do your own risk assessment, learn about heart disease, and change your behavior. Even without a partner's support, those things are not that hard to do."

Small Changes for a Big Change of Heart

Don't overlook all the small lifestyle changes that can help protect you from heart disease. "Exercise and diet work terrifically to reduce your risk factors, even after menopause," says Dr. Castelli. Another incentive: "Women seem to be able to reverse heart disease more easily than men," says Dean Ornish, M.D., author of *Dr. Dean Ornish's Program for Reversing Heart Disease without Drugs or Surgery*. "Their bodies respond to changes in diet and lifestyle more dramatically than men's."

Focus first on the basics. The obvious steps may make the biggest difference.

If you smoke, quit. Smoking is the number one risk factor for heart disease. Women who smoke are two to four times more likely to develop heart disease than women who don't. Smoking lowers HDL cholesterol. Quitting is a proven way to raise HDL, notes JoAnn Manson, M.D., co-director of women's health at the Brigham and Women's Hospital in Boston.

If you're overweight, lose weight. Even if your ideal weight is miles away, a little weight loss can make a big difference, says Dr. Castelli. "I've seen people who lost just 5 to 25 pounds have dramatic improvements in their blood pressures, blood sugars, and HDL and LDL levels. I've even seen people who were able to go off blood pressure and diabetes medication by losing a relatively small amount of weight."

Get regular aerobic exercise. Exercise keeps weight down and HDL up. "You don't need to be a marathon runner," says Dr. Manson. Her research indicates that 3 hours a week of moderate-intensity exercise, like brisk walking, can reduce heart disease risk by 40 percent. "It's probably best to divide up the 3 hours so that you exercise at least 30 minutes every day," she adds. Although it's not conclusive, some research suggests that exercise may reduce women's risks more than it reduces men's risks.

Eat less fat, especially saturated fat. Your daily diet should contain no more than 25 percent of calories from fat.

CHAPTER 12

A Power Plan to Prevent Cancer

Imagine discoveries that reduce the threat of cancer by 50 percent. Amazing, right? Imagine that these miracle substances come from a rain forest somewhere. You know what would happen: Peter Jennings would be on the next plane, and everyone in America would be glued to their TV sets. But none of that will happen, simply because the miracle substances are...fruits and vegetables.

It's that simple, that convenient, that delicious. And now, a major study confirms more dramatically than ever the power of produce. Researchers in America and Germany reviewed more than 200 human diet studies from around the world, and they found consistent evidence that people who are high on the produce-consumption scale have about one-half the risk of developing a broad range of cancers compared with people who eat few fruits and vegetables.

Some of the research may have even underestimated the threat of cancer, believes Kristi Steinmetz, R.D., Ph.D., a nutritional epidemiologist in Forchheim, Germany, and one of the study's authors. So in reality, the reduction in cancer risk provided by eating fruits and vegetables may be even greater than first believed.

The study found that the strongest protection against cancer may come from raw vegetables, garlic and onions, legumes, carrots, green vegetables, cruciferous vegetables (the broccoli and cauliflower gang), tomatoes, and citrus fruits. But Dr. Steinmetz emphasizes that these particular foods are also the ones that people eat most often; other varieties of produce might be just as protective but wouldn't show up in studies because they're uncommon. Like most nutritional experts, she believes that all produce is likely to help us.

A New Clue for Preventing Ovarian Cancer

High cholesterol may be responsible for more than heart disease in women. In a recent study of 35 women with ovarian cancer and 67 women without cancer, researchers at Johns Hopkins University in Baltimore found that women with the highest cholesterol levels were more than three times as likely to get ovarian cancer as the women with the lowest cholesterol levels.

This is heartening news, since cholesterol levels are, to say the least, a little easier to control than other cancer risk factors, such as family history. Women with cholesterol levels above 200 were at highest risk. Whether lowering cholesterol can deflate risk has yet to be determined, but one study has linked cuts in dietary fat intake (subtracting 10 saturated fat grams a day) with a 20 percent reduction in ovarian cancer risk.

Researchers suspect that if there is a link between cholesterol and ovarian cancer, it could be because the fatty foods that increase cholesterol levels may also wreak havoc with hormone levels. Skewed hormone levels may offer an especially welcoming environment to gynecological cancers, including ovarian cancer.

Even if other studies confirm that high cholesterol is connected to this cancer, these blood fats aren't likely to be the biggest or the only cause of ovarian cancer, says study leader Kathy J. Helzlsouer, M.D., associate professor at Johns Hopkins University School of Hygiene and Public Health. Nonetheless, lowering cholesterol is one of the few roadblocks that research has begun to build in the path of this cunning cancer so far. While the threat of ovarian cancer doesn't begin to match that of, say, breast cancer, ovarian cancer is so stealthy that anything that can potentially stop it in its tracks is significant.

HEALTH FLASH

Flavorful Health Protectors

Fruits and vegetables deliver a legion of substances believed to fight cancer: essential vitamins like vitamin C, folate, and beta-carotene. Fiber. And dozens of natural substances called phytochemicals that scientists are just beginning to identify—like lycopene in tomatoes and ellagic acid in strawberries.

Speaking of strawberries, it appears that they're the fruits that nasty, body-damaging free radicals fear most. Free radicals are renegade oxygen particles left over from various activities in your cells. These renegades can damage cells, leading to cancer and other problems (like heart disease) unless they're mopped up by substances called antioxidants. Among popular fruits, strawberries turn out to be the highest in total antioxidant power. What that means is that strawberries may be the meanest fruits at helping our bodies mop up free radicals. Other members of the antioxidant "A-team" are plums, oranges, and red grapes, according to research.

All fruits provide some antioxidants (vitamins C and E, carotenoids like beta-carotene, flavonoids, and a slew of other compounds). But when scientists measured total free-radical zapping power from the combined antioxidants in each of 12 common fruits, they found that, ounce for ounce, strawberries are up to 2 times stronger than plums, oranges, and red grapes; 3 times stronger than kiwifruit and pink and white grapefruit; 7 times stronger than bananas, apples, and tomatoes (technically fruits); and 15 times stronger than pears and honeydews.

Scientists also analyzed five commercial fruit juices. The results? Bottled Concord grape juice had about five times the total antioxidant punch of red grapefruit juice, orange juice, tomato juice, or apple juice. Does this mean sipping apple juice or eating grapefruit is pointless? "Positively not," says researcher Ronald Prior, Ph.D., of the U.S. Department of Agriculture Human Nutrition Research Center on Aging at Tufts University in Boston. "Every fruit brings you benefits of some kind. But this study does suggest that some fruits give us extra help against free radicals and the associated diseases of aging."

And here's another potent cancer challenger from the plant kingdom: garlic. Chop some garlic, maybe sauté it a bit, and, along with a wonderful aroma, you release dozens of compounds that cancer researchers are scrutinizing. In studies one garlic compound, DATS, slowed the growth of—or even killed— human lung cancer cells grown in test tubes. DATS was just as effective against lung cancer cells as a common anticancer drug (5-fluorouracil) but was less toxic to healthy cells.

"These results have profound implications both for diet and drug therapy," says John Milner, Ph.D., who heads the department of nutrition at Pennsylvania State University in University Park. To develop DATS as a drug, we need to run more studies, he says, "but in the meantime, our results back up the idea that garlic should be a part of a healthy, anticancer diet." Deodorized garlic products typically don't contain DATS, though they have other potentially useful compounds that researchers are studying.

Putting Produce Power on Your Plate

Fortunately, no dietary heroics are necessary to gain the protective benefits that produce can give you. (In other words, nobody's making you eat 12 bowls of raw kale.) Dr. Steinmetz says raw produce may provide a slight edge over cooked in some cases, but your main concern should be getting enough of either. The same goes in the fresh versus frozen versus canned debate: In the end, it really doesn't matter all that much.

The National Cancer Institute's official dietary guideline, nationally promoted as the "5 a Day for Better Health" program, is a minimum of 5 servings of fruits and vegetables a day. Sadly, only one in four Americans really follows this advice. The average American woman eats fewer than 3.3 servings of fruits and vegetables per day (not counting potato products like french fries).

"There is no doubt in my mind," says Peter Greenwald, M.D., director of cancer prevention and control at the National Cancer Institute, "that Americans can substantially improve their long-term health outcomes if they simply get in the habit of eating fruits and vegetables more often."

For women who say they don't have time for fruits and vegetables, here are 20 produce-packed tips requiring almost zero extra time or effort. If you incorporate just a few of them into your daily diet, you'll meet your fruit and vegetable needs.

Give canned soup a boost. Heating canned soup in a microwave? Add to the bowl a cup of frozen peas, string beans, or carrots. You instantly boost vegetable content.

Sip your vegetables. Keep single-serving (6-ounce) cans of low-sodium tomato juice or vegetable juice cocktail at work, in the car, in your tote, or in your briefcase. They count as one instant serving.

Pile 'em on. Add more vegetables than your casserole recipe calls for. You're already investing time in slicing up something—celery, onions, carrots, peppers, mushrooms, zucchini, eggplant, whatever. It takes just seconds longer to slice twice as much.

Go Italian. Serving pasta sauce? Doctor it up with extra chunks of zucchini, onions, mushrooms, peppers, or carrots.

Try a fruity chicken salad. Make a humdrum chicken salad magnificent with chopped apples, grape halves, pineapple cubes, or diced mangoes. Aim for a ratio of half chicken, half fruit.

Add crunch to tuna. Making tuna salad? Add lots of chopped celery and onions. Or, add texture with chopped jícama—a mild, slightly sweet-tasting vegetable similar to a water chestnut. Shoot for half tuna, half vegetables.

Say olé to salsa. Indulge your salsa cravings. Each ½ cup counts as one serving of fruits and vegetables (most are tomato based). Try new varieties like mango salsa.

Explore citrus under glass. For instant grapefruit in the morning, keep a jar of grapefruit sections on hand.

Nibble on a new sweet. Instead of candy, reach for a bowl of dried fruit: only 2 tablespoons gets you one serving. Beyond raisins, consider dried cranberries, cherries, or papayas.

What, Exactly, Is a Serving?

The National Cancer Institute recommends eating five servings of fruits and vegetables a day (ideally, two fruits and three veggies). That sounds harder than it is. Have a banana on your cereal and a glass of orange juice in the morning, and you've finished your fruits. Add 2 cups of salad for lunch, a helping of broccoli with your dinner, and you're done. Here's what a "serving" really means.

❖ 1 cup raw leafy greens (spinach, romaine lettuce, kale)
❖ $1/2$ cup cooked, canned, or raw vegetables (sliced carrots, broccoli pieces)
❖ $1/2$ cup cut-up raw, cooked, or canned fruit (cubed melon, applesauce)
❖ 1 medium whole fruit or vegetable (orange, banana, peach, tomato, artichoke)
❖ $3/4$ cup (6 ounces) fruit or vegetable juice
❖ 2 tablespoons dried fruit (raisins)

Create vegaroni 'n' cheese. Making macaroni and cheese? Cook a box of frozen mixed vegetables to add it to your recipe. If you're in a cafeteria, take small side dishes of mac and cheese, broccoli, and carrots. Mix them together for an instant casserole.

Carry car cuisine. Grab an apple to munch on in the car. They're perfect for on-the-go dining—no drips or crumbs.

Delve into a can. No fresh fruit to pack for lunch? Keep single-serving cans of fruit cocktail on hand. Or open a can of tropical fruit cocktail and transfer some to a single-serving container.

Grab a handful of snackin' veggies. Look for Just Veggies snack mix of freeze-dried corn, peas, and pieces of tomatoes, carrots, and sweet peppers. It's lightly crunchy, lightly sweet, preservative-free, and addictive. Also super is Fruit Crunchies, a tart-sweet mix of freeze-dried apples, raisins, blueberries, sour cherries, mangoes, pineapples, and raspberries. Both snacks are available in health food stores.

Double the produce on your pie. Order every pizza with lots of "double" vegetables. If you don't order double, sometimes what you get is a token sprinkle.

Always order a vegetable. When eating out at a restaurant, ask whether your entrée comes with a vegetable side dish. If it doesn't, make sure you order an extra.

Trade up. If your restaurant entrée includes a salad, ask if it contains iceberg lettuce, which isn't as nutrient-rich as most leafy greens. If it is mostly iceberg, ask to trade it in for a vegetable, applesauce, or a fruit cup.

Order dessert early and often. Fine restaurants usually offer wonderful fresh fruits for dessert, no matter what season of the year it is. But why enjoy these delicacies only for dessert? Relish them as a luxurious appetizer. Another appetizer idea is to order one of the vegetables of the day.

Befriend the salad bar. Use salad bars to make a vegetable sandwich. Fill a sandwich roll or pita-half with your choice of shredded carrots, chopped peppers, tomato wedges, sprouts, and more. Top with a splash of olive oil or balsamic vinegar, if available.

Become the produce-meister of the party. When you're asked to bring contributions to parties or family dinners, become famous for the beautiful crudité trays you bring, complete with low-fat dip.

Double up. This one is so obvious that it's overlooked a lot: Instead of having a $1/2$ cup serving of vegetables, eat a full cup. It's only a few more bites, but you've racked up two servings.

14

The Natural Prescription for Healthy Bones

I f you think that it's too early (or too late) to think about preventing osteo-porosis—the brittle-bone disease that affects 20 million American women—it's time to think again. The good news is that this disease could eas-ily become yesterday's news if you focus on delicious, bone-building foods and easy, bone-toning physical activities.

"Osteoporosis is 100 percent preventable," says Susan Ward, M.D., clinical assistant professor of medicine at Jefferson Medical College of Thomas Jeffer-son University and associate director of the Jefferson Osteoporosis Center at Thomas Jefferson University Hospital, both in Philadelphia. Women's bodies were originally designed to last only until menopause, when estrogen produc-tion slows and finally ceases, or a little longer, according to Dr. Ward. Lack of estrogen triggers an increase in bone resorption—in other words, bone loss.

The earlier you start thinking about bone health, the better, says Susan Allen, M.D., Ph.D., associate professor of internal medicine at the University of Missouri—Columbia School of Medicine.

Boosting Your Bone "Savings Account"

Up to age 35, your body acts like a smart investor—if you follow a healthy lifestyle, your body makes more bone deposits to than withdrawals from your

Daily Calcium Investments Yield Big Payoffs

Yogurt and calcium-fortified orange juice for breakfast. A cheese dish at dinner. Instant hot cocoa as a nightcap. Even if you never touch a milk carton, this daily menu could keep you standing strong and straight for decades to come, according to research revealing the long-term benefits of fitting in calcium during a woman's middle years.

When a team of scientists from the Netherlands reviewed 33 studies of 4,000 18- to 50-year-old women, they found an encouraging pattern. Women who took in 1,000 milligrams of calcium a day hung on to 1 percent more bone every year in their hips and backs than those who didn't get that much of the mineral. One percent might not sound like much until you put it into perspective. "Think about your bank account. Would you like to have it going down 1 percent a year?" asks osteoporosis expert Robert Heaney, M.D., professor of medicine at Creighton University School of Medicine in Omaha, Nebraska.

For a fortysomething woman who hasn't yet met with the bone thievery of menopause, this means that she has plenty of time to build a defense against it. Twenty years from now, when declining hormones begin to cause a thinning of her bones, her daily nibbles of calcium may have saved 20 percent more bone thickness than she might have had. This could mean the difference between having brittle bones and robust ones.

HEALTH FLASH

skeleton. But from then on, withdrawals become more frequent while deposits remain the same. Once a woman enters menopause, those withdrawals escalate due to a lack of estrogen. For too many women the balance sheet goes deep into the red and osteoporosis is the result. And by the age of 50, a woman's lifetime odds of breaking a bone due to osteoporosis are almost one in two. Hip fractures are by far the most devastating consequence.

But no woman has to resign herself to Nature's bookkeeping. There's plenty you can do to deter or treat osteoporosis. Start with a food plan that lets you invest as much as possible in that precious commodity, your bones. Here's how.

Bone up on dairy. Premenopausal women need at least 1,000 milligrams of calcium a day, says Doris Gorka Bartuska, M.D., director of endocrinology, diabetes, and metabolism clinical services at Allegheny University of the Health

Sciences in Philadelphia. Once they're past menopause, women should get 1,200 to 1,500 milligrams a day, she advises.

The best sources of calcium? Low-fat dairy products. Topping the list are nonfat yogurt (1 cup has 452 milligrams), skim milk (1 cup has 302 milligrams), and part-skim mozzarella cheese (1 ounce has 181 milligrams).

If you can't tolerate the lactose in dairy products, try Lactaid calcium-fortified, lactose-reduced nonfat milk, which has 500 milligrams of calcium in every 8-ounce glass. If your daily calcium goal is 1,000 milligrams, just two glasses of Lactaid milk a day will fulfill your needs. For women over 50, who need 1,500 milligrams of calcium a day, drinking just one glass puts you one-third of the way there. Don't need milk that's lactose-reduced? It won't hurt you. And some people prefer the slightly sweeter, richer taste that naturally results when lactose in milk is broken down. Look for Lactaid milk in the dairy case at supermarkets nationally. Be sure the carton says "Calcium Fortified."

Go for calcium without the moo. If you're a vegetarian who doesn't eat dairy products, or if you simply don't have a taste for dairy products, there are other mealtime routes to better bones. Women can get most of their calcium from beans, green vegetables, nuts, and seeds (including sesame seeds and tahini butter made from sesame) as well as from calcium-fortified foods such as orange juice, soy milk, rice milk, and cereals, says Andrew Nicholson, M.D., of the Physicians' Committee for Responsible Medicine, a national organization of doctors that advocates preventive health care. While plant sources are not as loaded with calcium as milk or yogurt, they do provide significant amounts of the mineral.

In fact, some bone experts believe that nondairy sources of calcium are best. "Studies consistently show that countries where people eat the most dairy products also have the highest rates of osteoporosis," says T. Colin Campbell, Ph.D., professor of nutritional biochemistry at Cornell University in Ithaca, New York, and one of the architects of the China Project on Nutrition, Health, and Environment, a long-term study of the relationship between diet and health. "The more dairy products a population eats, the more osteoporosis there is." The problem with dairy products, experts say, is that they're high in animal protein, which has been shown to increase calcium excretion.

"Much of the calcium you get is probably counterbalanced by the protein that pulls it into the urine," says Dr. Nicholson. "If you get most of your calcium from dairy, you're already at a disadvantage compared to someone who gets less calcium but gets it from plant sources."

You could easily get 800 milligrams of calcium a day by choosing a cup of calcium-fortified soy milk and calcium-fortified breakfast cereal in the morning, 1/2 cup beans in your lunchtime chili, and 1/2 cup each of broccoli and bok choy in your Chinese stir-fry. Sneak in a glass of calcium-fortified orange juice and a calcium supplement, and you can easily consume the recommended amount of calcium.

Sip Supermilk

Mix $1/4$ cup nonfat dry milk with 1 cup nonfat liquid milk and what do you get? "Supermilk"—with 525 milligrams of calcium per glass and a richer taste than regular skim milk has. Drinking $2^1/2$ cups of this revved-up moo juice gives you slightly more than the 1,000 milligrams of calcium a day that most premenopausal women need and provides two-thirds of the calcium needs for women past menopause.

But here's an important note. If you take a multivitamin with 100 percent of the Daily Value (DV) of vitamin D, limit yourself to one to two glasses of supermilk a day to avoid getting more vitamin D than experts recommend. Why? Liquid and dry milk are fortified with vitamin D, so every glass of supermilk contains 45 percent of the DV of vitamin D.

Some experts caution that the calcium in beans and vegetables is a little harder for the body to absorb than that found in dairy products, so if you're depending on plant sources, it's important to make sure you get as much calcium from your food as possible. "To get to the calcium, you have to break down the cell walls of the plant, which contain fiber," says John J. B. Anderson, Ph.D., professor of nutrition at the University of North Carolina at Chapel Hill. "Cooking or even lightly steaming the foods will help, and it's important to chew very well so you get as much of the calcium as possible."

Include a supplement. Of course, taking calcium carbonate, calcium gluconate, calcium citrate, or other forms of calcium supplements is one way to ensure that you get what you need each and every day of the week.

Skip coffee and alcohol. "Put both alcohol and caffeine on your no-no list," says Dr. Bartuska. "Both are diuretics that leach calcium from your bones."

But there are even more compelling reasons to just say no to alcohol. Alcohol may be toxic to bone-forming cells and may interfere with intestinal absorption of calcium, say experts. Plus, drinking alcohol affects your balance and, as you get older, increases your chances of falling and breaking a bone.

Another lifestyle change your bones will love: If you smoke, join a smoking-cessation program. "Smoking cigarettes can lower estrogen levels," says Dr. Bartuska, "and it has a negative impact on bone density." A study of female twins suggested that a woman who smokes a pack of cigarettes a day may experience a 5 to 10 percent reduction in bone density at the time of menopause, a deficit that could increase the risk of bone fractures.

Bone-Friendly Moves

You already know that exercise conditions your heart and builds shapely muscles. But what about exercise to strengthen your bones? The right kind of workout can do just that. In fact, research hints that certain kinds of exercise can not only help a woman protect herself against the bone loss that comes with aging but may even increase her bone mass in particular areas as well.

Physical activity builds bones in two important ways. Impact exercises—from walking to step aerobics, from jogging to sports like tennis—signal your bones to add more bone mass and get stronger. Any and all impact moves—even descending a flight of stairs—have this beneficial effect. The skeletal impact is also greater when you leave the supermarket carrying bags of groceries than it was when you went in empty-handed.

Second, muscle contractions help build bones, too. Muscles are attached to bones. So, when your muscles contract, they pull on your bones. The bigger the muscles, the harder they pull. And the harder they pull, the more your bones are strengthened.

Based on your everyday activities, your skeleton settles in at a level of bone strength capable of withstanding the impacts and muscle contractions it's used to. So if you sit at a computer all day and regularly plop in front of the television after dinner, your bone strength will likely be lower than that of a waitress who's on her feet all day. In general, the more active you are, the stronger your bones are. "You want to add as much weight-bearing physical activity to your daily life as you can," says Gail Dalsky, Ph.D., director of the exercise research lab at the University of Connecticut Health Center's Osteoporosis Center in Farmington.

But there's more to exercising your way to stronger bones than that. To really do it right, you have to do the following.

Stay (or get) active. "Incorporate activity into your lifestyle now," says Susan A. Bloomfield, M.D., assistant professor of kinesiology at Texas A&M University in College Station. "The most important thing is to do something active every day." Dr. Bloomfield advises women to alter sedentary routines, for example, "never sit when you can stand or ride when you can walk. Any exercise is better than no exercise at all."

Take a walk. "Every woman should have a program that includes weight-bearing exercise," states Dr. Allen. "And one of the very best and easiest is walking."

"Schedule yourself for a daily 20-minute walk," suggests Dr. Ward.

Zero in on specific bones. There's no one activity that builds all bones. "To strengthen a bone, you have to do an exercise or activity that specifically targets that bone," says Dr. Dalsky. So, for example, while jogging may give your spine a jolt of strength, it does little for your wrists.

Surprise your bones. Research suggests that bones are strengthened the most when they're subjected to forces they're not used to, says Robert Marcus, M.D., professor of medicine and director of the aging study unit at Stanford University School of Medicine. For example, walking has always been an old standby in the fight against osteoporosis. But if you walk the same distance

Meet a Delicious Bone-Building Assistant

Orange chicken. Kiwifruit over yogurt. These menu items won't just get you raves. They might also get you stronger bones. Research suggests that oranges, kiwifruit, broccoli, and other foods rich in vitamin C might soon muscle in on calcium's bone-building stronghold.

When scientists at Loma Linda University in California looked at the bone densities and eating habits of 775 postmenopausal women, they saw that the heartiest bones belonged to the women who were getting some vitamin C along with their daily calcium. For every 100 milligrams of C that they were eating, the women's bone densities registered almost 2 percent higher than those of women who ate less C. An additional 2 percent bone density might not sound like much, but every bit of bone that's spared takes you one step further away from the debilitation that osteoporosis can bring.

One theory about what C might do for bones is that it helps build collagen, the framework around which bone is built. Without collagen, the crystals that form the hard part of the bone have no place to call home, and bone density is weakened, says study author Susan Hall, Ph.D., a researcher at Loma Linda University. Density also is weakened if calcium is missing. "We saw this effect only in women getting more than 500 milligrams of calcium a day," she says.

every day, day in and day out, your bones become accustomed to that level of activity. To stimulate an increase in bone density, you have to increase the amount of walking you do—or increase the load on your bones when you do your regular walking routine.

Another good way to give your bones a little surprise is to add activities to your exercise routine that are out of the norm. If you always walk, for example, mix in some step aerobics, racquetball, or rowing.

Stay in motion. Building bone isn't like erecting a building framework that, once it's built, is permanent. Left alone, a steel foundation lasts for centuries; but your bones need constant attention. "You have to continue your activity level long-term to keep up the strength of your bones," says Barbara Drinkwater, Ph.D., research physiologist at the Pacific Medical Center in Seattle. "On a practical level, this means choosing activities that are fun and that you will keep doing on a regular basis, and adding variety so you don't get bored."

Your Personal Bone-Construction Program

Let's be clear about the bone-exercise connection. Any physical activity can help maintain bone. But some forms of exercise may be better than others when it comes to boosting bone mass. And if you are vulnerable to bone loss in certain areas of your skeleton, it may be possible to give yourself an edge there. Some exercises are good at specifically targeting bones in fracture zones or those areas where osteoporosis hits hardest—the spine, hips, and wrists.

One type of exercise—resistance training—may actually increase bone density in certain areas of the skeleton. One of the studies showing specific-area increases through exercise was performed by Miriam Nelson, Ph.D., and colleagues at the U.S. Department of Agriculture Human Nutrition Research Center on Aging at Tufts University in Boston. The study put postmenopausal women, ages 50 to 70, who were not taking estrogen through a one-year program of resistance training two days a week for 40 minutes a session. Those who did five different resistance-training exercises maintained total-body bone density and actually increased density in two crucial areas: the hips and spine. In contrast, those who didn't participate tended to lose bone density.

"One of the most important outcomes from this study is that women greatly improved their strength—some got really strong—and their balance," Dr. Nelson says. "When you consider that falls are the number one cause of fractures, especially hip fractures, you can see how important improved balance really is."

Resistance training may also target two areas that few other activities can—the wrists and forearms. This is important because the wrists are likely to be the first fracture sites in women who develop osteoporosis. Racket sports like tennis can increase wrist and forearm density only in the arm used most.

If you have never worked out with weights before, or if you have osteoporosis or weak bones, get some advice from a sports-medicine doctor or certified personal trainer first. It's important to remember that some of the best bone-builders can be hard on the joints, and that some activities may increase your risk of fracture, so consult your doctor before beginning an exercise program.

Here are three basic bone-building moves you can do at home, with minimal equipment, that target a woman's at-risk bones.

Hip builder. You'll need a chair and adjustable ankle weights. Select a pair of weights that are comfortably padded and easy to adjust to fit the diameter of your lower leg, just above the ankle. Adjustable weights let you add or subtract the weight in $1/2$- or 1-pound increments.

Step 1: Put on the weights. Then sit on a chair or bench with your back straight and your feet firmly planted on the floor. Grasp the sides of the chair with your hands.

Step 2: Slightly raise one knee to lift your foot off the floor. Then raise and extend the lower part of your leg, straightening it until your entire leg is parallel to the floor. Hold for a count of 4 or 5.

Step 3: Hold the tension in your leg muscles as you slowly return the leg to the starting position.

Step 4: Do one set of 6 to 25 repetitions, depending on your level of fitness, with one leg. Then do an equal number with the other.

Wrist strengthener. You'll need a small dumbbell or a half-gallon milk jug, rinsed and partially filled with sand. With either, experiment to find the weight that's right for you—generally just heavy enough so that you can perform a dozen repetitions. (You can buy play sand at garden supply stores or larger toy stores.)

Step 1: Sit on an armless chair or bench.

Step 2: Holding a weight in one hand, slowly bring your forearm straight up toward your shoulder, keeping your elbow bent and your palm facing your shoulder.

Step 3: Slowly return to the starting position.

Step 4: After finishing a dozen repetitions on one side, move the weight to your other hand and do an equal number of repetitions.

Spine toner. You'll need an armless chair, a door, and a resistance band—a stretchy exercise band about 4 feet long.

Step 1: Open the door halfway and hang the band over the top, with the ends at an even length. Place the chair so the front almost touches the edge of the door into which the latch is set.

Step 2: Sit on the chair with your legs firmly planted on the floor on either side of the door. Grasp the ends of the exercise band.

Step 3: Pull back and down on the band firmly and slowly with both hands. Your elbows should be pointed to the ground and slightly outward. Hold, then slowly raise your arms to the starting position.

Step 4: Perform 5 to 10 repetitions.

Mistake-Proof Your Next Pap

15

You know the routine. The doctor scrapes cells from your cervix (the opening to your uterus). Then the cells are "fixed" on a slide. Finally, that slide is sent to a lab where a specially trained technician—a cytotechnologist—analyzes it under a microscope for signs of trouble.

And the results? Lifesaving. In the 40 years since Pap smears were introduced, cervical cancer has dropped from being a leading cancer killer among women to tenth place. No other cancer-screening test can boast that lifesaving record.

But what every woman fears is the small minority of Pap tests called false negatives. That means she is told that her results are "negative"—meaning no abnormal cells or disease are apparent—when, in fact, there are cancerous or precancerous cells present. In other words, potential or even full-blown cancer gets missed.

Fortunately, in many cases abnormal cells never develop into cancer. Or sometimes a precancerous or cancerous condition is missed one year but caught by the following year's Pap test. But when this doesn't happen, a false negative can be devastating. Experts agree that every year, some cervical-cancer deaths—although the number may be small—result from false-negative Pap smears that could have been prevented.

Clearly, reducing the rate of false-negative Pap tests can spare women's tears and lives. And now there's something you can do to spare yourself. Follow these steps, recommended by cancer experts, and you will increase the odds of an accurate Pap test in your healthy favor.

Cutting the Risk of Cervical Cancer

Estimates suggest that 10 to 20 million American women carry traces of human papillomavirus (HPV), a particularly potent risk factor for cervical cancer, says Diane Solomon, M.D., cytopathologist and director of the cervical cytology trial at the National Cancer Institute in Bethesda, Maryland. But most of these women don't know that they're infected.

Certain strains of HPV are implicated in 93 percent of all cervical cancers. And while having HPV may raise your risk, be reassured. It doesn't mean that you're bound to get cancer. "HPV is a necessary—but insufficient—cause of cervical cancer. In other words, in order to get cervical cancer, you need HPV infection. But infection in and of itself doesn't mean that you're going to get cancer, because other factors come into play," says Robert Kurman, M.D., professor of gynecology, obstetrics, and pathology and director of gynecologic pathology at Johns Hopkins University School of Medicine in Baltimore.

Those factors include smoking and multiple childbirths. Minor risk factors now under investigation are long-term use of birth control pills and low dietary intake of nutrients like vitamin C, beta-carotene, and folate.

Happily, you can reduce your chances of contracting HPV during sexual intercourse. If you're in a relationship, use condoms until you're certain about your partner's sexual history. "Condoms aren't 100 percent effective in preventing the transmission of sexually transmitted diseases, but they still provide a very high degree of protection," says Dr. Kurman.

To lower your risk of cervical cancer further, eat your fruits and vegetables every day, and don't smoke, says Charles Levenback, M.D., associate professor in the department of gynecologic oncology at the University of Texas M. D. Anderson Cancer Center in Houston.

HEALTH FLASH

Find a Professional Skilled at Sampling

Most faulty Paps happen when your feet are in the stirrups. "More than 60 percent of erroneous Pap smears go wrong when the doctor takes cells from the woman's cervix and puts them on the slide," says Ellen Sheets, M.D., gynecologic cancer specialist and director of the Pap Smear Evaluation Center at

Brigham and Women's Hospital in Boston. If the doctor is rushed or inexperienced, for example, she may not collect cells from the whole cervical area. Or the sampling tools may miss an abnormal area that is unusually high in the cervix. These are called sampling errors—and even the most careful lab screening is pointless once they're made.

Keep sampling errors to a minimum by going to someone skilled in taking Paps, experts say. Here's how to find the best Pap pro around.

Go to a gynecologist. "The medical literature clearly shows that gynecologists take better smears than family doctors, general practitioners, or internists," says David Wilbur, M.D., director of cytology at the University of Rochester Medical Center in New York. Data show that nurse clinicians in busy gynecology practices may actually take the best samples. "In both cases that's probably because they do more of them and are better trained," explains Dr. Wilbur.

This doesn't mean that no other doctors or nurse-practitioners take careful Paps, however. Some undoubtedly do.

If you want to see a gynecologist for Pap smears but you're in a health maintenance organization (HMO) with rules that call for general practitioners to do Paps, you might have to pay for the visit yourself...or perhaps you won't. Complain; when people make a fuss, they can win.

Watch the tools. Your doctor should be using two tools to remove cells for testing: a small wooden or plastic spatula for the outside of the cervix and a small brush that looks like a pipe cleaner or a mascara brush for the inside.

"If you see a doctor coming at you with a cotton swab, just say, 'No, thank you,'" says Dorothy Rosenthal, M.D., professor of pathology and oncology at Johns Hopkins University School of Medicine in Baltimore. "It's worthless."

Ask about ThinPrep. It's an extra-good sign if, after taking your sample, the doctor immediately dunks her sampling tools in a little fluid-filled vial instead of smearing them on glass slides. That means she's using ThinPrep, approved recently by the Food and Drug Administration (FDA). This method results in a larger collection of cells and helps make cells more readable.

Insist on the Best Lab

Assuming that your doctor has taken a good sample, the next vital link in getting an accurate Pap is the laboratory where the doctor sends your sample. The cytotechnologists who analyze smears spend their days peering through microscopes at Pap slides covered with thousands of cells that look like tiny dots. A given slide can hold 50,000 to a half-million cells each, and the cytotechnologist is looking for perhaps one or two abnormal cells among all of them.

"Having done this job myself," says Leopold G. Koss, M.D., professor and chairman emeritus of pathology at Montefiore Medical Center in New York

Prepare for Your Pap

You can increase your chances of an getting an accurate Pap by taking the following steps at home, says Dorothy Rosenthal, M.D., professor of pathology and oncology at Johns Hopkins University School of Medicine in Baltimore.

❖ Avoid sexual intercourse in the 24 hours before your test. Semen can interfere with test results.

❖ Schedule your Pap for about two weeks after the start of your menstrual period so that you can avoid having it done during your period. The background blood can obscure cells on the slide.

❖ Don't wear a tampon for at least 24 hours before your Pap. You may reduce the cells available for sampling.

❖ Postpone your Pap test if you have an active yeast infection. Inflammation can mask abnormal cells on your cervix.

❖ Don't douche or use intravaginal lubricants or medications for 48 hours before you have a Pap smear taken. You may wash away or hide the cells of greatest interest.

City, "I can tell you it is one of the most tedious, demanding occupations ever invented." Even the best cytotechnologist, being human, sometimes makes mistakes.

Unfortunately, some labs make more mistakes than others. "And in this day of managed health care, some medical practitioners use the cheapest labs they can, and those labs may be forced to cut corners," says Martha Hutchinson, M.D., Ph.D., director of cytopathology at New England Medical Center Hospital in Boston.

Since 1992, the federal government has enforced minimum lab standards under the Clinical Laboratory Improvement Amendments of 1988 (CLIA)—but minimum standards don't mean all labs are great. Here's how to find out what's going on at the lab that will read your Pap smear.

Talk with your doctor. Ask the following questions:

❖ "What's the name of the lab you use? Where is it?" (At the very least, your doctor should be aware of this.)

❖ "Do you talk to the lab a lot? Do they tell you if a smear is inadequate for evaluation and if you need to do it over again?"

❖ "How much confidence do you have in your lab?" Ideally, your doctor will be so enthusiastic about the lab that she'll be delighted you asked. For example, Jonathan Berek, M.D., chief of gynecologic oncology at University of California, Los Angeles, Medical Center, tells patients, "We have a very good lab. I know the people there, and if anything is questionable at all, they call me."

❖ "In one day, how many slides does a cytotechnologist at your lab screen?" Good answer: 60 or fewer. Disaster (and illegal under CLIA): more than 100. And in between? In most cases more than 70 or 80 slides on a daily basis is a strain on most cytotechnologists, according to Patricia E. Saigo, chief of the cytology service at Memorial Sloan-Kettering Cancer Center in New York City. Screener fatigue is considered the number one cause of lab error. If your doctor doesn't know the answer to this question, it's worth your time to call the lab directly.

Change labs. If you don't like the answers you get to these questions, maybe you should consider changing doctors. Or ask your doctor or insurer to send your slide to another lab. Request a lab at a teaching hospital or a major medical center, suggests Beth Y. Karlan, M.D., director of gynecologic oncology at Cedars Sinai Medical Center in Los Angeles. "Often, all of the slides are looked at by more than one knowledgeable person, including residents, pathologists, and technicians." Be aware that you may have to pay out of pocket to use another lab, around $10 to $30, but this may vary.

Have Your Pap Checked Twice

If every negative slide were examined twice, the rate of false negatives would go down. In a good lab, rescreening might drop the false-negative rate from 5 to 10 percent to 3 to 7 percent. In a not-so-good lab, the decrease might be even greater.

But under CLIA law all labs must recheck only 10 percent of negatives. So chances are your negative slide won't get that second look. Still, if you want extra insurance against a false negative, ask your doctor to have your negative slide rescreened. You will probably have to pay for this out of your own pocket, but it might be worth it.

Right now there's a raging debate among experts about whether humans or humans aided by computers recheck Pap smears best—with evidence for superior results on both sides. With computerized checking systems now available, you may be able to choose whether a human or a human helped by a machine will do this vital work. "This technology is in its infancy, and there is tremendous potential for future applications," predicts Diane Solomon, M.D., cytopathologist and director of the cervical cytology trial at the National Cancer Institute in Bethesda, Maryland. Dr. Solomon thinks that, as the technology evolves, computer-assisted screening will reach a point where it is clearly better than human screening alone.

Either way, here's how to arrange to have your Pap rechecked.

Have the same lab read it twice. If you're confident in your doctor's lab, you can ask your doctor to have the lab staff look at your slide twice. Probable fee: about $20.

If your doctor has agreed to send your slide to a university or medical-center lab, ask for your slide to be screened twice there. Probable fee: about $25 to $30, but it may vary.

Call in computer technology. If you still have questions about the quality of the lab your doctor uses, you may want to ask your doctor to send your Pap smear for a computer-assisted rescreening, technology recently approved by the FDA.

One procedure, called Papnet, works like this: Your Pap smear is taken at your doctor's office, and then at your request is sent to a local lab that offers Papnet testing. After this lab does a first screening and your slide is negative, it is sent to the Papnet scanning center at Neuromedical Systems in Suffern, New York. Papnet's automated microscopes scan your cells, and a supercomputer identifies cells most likely to be abnormal. Magnified images of these cells are sent back to the originating lab for another look.

For more information about a Papnet rescreen, you can call the company at (800) 727-6384. A Papnet recheck costs $35 to $40, and your insurer probably will not pay for it.

Another computer rescreening system recently approved by the FDA is AutoPap QC, made by Neopath in Redmond, Washington. Unlike labs with Papnet, labs equipped with AutoPap can offer computer rescreening on-site. Although AutoPap uses slightly different technology, as with Papnet, accuracy trials are encouraging.

After the initial screening by a cytotechnologist, your negative slide goes through the AutoPap system and is "scored." If the score indicates the possibility of abnormal cells, the cells on your slide get another look by a cytopathologist or pathologist.

A lab that uses AutoPap automatically rescreens all negative slides. You don't need to request it. But if your doctor's lab doesn't have AutoPap, he or she can arrange to have your slide sent to a lab that does. To find out more about AutoPap, you can call (800) 636-7284. The cost may vary from lab to lab, but averages around $20.

Go Back Every Year

Fabulous fact: The more Paps you get, the safer you are. The chance of finding abnormal cervical cells on a single Pap smear is higher than 80 percent. But if you get Pap smears three years in a row and they all turn up negative, there's a 99 percent chance that you really have no cervical cancer or precancer, says Dr. Hutchinson. That's tremendous peace of mind. (But you should still continue to get Paps every year.)

The vast majority of cervical cancers—90 percent—grow very slowly and are curable in the early stages. A cancer missed by one year's Pap (a false negative) will likely be caught next year or two years later, in time for successful treatment. But three or more years later, it may be too late.

So instead of skipping a few years (as some organizations, including the American Cancer Society, allow under certain circumstances), get a Pap every year. Some insurers don't pay for annual Paps, so you may have to pick up the tab, but it's worth it. Fee range: $15 to $30, plus the charge for the office visit.

For a blue-ribbon Pap every time, here are more expert tips.

Don't wait by the phone for results. Call your doctor for Pap results. Better still, ask her to send them to you.

Know the symptoms of cervical cancer. Symptoms include bleeding between periods, bleeding after intercourse, and abnormal vaginal discharge. Even if your Pap comes back negative, such symptoms are cause for concern, and you should get another look.

Choose yearly Paps first. Suppose you have to choose between paying for a Pap test every year or paying for a Pap test and a rescreening every other year? Go for the yearly Pap tests. Until computerized systems are perfected and proven, experts agree that annual Pap tests, taken by competent doctors who use excellent labs, are your best safeguard for the most reliable Paps possible.

16

The Right Way to Tame High Blood Pressure

Blame it on hormones, genetics, and diet: One in 10 women between the ages of 35 and 44 has high blood pressure. By age 55, one in four has this silent but serious condition that, if ignored, leaves you 12 times more likely to suffer a stroke, 6 times more likely to have a heart attack, and 5 times more likely to die of congestive heart failure.

When you have hypertension, blood rushes through your blood vessels like a soundless speedboat. You don't feel it, but over time the force of that ride damages the vessels' surfaces. Fatty debris begins to stick easily to rough walls. The vessels narrow. Clots can form and break loose, causing a heart attack or stroke. Even if that doesn't happen, the heart labors and strains, weakening and enlarging. For all the drama, it's mute theater. A stubbed toe causes more pain than blood vessel damage. That's why one-third of women with high blood pressure don't even know they have it.

Sobering news, but even more sobering are the reports from doctors who treat high blood pressure. Members of the American College of Cardiology, the American College of Preventive Medicine, and six other health-care groups took a look at the treatment of high blood pressure in this country and found it wanting. They gave it a C-minus. Go to the back of the class.

That wasn't the only dunce cap issued. The National Heart, Lung, and Blood Institute also released a statement saying that 50 percent of the hyper-

Easing High Blood Pressure— At Home and at Work

Your report is overdue, the meeting has already started, and the copier has rebelled again. This evening, you have to ferry the kids to soccer practice, cook dinner, do two loads of laundry, and find a birthday present for your mother. You mutter that it's a good thing that your blood pressure isn't being checked right now. In an important study of women's blood pressure levels, researchers at Duke University in Durham, North Carolina, have discovered that not only work but also home life can make women's blood boil. And they've discovered a simple way to ease it.

The Duke study looked at 24 women whose average age was 47. All were somewhat sedentary, somewhat overweight, and had slightly elevated blood pressures. Each wore a portable blood pressure monitor that automatically recorded her blood pressure four times an hour throughout a working day and that evening, until bedtime.

This continual monitoring showed that women's pressures went up at work, as expected. But their pressures also remained up when they went home. Researchers speculate that this may reflect women's responses to their multiple roles of employees, homemakers, and caregivers.

While most studies have examined the effects of job stress on men, "few have looked at stress and blood pressure during women's workdays," says James Blumenthal, Ph.D., study co-author and director of the Behavioral Medicine Program at Duke University's Center for Living. "And women may have different or additional job stressors than men."

Regardless of the cause of stress, physical fitness appeared to offer protection during the day and during "second shifts." When blood pressures were reexamined according to fitness levels, the least fit were found to have the biggest rises at work and at home, while the fitter women's pressures remained relatively stable.

The message is that you should make a habit of kicking up your heels—after slipping out of them. Walking, bicycling, and swimming are just a few examples of activities that build aerobic capacity, the type of fitness measured in the study. Scientists aren't sure how exercise short-circuits the body's response to stress, but they've seen enough evidence of its benefits to recommend it heartily.

HEALTH FLASH

tension in the United States is undetected or—even after the condition is discovered in a person—is inadequately treated.

Other experts say the statistics are even worse. Thirty-five percent of people with high blood pressure don't even know that they have the problem, according to Harry Gavras, M.D., vice-chairman of the American Heart Association's Council for High Blood Pressure Research and chief of the hypertension and atherosclerosis section of Boston University Medical Center, and 27 percent are inadequately treated. Only 25 percent are adequately or well-treated.

That's why women need yearly blood pressure checks—and a strategy for ensuring proper treatment. Read on for easy techniques that will help you keep hypertension in check.

The Case for Frequent Readings

What usually happens is that "patients get one high blood pressure reading. Their doctors put them on medication. The next time the patients see their doctors, they're fine; the doctors say the medication has done the trick. But in many cases these people would have been fine even without medication," says Thomas G. Pickering, M.D., professor of medicine at the hypertension center at New York Hospital–Cornell Medical Center in New York City and author of *Good News about High Blood Pressure.*

That's because a single blood pressure reading is just one brief moment in time. One reading may not at all represent what's going on most days. Government guidelines for treatment suggest multiple readings during each doctor's visit.

"Even then, our research has shown that for some people, doctors' readings are often the least representative of their overall levels of blood pressure," says Dr. Pickering. The reason is that about 20 percent of people with high blood pressure suffer from "white-coat hypertension." Doctors' offices make them nervous. Their blood pressures spike. But they don't usually need to be medicated. Here's how to get around this problem.

Skip the doctor. One way to bypass white-coat hypertension is to ask the doctor's nurse or technician to take your blood pressure reading, says Dr. Pickering. Dealing with someone other than the doctor may help you feel less nervous.

Take it yourself. There's a big movement for home monitoring of blood pressure, says Dr. Pickering. You can buy manual or electronic home units that provide fairly reliable readings.

With a home monitor you can average out various readings taken during the course of a day. Your measurements may very well be different in the morning and evening, at work, and after exercise. But you'll be able to get the total picture, especially if you track your pressure for a few weeks and average out all the different readings.

One home blood pressure unit that Dr. Pickering likes incorporates the stethoscope on the blood pressure cuff. "It's reliable, but still requires a certain degree of skill and hearing ability. So not everybody can use it."

Most people find electronic home units the easiest systems to manage. They read blood pressure via sensors and print out the reading. Avoid the units that measure pressure from your finger or wrist—they're not reliable, says Dr. Pickering. Home monitors should be taken to a doctor's office to make sure that they're accurate, he says. No matter which kind of monitor you purchase, test the new machine alongside your doctor's to make sure that they're in sync. Then take it in once a year for an accuracy checkup. (The manual models aren't as touchy.)

Is Your Doctor Paying Attention?

Too often, high blood pressure gets short shrift in doctors' offices—for two big reasons. "Part of the problem is that even though hypertension is extremely common, its treatment is not generally recognized as a medical specialty," explains Dr. Pickering. "There are no board examinations to qualify as a specialist. And, for most physicians, it's not their prime interest. So hypertension frequently doesn't get the professional scrutiny it requires. It is treated mostly by family practitioners, internists, nephrologists, and cardiologists," he says.

The other part of the problem is the sheer amount of time that treatment of hypertension demands. "You have to give patients tender loving care. But that's hard to do on a 15-minute schedule. If you don't, though, you're doomed to failure," says Ray W. Gifford Jr., M.D., professor of internal medicine at Ohio State University College of Medicine in Columbus and consulting physician in the department of nephrology and hypertension at the Cleveland Clinic Foundation. "One of the most common mistakes is that doctors don't spend enough time convincing patients that the way to reduce their risk of stroke and heart attack is to lower their blood pressures. Doctors need to talk to their patients in order to make lifestyle changes tempting, because people tend to resist such changes. Doctors have to make sure that patients know that those changes are almost sure to bring blood pressure down so they may not need medication," Dr. Gifford explains.

"Doctors can't just tell patients to start low-salt diets and exercise programs and to come back in six months," Dr. Gifford adds. "Patients need to come in three times during those six months to reinforce lifestyle modifications. They need physicians who spend the time to keep evaluating them once they're on treatment programs."

But how do you find a dedicated doctor if you can't look under "Hypertension Specialist, Long Hours" in the yellow pages? Try these suggestions.

Shop for a doc online or by mail. Dr. Pickering has formed the Hypertension Network, which makes use of the Internet to provide people with up-to-date information about hypertension, including question-and-answer forums. It also provides a list of physicians who have a special interest in treating hypertension. Write to the Hypertension Network at P.O. Box 302, Wingdale, NY 12594.

Have a heart-to-heart with your family doctor. If you already have a long-time family doctor whom you like, make an appointment to talk with her. Go prepared: Write down your questions and refer to them. If you've read up on hypertension and made notes for discussion, take them in, too. Tell your doctor your concerns about your blood pressure and its treatment. Let her know that you're willing to take an active role in managing your condition by recording your blood pressure and by making appropriate lifestyle changes.

Don't Play the Waiting Game

"This is a common problem—physicians often don't initiate therapy in patients with mild hypertension. They wait until the hypertension is worse. But experts consider this waiting game a major public-health concern," says William B. White, M.D., chief of the hypertension section at University of Connecticut Health Center in Farmington.

The fact is, even mild hypertension increases your risk of stroke and heart attack. Stage 1 (mild) hypertension means that your systolic reading (the top figure, which measures how hard your heart has to pump) is between 140 and 159. And your diastolic pressure (which measures the amount of pressure produced by your heart between beats) is between 90 and 99.

Dr. White thinks that doctors just fail to see mild hypertension as a significant problem in the vigorous people sitting across from them. "A doctor may think, 'Okay, this person is 40 years old, and pretty healthy otherwise, with a blood pressure of 140/90,'" says Dr. White. "So she thinks that hypertension isn't very serious. The patient thinks she's healthy because she doesn't have something bad enough to get medicine for. But mildly elevated blood pressure is likely to become even higher over time," Dr. White warns. "So the patient resurfaces five years later, when her blood pressure is 160/110. During that interval, damage has occurred, such as cardiac changes associated with blood pressure elevation or kidney problems."

Dr. Gifford believes in very early intervention—when blood pressure is high-normal, in the range of 130 to 139 over 85 to 89. "But doctors don't tend to make much fuss if blood pressure is 135/85. The message doesn't come across that it might be risky. But the high-normal stage is the time to get to it.

More Savvy Strategies to Lower a Woman's Blood Pressure

Ultimately, the power to lower high blood pressure is in your hands—whether it's by sticking with a healthy lifestyle or being smart about taking medication on time, every day. Here's how to keep yourself on track.

❖ Ask your medical insurer or local hospitals and health groups where you can find hypertension support groups.

❖ Look in your local newspaper for heart-healthy cooking classes. They're cropping up all over.

❖ Use a home blood pressure monitor regularly to get feedback on how well lifestyle changes are working for you.

❖ Join a health club or a gym. Or find a buddy to work out with.

If the idea of taking a pill every day of your life turns you off, you need to do a little research on why blood pressure–lowering medication is necessary for you. Ask your doctor to point you in the direction of information. If side effects have understandably put you off pill taking, be aware that there are six very different classes of drugs for high blood pressure and many medications in each class. "You really need to try a different medication. You shouldn't take a hypertension drug that produces side effects," says Thomas G. Pickering, M.D., professor of medicine at the hypertension center at New York Hospital–Cornell Medical Center in New York City and author of *Good News about High Blood Pressure*.

There's really good evidence that you can prevent high blood pressure then, before it gets worse," he says.

Unless blood pressure is high—above 160/105, says Dr. Gifford—or is complicated by a condition like diabetes, prompt treatment means initiating lifestyle changes.

"Lifestyle changes are very important," says Dr. Gavras. "Your doctor should educate you to eat less sodium, lose weight, and exercise with activities like walking." Just by decreasing sodium intake and losing weight, one-third of those with hypertension can control their blood pressures.

But doctors seem more at ease with drugs than with eating or exercise regimens, says Dr. White. "We have a much harder time educating patients about lifestyle changes. Changes are hard to implement because physicians don't have the time or the background information on how to educate patients during short office visits," he says.

So when doctors finally nab blood pressure at Stage 1, they often do so with medication. "When a doctor doesn't have much time, it's easy to just say to the patient, 'You have high blood pressure—I'll give you a prescription,'" says Sheldon G. Sheps, M.D., chief of the hypertension division at the Mayo Clinic in Rochester, Minnesota. If you find yourself as a patient in that position, and your hypertension is mild and uncomplicated, Dr. Sheps says, "then it's all right for you to say, 'I've been reading that I might be able to help my blood pressure by losing 10 pounds, and I'd like to try that first. Is it okay? If it doesn't work in three months, I'll consider medication.'"

But if your blood pressure is high-normal, and you'd like to take it down a notch even though your doctor seems unconcerned, ask her about lifestyle changes. "It's always a good idea to ask about ways to change your diet and exercise," says Dr. White. "I also think it's a good idea to ask if you should have a medical evaluation before you start an exercise program." Here are the top lifestyle changes our experts recommend.

If you're overweight, lose some pounds. "You get the biggest bang for your buck right here," says Dr. Gifford. Even 10 pounds may be enough to give you the blood pressure control you need. Why is your weight so important? Extra fatty tissue makes your heart pump harder.

Control your salt intake. Give up table salt and cooking salt, advises Dr. Gifford. And rely more on fresh foods than salty processed ones, he says. Half the folks who have high blood pressure are sensitive to sodium. Excess salt makes them retain water, which waterlogs blood vessels, narrows them, and makes the heart work too hard. (Talk to your doctor before making major dietary changes.)

Get moving. Aerobic exercise has been shown to reduce blood pressure if it's done for 40 minutes three times a week or more. The effect is greatest on the top, systolic number. Aerobic activities include walking, biking, and swimming. Whether or not weight is a problem, working out tones your heart as well as your muscles, studies show. Weight training (when done properly—making sure not to hold your breath, avoiding prolonged gripping, and using weights that you can easily handle) can also reduce blood pressure.

Cut down on alcohol. Two drinks a day is the absolute maximum.

Stop smoking. It's the major risk factor for heart disease.

Just Say No to Drug Overload

"There's a tendency among physicians to just prescribe additional blood pressure medication when one isn't working adequately, rather than to try substituting them," says Dr. Pickering. "Some medications simply don't work on particular patients. For those people it would make more sense to substitute something that does work, not pile one drug on top of another."

Part of the problem, Dr. Pickering explains, is that trying to find out whether a medication is working involves taking many blood pressure measurements. But if you get only three readings at a doctor's visit, and you have only one visit every few weeks, it's difficult for your doctor to get enough data to make a good decision about medication. If you're trying a series of drugs to see which is best, it's cumbersome and expensive to do it by going to the doctor every week.

One thing a patient can do, Dr. Pickering says, "is self-monitor your blood pressure. It's economical and easy to tell if medication seems to be working by using a home monitor. Then you can phone in or fax in your readings to your doctor. Your doctor can get a feel for whether the drug is working. It's a valuable way to assess medication."

Relief from Fibroids— With or without Surgery

Karen Tursi had a hysterectomy on Day 57 of her last menstrual period. "I was ready to go out and buy stock in tampons," the marketing manager from Chicago says wryly.

She had experienced pain and bleeding from uterine fibroids and endometriosis since college. The two years before her hysterectomy were particularly bad. "From the day before my period to two days after it began, the pain was sometimes so intense that I could not stand up," she says. Yet some relatives and friends—not to mention a series of doctors—couldn't understand why a woman in her thirties would even consider having her uterus removed.

Her regular gynecologist advised against the operation. So did three other doctors to whom she turned for help. All argued that she was too young to become infertile, even though she had no desire to become a mother. "Some people cannot fathom a woman not wanting to have children," Tursi says. Finally, she convinced a fifth doctor that she was of sound mind and wanted a sound body. So, six weeks after her 36th birthday, Tursi had her uterus removed. "A week after surgery, I was actually feeling better than I'd felt during the previous two years," she says.

Acupuncture Relieves Fibroid Pain

More and more American women are easing symptoms associated with fibroid tumors, such as bleeding, urinary incontinence, and infertility, with a new alternative—the ancient Chinese healing art of acupuncture, says Sharon Weizenbaum, a certified acupuncturist and director of Traditional Asian Healing Arts in Amherst, Massachusetts.

In some cases acupuncture may even reduce the size of these benign growths that arise from the walls of the uterus, says Patrick J. LaRiccia, M.D., who has a private practice in alternative medicine at the Presbyterian Medical Center and who is director of the Acupuncture Pain Clinic at the Hospital of the University of Pennsylvania, both in Philadelphia.

"With acupuncture, most women find relief from symptoms associated with fibroids after the first two or three treatments," says Weizenbaum. "Many of the women who come to me were told that they needed hysterectomies because of their fibroids. But after acupuncture, many felt relief from their symptoms and did not need surgery."

This form of alternative medicine may not work for all women with fibroids. If a woman is unresponsive to acupuncture or has severe menstrual bleeding, the fibroids can be surgically removed, says Dr. LaRiccia.

Acupuncture uses tiny needles to stimulate what Chinese medical practitioners call *chi*—the body's basic healing energy. A trained acupuncturist inserts the needles, painlessly, at specific points on the body where this energy may be blocked. "On average, I insert about 12 needles at various locations on the body," explains Weizenbaum.

Usually, a woman would undergo a trial of eight treatments, says Dr. LaRiccia. After that, she may need occasional or periodic booster sessions.

If you are thinking of consulting an acupuncturist for fibroids, contact the National Certification Commission for Acupuncture and Oriental Medicine, Department No. 0595, Washington, DC 20073-0595. For $3 they will send you a list of certified acupuncturists in your state.

For a referral to a physician acupuncturist, call the American Academy of Medical Acupuncture physician referral line at (800) 521-2262.

HEALTH FLASH

Needless Surgery or Necessary Relief?

Tursi isn't the only woman to maintain that a hysterectomy has improved the quality of her life. A small but growing body of research is challenging the notion that most hysterectomies are needlessly foisted upon women by paternalistic doctors. New studies suggest that what may seem to be a politically incorrect operation is the physiologically correct choice for many women.

Hysterectomies began developing a bad name in the 1970s, when feminists and consumer advocates sounded the alarm about unnecessary operations. Nearly 600,000 hysterectomies—a third of the world's total—are done in the United States each year. Although the U.S. rate has fallen since its mid-1970s high, it remains several times greater than the rate of hysterectomies in Europe. A third of American women have had their uteruses removed by the time they're 60. Only 8 to 12 percent of them have the operation because of cancer or a life-threatening infection. The rest have the surgery to treat a variety of lesser ills. These include unexplained heavy vaginal bleeding, which can cause anemia; a prolapsed (drooping) uterus, which can press on the bladder and lead to incontinence; and endometriosis, in which the uterine lining grows outside the uterus, causing pain and heavy bleeding.

But the most common reason for having hysterectomies—accounting for more than a quarter of such operations—is fibroid tumors, whorled masses of muscle and fibrous tissue that grow out of the uterine walls, fed by the female hormone estrogen. It's estimated that at least 40 percent of all women will develop fibroids at some point in their lives, usually between the ages of 30 and 50. Often, women don't know that they have them. But when a fibroid grows as large as a plum or an orange, it can cause heavy menstrual bleeding, pelvic pain, and uncomfortable pressure on the bladder or bowels.

The symptoms rarely threaten a woman's life, but they can make her miserable. Despite the huge number of elective hysterectomies in the United States each year, until recently few researchers had carefully asked women what they thought about the operation. When two finally did, they were surprised. Karen Carlson, M.D., a primary-care doctor at Massachusetts General Hospital in Boston, had read plenty about doctors' overreliance on the operation and about its effects on quality of life. Some studies, usually based on surveys of doctors, had found that hysterectomy reduces sexual responsiveness in a quarter of women. Other problems reported by doctors and dissatisfied patients included fatigue and depression.

Worse, unless they take hormone-replacement therapy (HRT), the 40 percent of hysterectomy patients who have their ovaries removed along with their uteruses are plunged into premature menopause. Their bodies suddenly stop producing estrogen, which leads to hot flashes, mood swings, night sweats, and other menopausal symptoms. A lack of estrogen also puts them at higher risk for osteoporosis, heart disease, perhaps even Alzheimer's disease. Yet gynecologists kept telling Dr. Carlson, " 'Look, my patients thanked me for doing these procedures.' So we went into our research trying to be unbiased," she says.

Even so, Dr. Carlson did not expect the level of satisfaction she discovered when she interviewed 418 women before their hysterectomy, then 3, 6, and 12 months later. "Symptom relief following hysterectomy is associated with a marked improvement in quality of life," Dr. Carlson and her colleagues concluded. In Dr. Carlson's interviews few women reported problems as a result of hysterectomies. Only 7 percent felt any loss of sexual responsiveness, and just 8 percent experienced depression—rates far lower than previous estimates. What's more, the operation alleviated preexisting sexual problems as well as fatigue, urinary incontinence, and pelvic pain in most women.

In related research Dr. Carlson's team found that women who opted for drug treatments (either hormones or anti-inflammatory medicine) instead of hysterectomies frequently reported that their pelvic pain, bleeding, or incontinence persisted after a year. Of those with severe pelvic pain, half still suffered. Of those with heavy menstrual bleeding, a quarter got no relief from drugs. Hence, nearly a fourth of the 380 women in this study went on to have hysterectomies.

Gentler Alternatives

A more recent study of 1,300 hysterectomy patients in Maryland backs up Dr. Carlson's findings. Kristen Kjerulff, Ph.D., associate professor of epidemiology and preventive medicine at the University of Maryland Medical Center in Baltimore, found that these women, all of whom had severe symptoms for at least two years, decided that hysterectomies were their best options. And more than 95 percent were generally happy with the results even two years later, when memories of their symptoms had dimmed.

These startling findings do not mean that women shouldn't be concerned about the overuse of hysterectomies. Women today have a growing number of less drastic surgical alternatives in which surgeons remove either the fibroids alone or the uterine linings. And no one has yet compared women's satisfaction with those treatments to their feelings after hysterectomies.

"There are other good options available 80 percent of the time," says Joseph Gambone, D.O., head of reproductive endocrinology at the University of California, Los Angeles, UCLA School of Medicine. "If nothing else has been tried, and you're told that you need a hysterectomy, you should be suspicious, unless, of course, it's an emergency or cancer."

Dr. Carlson's research doesn't mean that hysterectomy is the right answer for every woman, but that the operation should remain an option. Women needn't feel as though they've betrayed their sex if they choose to have hysterectomies.

What follows are the stories of three women with fibroids. None wanted to bear more children, so hysterectomies were among the possibilities for them. Each made a choice that she believes was right for her.

"The Smartest Thing I've Ever Done"

Between sick days and doctor's appointments, Tursi missed three weeks of work the year before her hysterectomy. On the worst days, she was in such agony that she had to crawl to the bathroom. Her menstrual cycle was dictating every part of her life.

Tursi had about a half-dozen fibroids; the biggest was nearly 3 inches thick. They crowded her cervix. They grew into the lining of her uterus. Birth control pills did lighten the flow of Tursi's periods for a while, but during the four years before her hysterectomy she switched pill formulas every six months, searching for one that would relieve her increasing torment. She didn't want to try the medication Lupron because it shuts down estrogen production abruptly and can cause severe mood swings. Finally, on her doctor's advice, she injected Depo-Provera, the long-acting contraceptive that suppresses natural estrogen. For two months, she had no period, but when she did get her period it lasted 57 days.

Throughout these years, Tursi relied on powerful painkillers (Darvocet and Tylenol with codeine) to get through difficult days. As each analgesic gradually lost its effectiveness, she thought more seriously about a hysterectomy. "I know my body better than anyone does," she says. "I wanted a life. I was tired of being in pain." Tursi wanted a permanent solution. And only a hysterectomy could ensure that she would remain free of fibroids, uterine pain, and excessive bleeding.

So Tursi's doctor removed the organ most identified with womanhood, but didn't remove her ovaries, which continue to produce estrogen. "I feel fantastic," she says. "It is the smartest thing I've ever done."

"I Didn't Want a Scar"

Doctors often advise women like Barbara Piccoli to ride out the inconvenience of fibroids until menopause, when ovaries stop producing the estrogen that feeds fibroids. Piccoli, a mother of two who lives in New Jersey, was untroubled by pain or heavy bleeding. She didn't even realize that she had fibroids until her doctor felt them during a routine exam. But as her fibroids grew, so did her concern.

A dance teacher and choreographer, Piccoli wears form-fitting leotards almost every day. Her fibroids bothered her mainly because they were expanding her usually flat abdomen. And since her body was giving her no indication that menopause was near, waiting it out meant having a bloated tummy protruding from her trim figure for years. She wanted a solution, but she didn't want a hysterectomy. Yet five doctors, over a span of 18 months, offered just two options: Wait it out or yank it out.

"Doctors are extremely condescending when you're 49 years old," says Piccoli, now 52. "The physicians asked me, 'What would you need your uterus for?' " Their attitude incensed her. "If they had warts on their penises, would they want their penises removed? I don't think so. But if we have fibroids on our uteruses, they tell us to get rid of everything."

In Piccoli's case doctors wanted to remove her ovaries as well as her uterus, a common combination for women over the age of 40. The medical reasoning goes like this: Ovaries almost completely stop producing estrogen at menopause anyway, but they remain a risk for ovarian cancer, which kills nearly 15,000 American women each year. That didn't persuade Piccoli, who feared the mood swings, bone loss, and aging associated with menopause. Finally, she was concerned about the operation itself. "I'm extremely vain, so I didn't want a scar," she says. "I didn't want to be cut from stem to stern."

The Hysterectomy Education and Referral Service (HERS), which tends to steer women away from hysterectomies, directed Piccoli to a doctor in Philadelphia who performs myolysis. In myolysis a surgeon makes a small cut in the navel and one to three more in the abdomen. The doctor slips a narrow viewing tube through the cut in the navel and puts a laser or electrified needle through the other incisions to burn the tissue connecting a fibroid to the uterus. Cut off from its blood supply, the fibroid gradually withers away.

Because burns on the uterine wall might affect fertility, doctors don't recommend myolysis for women who want to bear children. Nor is it suggested for women with more than four fibroids or with a fibroid larger than an orange. All women who consider having myolysis should be aware that there is a possibility that the fibroids will grow back.

"There was some discomfort," Piccoli says. "After all, your body is being invaded. No matter what procedure you have, there is going to be a recuperation period." Still, she was back at work two weeks later (recovery from hysterectomy takes five weeks), and she has just two tiny scars, one on each side of her pelvis.

Would Her Sex Life Suffer?

For 3 to 4 hours every month, Theresa O'Rourke bled so heavily because of fibroids that she couldn't leave the bathroom. At 46, though, she would not consider a hysterectomy. She felt no pain, and as a nurse-midwife in solo practice, she didn't have time for major surgery.

In the back of her mind she also worried that her sex life would suffer. The uterus often contracts during orgasm, heightening the experience. "I think this is one area that isn't adequately discussed with patients," she says. "I had one

New Ways to Be Free of Fibroids

Short of hysterectomy, there are many surgical procedures available for removing fibroids and for easing the pain and stopping the excessive bleeding that they cause. For women who want to preserve their fertility, the following techniques are worth consideration.

Electrosurgical vaporization. This option is the least risky, least complicated way to remove fibroids without removing the uterus. A long, thin electrode is inserted into the uterus through the vagina, and its high heat melts the fibroid cells and seals blood vessels at the same time. Vaporization works even for women with large fibroids growing on the surface of the uterus, though not for fibroids embedded in the uterine wall.

Laparoscopic myomectomy. This procedure allows doctors to remove the most embedded fibroids without major abdominal scarring. A surgeon makes a slit in the navel and inserts a hollow tube and a viewing instrument called a laparoscope into the uterus. The doctor then slides a tiny laser or scalpel through the laparoscope, chops up the fibroid, and removes the bits through the tube. Because sewing up the incisions in the uterine wall through the laparoscope's small opening can be difficult, sometimes doctors must make a second, 2-inch incision to finish the operation. Some surgeons are using a new laparoscopic "sewing machine" to solve the problem.

For women who don't plan to bear children, these additional techniques are recommended by doctors.

Myolysis. By cauterizing the tissue between the uterus and the fibroids, thereby cutting off the blood supply, myolysis can shrink all but the largest fibroids enough to relieve symptoms. When performed by a skilled physician using two electric needles and a laparoscope, this surgery can be the safest option. But uterine scarring from myolysis can cause pain

---

woman friend tell me that having a hysterectomy was a terrible mistake. I had other women tell me that it made no difference."

O'Rourke happened to work with Milton Goldrath, M.D., director of gynecology at Sinai Hospital in Detroit and a pioneer of endometrial ablation, a technique of burning or cutting away the uterine lining (called the endometrium), which is the primary source of menstrual bleeding. Ablation is done without an incision. A doctor inserts a thin scope through the vagina into the uterus, then uses a laser or an electrified needle to destroy the lining. Women with small fibroids are good candidates for ablation; so are those with endometriosis and excessive bleeding. But because this technique permanently destroys part of the uterine lining, it is not a choice for women who want to become pregnant.

With a daughter approaching college age, however, O'Rourke was far more concerned with preserving her romantic life with her husband than with child-

and other complications, including infertility. Doctors at Yale University are experimenting with myolysis equipment that freezes—rather than burns—fibroids, which could someday make the procedure also an option for women who plan to have children.

Drug therapy. Drugs called Gn-RH agonists are sometimes prescribed to shrink fibroids until a woman reaches menopause, when the growths often get smaller on their own. The drugs can be taken only for six months, however, because they block estrogen production, making women vulnerable to osteoporosis. Unfortunately, the fibroids usually begin to grow back about six months after the drugs are discontinued. To avoid this problem, doctors are now offering Gn-RH agonists along with low-dose hormone-replacement therapy (HRT) to keep bones from thinning. But this treatment is expensive ($400 a month) and rarely covered by health insurance. Thus it may be a realistic option for older women who won't need the drugs for long because they don't intend to take hormones after menopause.

Vaginal hysterectomy. This procedure is less invasive than abdominal hysterectomy, requires less than half the hospital stay and recuperation time, and causes little scarring. Yet only 25 percent of hysterectomy patients have the simpler procedure, even though studies suggest up to 80 percent could. The problem is that many doctors are still inexperienced with the technique, in which the surgeon slides a scalpel through the vagina, cuts the uterus free, and removes it through the vagina. To make the process easier, doctors have begun performing part of the surgery through a laparoscope inserted into the uterus through an incision in the navel. Vaginal hysterectomy is the best option for any woman who needs her uterus removed, unless she has severe endometriosis, dense uterine scar tissue, or very large fibroids.

bearing. Her fibroids, Dr. Goldrath told her, were small enough to qualify for an endometrial ablation, though he cautioned her that the procedure ends bleeding in just 30 to 40 percent of women and merely reduces it in the rest. As with myolysis, the fibroids could grow back. Still, for many women the procedure turns torturous symptoms into manageable ones. O'Rourke figured, "Why go in and have a major operation when this is far less traumatic to the body?" On a Thursday afternoon, she checked into the hospital. She went home the next morning and, after resting over the weekend, returned to work on Monday. "I had one year with no periods at all," recalls O'Rourke, now 56. "Then a year later, I started having a very light menses that was more than acceptable."

A few years after the ablation, however, O'Rourke felt the hot flashes of menopause. Heart disease runs in her family, and she had read about the studies showing that HRT seems to protect women against heart attacks. Trying to avoid her family's fatal path, she began taking estrogen. Consequently, her remaining fibroids grew, until her uterus swelled to the size of an 18-week pregnancy. "It began to ache and hurt. It was sticking up halfway to my belly button," she says. Her uterus, once essential to her sex life, became too painful to keep.

So eight years after undergoing endometrial ablation, O'Rourke had a hysterectomy. She does find it harder to achieve an orgasm these days, although she wonders whether that change might have followed menopause anyway. Regardless, she says that the trade-off is now worthwhile. She believes that she'll live longer and better by taking the hormones that help keep her bones strong and her arteries clear.

Is Hysterectomy the Right Choice for You?

If heavy menstrual bleeding and pain caused by fibroids are taking over your life, you have many options. The best one for you depends on your age, your symptoms, the size of the growths, and, most of all, how you feel about the consequences. Before you say yes or no, ask yourself the following questions.

How important is it to you to keep your uterus? Even a woman who doesn't intend to have children may feel that keeping her uterus is a priority—either for emotional or sexual reasons. Some women report that the removal of their uteruses makes it more difficult to achieve orgasm. Others say they simply feel less feminine. For others, however, heavy bleeding so disrupts their sex lives that having hysterectomies is actually liberating.

Are you close to menopause? If so, consider a procedure that removes or shrinks your fibroids; they rarely return after the body stops producing estrogen. But there's a caveat. If you plan on taking HRT to protect your heart and bones, only a hysterectomy will ensure that your fibroids won't grow back.

How do you feel about surgery? You may not think that having heavy periods warrants major surgery that will require weeks of recovery and leave a big scar on your abdomen. The alternative procedures are less traumatic, though sometimes temporary, solutions. If your symptoms are severe, however, you may decide that you need the immediate and permanent relief that only a hysterectomy can provide.

The Simple Cure for "Killer" Fatigue

Y ou feel a little blue; you've gained a little weight; your energy's a little low. You have dry skin, thinning hair, a nonstick memory. You ask yourself, "What's happening to me?"

Mary-Beth Hayden, a registered nurse from Long Island, New York, couldn't figure it out either. Her power walks were suddenly sapping her strength instead of giving her pep. "I felt like a snail," she says. That was so peculiar and went on for so long that she asked her doctor to check her thyroid. Sure enough, Hayden's problem wasn't change of life but change of hormones—not estrogen, but the thyroid gland's main elixir, thyroxine. Her thyroid wasn't producing enough thyroxine (a condition called hypothyroidism). This scarcity of thyroxine put her metabolism on s-l-o-w, which sapped her energy and caused a host of other menopause-like symptoms.

The solution was simple. Hormone medication bolstered Hayden's low supply. Her lazy thyroid started purring again.

The Great Imposter

Remember the movie *Zelig*, in which Woody Allen turned into an assortment of historical figures? Well, mild hypothyroid symptoms are the Zeligs of the diagnostic world. In women, who have thyroid problems three to eight

Yet Another Reason to Kick the Habit

If you have a sluggish thyroid, you have yet another reason to shun cigarettes. A European study has found higher levels of heart-damaging "bad" cholesterol among women smokers with slightly underactive thyroid glands.

"If you're a smoker and you have a slightly underactive thyroid, your cholesterol levels probably will be worse than if you didn't smoke," says David Cooper, M.D., director of endocrinology at Sinai Hospital of Baltimore.

Researchers from the University Hospital in Basel, Switzerland, and Queen Elizabeth Medical Centre in Birmingham, England, looked at cholesterol levels of 273 women—about half with mildly underactive thyroids and half with normally functioning thyroids. Among the women with mildly underactive thyroids, levels of low-density lipoproteins (LDLs)—the "bad" cholesterol—were 28 percent higher for smokers than for nonsmokers. Smokers also had total cholesterol levels 16 percent higher than did the nonsmokers.

Thyroid problems are more common in women than in men—yet many women don't know that they have this "silent" condition that slows metabolism to a crawl. The only way to know for sure is to have a thyroid function test. Meanwhile, smoking cigarettes only further compromises your health, says Dr. Cooper.

"The best advice, as usual, is if you smoke, stop smoking," says Martin Surks, M.D., director of endocrinology at Montefiore Medical Center in New York City. "But if you must smoke, this is even more reason to have your doctor check your thyroid."

HEALTH FLASH

times more often than men, they can mimic many conditions and are often mistaken for signs of stress, aging, or even menopause.

The list of possible symptoms is as long as the credits of a movie, too. "The fact is, almost any symptom that somebody has could theoretically be related to thyroid," says Gilbert H. Daniels, M.D., co-director of Thyroid Associates at Massachusetts General Hospital in Boston. Fatigue, weakness, irregular menstrual periods, infertility, dry hair, loss of hair, dry skin, coarse skin, hoarse voice, constipation, intolerance of cold, depression, mood swings, memory loss, decreased concentration, sore muscles, painful joints, muscle cramps, and more—you might have one; you might have many. You might notice nothing at all. In any case, an underactive thyroid can produce so many symptoms that researchers at Johns Hopkins University School of Medicine in Baltimore are now developing a kind of symptom index to sort them out.

The slipperiest signs of mild hypothyroidism can fool you and your doctors alike. If you've been struggling with any of the following, make an appointment to ask your physician for a thyroid check.

❖ You feel tired and depressed. If fatigue and depression have been bothering you for what seems like too long, don't automatically blame them on stress or the hormonal shifts of your menstrual cycle or menopause. Remember that fatigue and depression can be symptoms of a slow thyroid. You and your doctor should also rule out serious depression—and have your thyroid tested. If your stress level is high and your thyroid hormone is low, getting the gland treated would very likely make you better able to tackle the stress.

❖ You're having reproductive problems. A slow thyroid can interfere with the brain and pituitary gland's control of the menstrual cycle, says Paul W. Ladenson, M.D., director of endocrinology and metabolism at Johns Hopkins University School of Medicine. And that can lead to all kinds of trouble, including miscarriage, infertility, and heavy periods. If any of those problems have been plaguing you, they may be symptoms of low thyroid function. So explore the thyroid connection with your gynecologist.

The sneakiest, most serious effect of mild thyroid failure is symptom-free: "An elevation of cholesterol is one of the characteristic features of an underactive thyroid gland," says Dr. Ladenson.

This increased cholesterol level comes with incredible stealth, agrees Lawrence C. Wood, M.D., president and medical director of the Thyroid Foundation of America, an educational organization in Boston. High cholesterol puts you at risk for atherosclerosis—hardening of the arteries—and heart disease. The Thyroid Foundation estimates that almost seven million Americans walk around with no idea that they have underactive thyroids that may be hiking their cholesterol levels and harming their hearts.

Thyroid 101

It's all hormones. People use that popular piece of folk wisdom to explain almost everything that happens in the body. With thyroid hormone, though, it's just about true. The thyroid gland, which looks like a butterfly hugging your windpipe, culls the nutrient iodine out of the bloodstream and makes the hormone thyroxine out of it. Thyroxine seeps into almost every cell of every organ, regulating growth, metabolism, digestion, body temperature, and the very beating of your heart. That's why too little thyroxine (or too much) can produce such

Rescue Remedy

If your thyroid gland doesn't put out enough of the hormone thyroxine, your whole system can get put on "snooze." But the condition can be corrected easily with a form of thyroxine called levothyroxine sodium. As drugs go, levothyroxine is pretty benign, although you'll probably need to continue using it for life.

"It's exactly what the body makes," says Gilbert H. Daniels, M.D., a thyroid expert and associate professor at Harvard Medical School and co-director of Thyroid Associates at Massachsetts General Hospital in Boston. "So essentially, you can't be allergic to the medicine. In rare cases people have allergic reactions to the dye in the pills—and then they can be prescribed medicines that don't have the dye." Still, if you take a thyroid pill every day, there are a couple of things that you should do.

Make sure you get an annual thyroid-stimulating hormone test. Your doctor needs to monitor your medication to be certain that your dosage requirements haven't changed during the year. If you have too much or too little hormone swimming through your bloodstream, your doctor needs to decrease or increase your prescription. The main danger is too much hormone, which can weaken bones or cause serious heart rhythm problems.

Take your thyroid medication at the same time each day. But don't take it at the same time that you take other medicine or vitamins. Some substances can stick to levothyroxine and interfere with its absorption—iron in vitamin pills, for example, and aluminum hydroxide in antacids.

For free information, call the Thyroid Foundation of America at (800) 832-8321 or write them at Ruth Sleeper Hall 350, 40 Parkman Street, Box T, Boston, MA 02114-2698 (include a self-addressed stamped envelope).

a large number of symptoms. But nobody knows for sure what sickens and slows the thyroid. They do know that hypothyroidism is an autoimmune disease, like rheumatoid arthritis or diabetes. Autoimmune conditions, for mysterious reasons, cause the body to turn against itself; in the case of the thyroid, the body wages war on its own gland.

When levels of thyroxine are out of whack, it's usually a sign that there's trouble brewing with another important hormone called thyroid-stimulating hormone (TSH), a substance made by the pituitary gland at the base of the brain that directs the production of thyroxine. When the thyroid starts to fail, the pituitary pumps up the level of TSH to stimulate more hormone production. So a higher than normal level of the hormone is the first clue to a slowing thyroid. (A lower than normal level of TSH warns about the opposite disorder—called hyperthyroidism. It's less common than its hypothyroid cousin. And its symptoms, which include jitteriness, sleeplessness, and a rapid heartbeat, are usually more obvious.)

Until the 1970s, labs had no way of pinpointing TSH levels precisely. Then a supersensitive TSH test was developed to measure the amount of thyroid-stimulating hormone in the blood. Now physicians who order the test can detect even the most furtive case of thyroid dysfunction. But many doctors don't order it until symptoms rear up and bite their patients. Even then, TSH may be one of the last tests ordered—after all other diagnoses have been discarded. But it's a simple blood test like the cholesterol test. They both can be done from the same blood sample. The TSH test is also less expensive than a mammogram or a cholesterol test.

So shouldn't everyone be tested? Shouldn't you be tested? Technically, testing large groups of women even if no symptoms are present is known as screening, and testing only those who do have symptoms is testing. Right now, despite the relatively low cost of the TSH test and the impact that hypothyroidism can have on people's lives, there are no national, generally recognized guidelines for thyroid screening, as there are for cholesterol screening.

Doctors disagree on when and whether to screen people for underlying thyroid disease. The U.S. Preventive Services Task Force of the Department of Health and Human Services does not recommend routine screening for people without symptoms, with a few exceptions. Endocrinologists and thyroid specialists, however, usually recommend screening anyone with certain risk factors. Depending on whom you ask, the recommended age for initial screening may be 40 or 45 or 50. A TSH test may also be recommended when a woman is pregnant or after she delivers a child. Risk factors for mild thyroid failure include being over 50 if you're a woman, having a family history of thyroid problems or autoimmune disease, having an autoimmune disease yourself, past treatment of the head or neck with radioactive iodine or radiation, thyroid surgery, and current treatment with certain drugs. Considering what top thyroid experts say, plus all available scientific data, it seems to be in women's best interests to be screened for thyroid trouble.

Early Screening Pays Off

All women (and men) should be screened for mild thyroid failure when they get their cholesterol checked—that is, every five years from the age of 20, experts advise.

Why this sweeping recommendation? Getting both cholesterol and thyroid checked at the same time is simple. The doctor, nurse, or technician takes one blood sample and does two tests. The National Cholesterol Education Program (NCEP) recommends that you start being screened for cholesterol at the age of 20, and that you get rescreened every five years as long as levels are normal.

At Risk? Time for a Test

There are situations in which you need to speed up screening or testing for thyroid trouble—if you know for sure that Mom was on thyroid hormone, for instance, or your cholesterol is high. These circumstances suggest that you're at higher risk for thyroid trouble. Here's a list of what those special factors are and information on how often to screen.

❖ *You've reached age 50.* Three to eight women develop thyroid disease for every one man. By the time they've reached the half-century mark, 10 percent of American women show elevated levels of thyroid-stimulating hormone (TSH). When you celebrate that birthday, start checking your TSH levels every three years.

❖ *You have a family history of thyroid problems.* If you're sure that Mom or Dad or Sis was treated for thyroid disease, get your TSH level checked every three years no matter what your age. Even if your TSH is normal, your doctor may also test you for the presence of thyroid antibodies in order to see if the gland has actually started the process of attacking itself. If you are producing antibodies, you'll probably need to be retested once a year.

❖ *You have an autoimmune disease.* There are 70 or so autoimmune diseases, among the most common of which are diabetes, rheumatoid arthritis, vitiligo (which leaves white patches on your skin), and prematurely gray hair (graying before the age of 30). If you're diagnosed with such a disorder, ask to have your thyroid checked. Then get a TSH test whenever you have a physical—once every two to three years.

❖ *You were treated for cancer with radiation to the head or neck, or with radioactive iodine for hyperthyroidism, or you had thyroid surgery.* Any one of these circumstances may have predisposed you to develop an underactive thyroid gland. In that case consider having a TSH test done once a year.

❖ *You're taking certain drugs.* Lithium can do marvels for people who have certain forms of depression, especially manic depression. But it

The five-year schedule works with thyroid screening, too, says Dr. Ladenson. Hypothyroidism is a slow-growing disease. And, of course, because the link between high cholesterol and thyroid disease is so strong, it makes even more sense to get your thyroid checked along with your cholesterol, especially if you do have high cholesterol.

Screening for thyroid problems early is as reasonable as screening for cholesterol early. The incidence of hypothyroidism rises with age. So the numbers of young people detected with early hypothyroidism wouldn't be huge. But there are special reasons for women to consider screening. It's important to catch the disease before a woman's childbearing years are in full swing in order also increases the incidence of thyroid disease. So does the heart drug amiodarone (Cordarone) and many other drugs containing iodine. If you're taking lithium or amiodarone, be sure that your doctor is monitoring your thyroid function with TSH tests six weeks after your first treatment, then at three months, and then once a year.

❖ *Your cholesterol is high.* A hidden thyroid problem can thwart all of your efforts to lower cholesterol with diet and exercise, according to Paul W. Ladenson, M.D., director of endocrinology and metabolism at Johns Hopkins University School of Medicine in Baltimore. So it's crucial to test for thyroid failure if your cholesterol numbers are high. Dr. Ladenson suggests taking this step if your total cholesterol is above 200 milligrams per deciliter and your low-density lipoproteins (LDLs) are 130 or above.

Why a thyroid disorder makes cholesterol rise is only partially understood, says Dr. Ladenson. "Thyroid hormone regulates to some extent how quickly the liver takes cholesterol out of the blood. When there's not enough hormone, the liver removes cholesterol less efficiently and your cholesterol rises.

"Most studies have shown that patients with underactive thyroid glands have a level of LDL cholesterol (the so-called bad cholesterol) that's about 30 points higher than it is when their thyroid conditions are corrected," says Dr. Ladenson. That means a 60 percent increased risk of heart attack, he explains.

If you have high cholesterol and low thyroid function, your thyroid should be treated first, he says. "You may not need cholesterol-lowering drugs, with all their side effects and expense, if everything's straightened out with thyroid medication alone, which has no side effects when used in the proper dosage. It's better to get treatment and dedicate yourself to a sensible diet—and then see if your cholesterol level is still high or not."

to thwart the conception problems, miscarriages, and low birth weights that a slow thyroid can bring in its wake. In addition, "by age 35, 5 percent to 7 percent of women have mild thyroid dysfunction," says Dr. Ladenson. "That's a large number of women."

There's also the problem of postpartum symptoms. "I think early screening is reasonable in part because it helps predict which women are going to have postpartum thyroid problems," says Dr. Daniels. Childbirth can cause temporary thyroid dysfunction. In about 5 percent of new mothers, the gland malfunctions. In most mothers, it goes into overdrive, producing too much hormone. Then it may kick back and not produce enough. In the meantime, a mother may suffer what she thinks is postpartum depression. The real problem—postpartum thyroiditis—usually goes away on its own, but for three to six months, just when a new mother needs maximum energy, she may not be feeling her best. "Somewhere between one-quarter and one-half of mothers who develop postpartum thyroiditis go on to have persistent thyroid dysfunction, too," says Dr. Daniels. "So we're talking about 2 to 3 percent of all the women who've ever had babies. That's a lot."

Finally, we know that many (if not most) physicians favor thyroid testing for people with a family history of thyroid problems. That's because such a history is an extremely strong risk factor for thyroid disease. But most people simply don't know their families' medical histories. A lot of us just don't know whether Mom or Dad had a sluggish thyroid—or whether Mom's arthritis was rheumatoid (an autoimmune disease) or the osteoarthritis that comes with age. She may not have known herself. So thyroid screening would help those who aren't aware of their families' medical histories.

Your insurance company may not pay for screening (although it will pay for testing if you've already developed symptoms). But for all of the above reasons, the test is worth the $25 to $50 that it costs. And the cost may actually decrease in two to three years. That's when Franklin Diagnostics in Cedar Knoll, New Jersey, expects to introduce its $20 home TSH test. Called ThyroChek, it has recently been introduced to primary-care doctors as an office test.

Essential Medical Tests That Can Save Your Life

19

Want to do something really nice for yourself? Don't buy yourself a new silk scarf, a bouquet of tulips, or even a bottle of scented bubble bath. Go get the health tests you need—on schedule. Despite the inconvenience— you may have to make an appointment for the evening or for a Saturday morning or you may even have to take off part of a workday—and despite some minor discomfort, the truth is that medical tests can be lifesavers for women.

If every woman followed established guidelines for breast cancer screening, for instance, doctors estimate that some 15,000 lives would be spared each year. Similarly, screening for colon cancer could prevent many thousands of deaths annually. Even simple things such as having your blood pressure checked and your blood cholesterol levels measured regularly could help prevent up to half of the 250,000 heart attack deaths and the 100,000 stroke deaths among women each year.

Each woman's needs are different, based on age, genetics, medical history, and lifestyle. But some basic information, along with the advice of your doctor, can help you to determine the screening schedule that's best for you. The following general guidelines for women are approved by physicians representing the American Medical Women's Association.

One note: In addition to these tests, you may want to have the testing for AIDS and other sexually transmitted diseases that is recommended by many doctors.

A Better Heart Test for Women

Women running on treadmills may be going nowhere fast when doing the standard exercise stress test to screen for heart disease. That's because the test, for women, is almost as likely to produce misleading results as it is to pinpoint a diagnosis. But now, women have an alternative to the exercise stress test—a heart check called exercise echocardiography. And research suggests that it's more accurate.

In the standard exercise stress test, which produces electrocardiograms (ECGs), anywhere from 30 percent to more than 50 percent of women are mistakenly suspected of having heart disease, explains Thomas H. Marwick, M.D., director of cardiac stress imaging at the Cleveland Clinic in Ohio. These women may unnecessarily wind up taking the next diagnostic step, angiography, an x-ray look at the heart.

Researchers at the Cleveland Clinic evaluated 161 women with symptoms of heart disease, using the standard ECG simultaneously with stress echocardiography. (A heart catheter was used to confirm the accuracy of each.) While ECGs caused false alarms more than half (55 percent) of the time in women at moderate-to-high risk of heart disease, the false-alarm rate for stress echocardiography was only 20 percent.

The usual treadmill test used in ECG measures electrical conductivity—that is, the "wiring" of the heart. Electrical patterns are usually disturbed where heart disease exists. Not all electrical irregularities indicate heart disease, however, especially in women. Exercise echocardiography, on the other hand, looks at the actual motion of the heart, which is a better indicator of heart disease in women. Both tests can be done during a single session on the treadmill.

First Things First: Blood Tests

Heart disease is the leading cause of death in American women, striking down half a million each year. You can detect heart disease early and take steps to reverse it if you follow the guidelines below.

Blood pressure test. This measurement of blood pressure is performed with an inflatable cuff called a sphygmomanometer. If you have a healthy blood pressure, the reading should be less than 140 systolic over less than 90 diastolic. (The first number is a measure of the pressure when your heart contracts; the second, when it expands.) Have one once a year if all of the following apply to you.

❖ You are between the ages of 19 and 40.

❖ You have no heart disease factors.

❖ You are not taking oral contraceptives.

Have one twice each year or more often if any of the following apply to you.

❖ You are over age 40.

❖ You take oral contraceptives.

❖ You have borderline high blood pressure (140/90 or greater).

❖ You have a personal or family history of high blood pressure or heart disease.

❖ You are on blood pressure–control medication.

❖ You smoke.

❖ You are overweight.

❖ You regularly take over-the-counter nonsteroidal anti-inflammatory drugs (NSAIDs) such as aspirin or ibuprofen.

❖ You have a physician's recommendation to take the test more than once a year.

For more information on high blood pressure, please see chapter 16.

Blood cholesterol test. A small blood sample is analyzed at the doctor's office or in a laboratory. The results tell you your total cholesterol, plus the levels of "good" high-density lipoproteins (HDLs) and "bad" low-density lipoproteins (LDLs) as well as the levels of fatty triglycerides in your blood. The test should be taken after a 12-hour fast because triglycerides are very sensitive to diet. For women, healthy readings should be in the range of 160 milligrams per deciliter for total cholesterol, 50 milligrams per deciliter or higher for HDL, 120 milligrams per deciliter or lower for LDL, and 110 milligrams per deciliter or lower for triglycerides. Most women should be checked once a year. Have the test twice a year or more often if any of the following apply to you.

❖ You have recently gained a lot of weight.

❖ You have become sedentary.

❖ You have become ill.

❖ You have borderline high cholesterol (about 200 to 240 milligrams per deciliter).

❖ You have high cholesterol (above 240 milligrams per deciliter).

❖ You are on cholesterol-lowering medication.

❖ You have diabetes or kidney disease.

❖ You have HDL levels below 35 milligrams per deciliter.

❖ You have had your ovaries removed.

❖ You have recently gone through menopause.

❖ You have heart disease or symptoms of heart disease.

❖ You have a physician's recommendation to have it done more often than once a year.

How Fit Is Your Heart?

An exercise stress test is valuable because it shows how your heart performs when you're actually exercising. About 40 percent of the tests come back with false-positives—that is, the tests indicate problems when there are none. But your doctor has an arsenal of more sensitive tests that can be given as follow-ups. When the finding is abnormal, your doctor may give you a stress echocardiogram, which uses ultrasound to measure your heart's performance during exercise, or a nuclear medicine test, which involves injection of a radioactive tracing material. In fact, if you're at high risk for heart disease because of family history or a prior record of heart problems, a physician might skip the exercise stress test and go directly to a more sensitive test.

Exercise stress test. For this test of coronary fitness, you will perform some exercise, such as walking on a treadmill or pedaling a stationary bike, while your heart is monitored with a device called an electrocardiogram. This test can help reveal coronary artery disease. Have the test every two to five years if any of the following apply to you.

- ❖ You are over age 40.
- ❖ You are over age 30 and have strong risk factors for heart disease such as high blood pressure, diabetes, obesity, smoking, or family history of heart disease.
- ❖ You have had your ovaries removed.
- ❖ You have high cholesterol.
- ❖ You have symptoms of heart disease.
- ❖ You have a physician's recommendation.

Gynecological Checkups That You Really Need

We're all susceptible to a wide range of gynecological problems, from vaginal infections and uterine fibroids to cervical abnormalities and ovarian growths. You should be aware of some of the screening tests that are available to women. Here's a summary.

Pelvic exam. This manual examination of your vaginal area checks for abnormalities of your uterus and ovaries. Every woman should have one every year once she is over age 18.

Pap test. For this cervical cancer test, the doctor takes a scraping of cells from your cervix and cervical canal and smears it on a slide. The sample is then sent to a laboratory for analysis. For greatest reliability you need a skilled medical professional and analysis from a well-qualified laboratory. Seek a board-certified health practitioner for your test. Have one every year if you are over age 18. (For more information on Pap tests, see chapter 15.)

Transvaginal ultrasound. This test screens for changes in the lining of your uterus and ovaries that might suggest cancer. An ultrasound probe is inserted into your vagina, and the probe transmits images of your uterus and ovaries to a monitoring screen. You will need one if your physician recommends one, or if any of the following apply to you.

- ❖ You are at or past menopause.
- ❖ You have risk factors for endometrial cancer.
- ❖ You have a strong family history or other significant risk factors for ovarian cancer.

Endometrial tissue sample. A tiny piece of tissue from the lining of your uterus, called the endometrium, is removed and checked for the development of cancer. To perform this test, a thin instrument is inserted through your vagina and cervical opening to remove the tissue sample from your uterus. This procedure, also called an endometrial biopsy or aspiration, can cause cramping. Have one screening test, possibly followed by others, as recommended by a doctor, if any of the following apply to you.

- ❖ You are past menopause and are considering getting—or are currently re-ceiving—hormone-replacement therapy (HRT).
- ❖ You are taking the breast cancer medication tamoxifen (Nolvadex).
- ❖ You eat a very high fat diet.
- ❖ You have a history of infertility.
- ❖ You have a history of not ovulating.
- ❖ You are very overweight.
- ❖ You have a family history of endometrial cancer.
- ❖ You experience abnormal uterine bleeding.

Three Easy Steps to Breast Health

More than 180,000 women are diagnosed with breast cancer every year, and as many as 46,000 die prematurely as a result of this disease. If all women fol-lowed the guidelines below, one-third of those deaths could probably be avoided.

Breast self-examination. Perform this monthly test at home by carefully and methodically touching each breast, and the area between your breasts and armpits, for unusual lumps or masses. Many doctors say that breast self-exam should be a lifelong habit. To learn how to perform a thorough self-exam, ask your physician for guidance or take classes at your community hospital or at a woman's health clinic. Your local American Cancer Society office should also have information. Every women over the age of 16 should do a breast self-exam every month, preferably in the week after her period, when breasts are not tender or swollen.

Breast examination by a health professional. This visual and manual examination of your breasts and underarms by a qualified doctor or health professional should be done while you are sitting up, and again when you are lying down. Have one every two to three years if you are under age 39 and have no risk factors or symptoms for breast cancer. Have one annually, as part of your regular gynecological exam, or even more often, if any of the following apply to you.

❖ You are over age 40.
❖ You have lumpy breasts that are difficult to self-examine.
❖ You do not perform monthly breast self-exams.
❖ You have risk factors for breast cancer such as a family history of the disease, no children before age 30, breast biopsies that show atypical growths, or a personal history of breast cancer.

Mammography. For this low-dose breast x-ray, your breasts are pressed firmly between two plates for each x-ray view. Usually two or three views per breast are required for a complete screening. Most doctors recommend that you schedule your mammogram the week after your menstrual period to minimize discomfort.

If the doctor does find a suspicious lump, she should perform a biopsy to make a definite diagnosis. There is a 15 percent false-negative rate for mammography. The biopsy is therefore an important and necessary backup to verify the mammography.

You should have mammograms annually. (For more information on mammograms, see chapter 11.)

Next, Look at Your Bones

If you're an American woman, you have a one in two chance of developing fractures from osteoporosis sometime during your lifetime—most likely after menopause. Complications resulting from hip fractures account for 50,000 deaths every year. Many of these deaths may be preventable.

"There is no reason that we can't prevent most hip fractures and deaths from osteoporosis if we combine early detection and treatment," says Sydney Lou Bonnick, M.D., director of osteoporosis services at the Texas Woman's University in Denton and author of *The Osteoporosis Handbook.*

Many tests for osteoporosis are available, and all of the techniques are capable of detecting low bone mass and diagnosing the condition, according to Sandra C. Raymond, executive director of the National Osteoporosis Foundation. But some experts believe "that for predicting fracture risk, the specific bone at risk of fracturing should be measured," says Raymond. That means that your doctor may choose to focus on a particular area of bone, such as the hip, where fractures are likely to happen.

Many doctors recommend that you have a bone scan before you reach menopause. This first test provides a baseline measurement that your doctor can interpret to find out whether you should take estrogen or another medication (such as salmon calcitonin or etidronate) to prevent further bone weakening. By repeating the scan 12 to 18 months past menopause, your doctor can determine whether you have lost too much bone. Based on the results, she may recommend that you begin to take medication or adjust your current dosage.

Not all tests are accurately interpreted, however. "It's a problem that all of us recognize and are trying to improve," says Dr. Bonnick. He recommends that before having the test, you ask the technician whether she's had several years of experience with bone scans. Make sure that your physician will be reviewing the test and providing a written interpretation. Don't settle for a computer printout–based diagnosis, Dr. Bonnick cautions.

Bone scan. This is a painless procedure in which you sit or lie on a table, while a machine uses low-dose radiation to read your bone mass. Several different scanning techniques are available, including the dual energy x-ray absorptiometry (DEXA) test that's considered the best by many bone experts as well as dual photon absorptiometry, quantitative computed tomography, single energy x-ray absorptiometry, and more. To find a bone-testing facility near you, call the National Osteoporosis Foundation at (800) 464-6700.

The test usually takes up to 30 minutes. Have one baseline test just before menopause or very early in menopause, then a second test 12 to 18 months after menopause. You may need more follow-up tests, at the recommendation of your doctor, if any of the following apply to you.

- ❖ You have risk factors for osteoporosis based on your family history.
- ❖ You use steroids.
- ❖ You have a low-calcium diet.
- ❖ You lead a sedentary lifestyle.

Easing Worries about Colon Cancer

Colon cancer is the third leading cancer among women, after breast cancer and lung cancer—and more women than men get it every year. If you follow the screening recommendations below, you may be able to detect precancerous changes and early cancer. When it's caught early, colon cancer can usually be treated very effectively.

Digital rectal exam. This examination of the rectum with a gloved finger detects abnormalities. Have one every year if you are 40 or over.

Fecal occult blood test. A lab analyzes a stool sample, obtained at home or at the physician's office, for the presence of blood, which is a possible symptom of colorectal cancer. This test has been criticized because of the high rate of false-positives (wrongly indicating a possibility of cancer) and false-negatives (missing cancer that's really there). A positive result might indicate ulcers, hemorrhoids, or other problems. Follow-up tests can be used to confirm the results of this test. Have a fecal occult blood test yearly if you are 50 or older.

Sigmoidoscopy. With a thin, hollow, lighted tube, your physician looks for precancerous polyps in the lower part of your colon. Flexible sigmoidoscopes are preferred because they cause less discomfort than rigid scopes. Have a sigmoidoscopy every three to five years if you are age 50 or over and have no colorectal cancer risk factors or symptoms. Have one every three years, at the discretion of your doctor, if any of the following apply to you.

❖ You have a personal history of colon polyps, chronic inflammatory bowel disease, or colorectal cancer.
❖ You have a family history of these diseases—especially if your parents, siblings, or children developed colon cancer before age 50.
❖ You have symptoms of colorectal cancer, such as diarrhea, constipation, or both; blood in your stools; very narrow stools; unexplained weight loss; frequent gas pains; and general stomach discomfort.
❖ You feel as if your bowel does not empty completely.
❖ You have a history of breast, endometrial, or ovarian cancer.

New Tests on the Horizon

Doctors, researchers, and technicians are coming up with new medical tests so fast that it's hard to keep track of all the advances. But the general direction of the improved medical tests is toward less pain, more gain.

Among the new generation of medical tests is the "ouchless" variety. Some of these are noninvasive—that is, they involve no knives, needles, or tubes. Others are far less invasive or inconvenient than conventional procedures used previously. In many cases the new procedures are faster and more accurate. Here's a rundown of what these procedures have to offer.

Rotating delivery of excitation off-resonance (RODEO). This technique, which has been tested at Baylor University Medical Center in Dallas, may help many women with suspicious breast lumps avoid the wait, worry, and discomfort of breast biopsies. An improved form of magnetic resonance imaging (MRI), it involves simply placing a cone-shaped antenna over the breast for a few moments. While MRI combines magnetic fields and radio waves to produce an image of the inside of a breast, RODEO goes beyond that. It shows the contrast between normal breast tissue and cancerous tissue.

"Conventional MRI uses a contrasting agent that makes tumors appear as white," says Steven Harms, M.D., director of magnetic resonance at Baylor and co-developer of RODEO. "But since fatty tissue in the breast also shows up as white, finding a breast tumor on a standard MRI image can be like locating a snowman in a snowstorm. With RODEO, a special radio field blocks out the fat so cancerous tumors really stand out."

Bowel scintiscan. This test can complement routine blood tests and may even eliminate the need for complex endoscopic (internal) exams in the diagnosis of irritable bowel syndrome (IBS), a painful combination of cramping, diarrhea, and constipation that often is triggered by stress. Developed by doctors at the Mayo Clinic in Rochester, Minnesota, bowel scintiscan is as easy as taking an aspirin.

In IBS, problems in the stomach or small intestine can keep food from passing through the digestive system smoothly.

Bowel scintiscan is an outpatient procedure that involves swallowing a harmless radioactive capsule on an empty stomach and eating a small meal. Pictures, similar to x-rays, of the abdomen are taken immediately after the capsule and meal are swallowed and at intervals later. The pictures help a physician determine whether you have IBS or another disturbance of the intestinal contractions.

Bowel scintiscan has several advantages over older tests, according to Michael Camilleri, M.D., professor of medicine in the gastroenterology research unit at the Mayo Clinic. "It's painless for the patient, and it allows the doctor to test for IBS without inserting any tubes into the patient's body. It provides an extended exam that effectively assesses the entire digestive tract," he says.

First offered at the Mayo Clinic, the bowel scintiscan is expected to become increasingly available at other major research and treatment centers around the country.

Ulcer test. Conventional methods for detecting duodenal ulcers—ulcers in the upper section of the intestines, also known as peptic ulcers—may involve blood tests and endoscopic exams, which must often be conducted several weeks after treatment has started. But the latest innovation in ulcer testing not only eliminates the invasive procedures but also takes the guesswork out of diagnosis and can chart the healing process without lengthy and costly laboratory work.

The innovation is a breath test, developed at Baylor College of Medicine in Houston, to detect *Helicobacter pylori* (*H. pylori*), a type of bacteria that lives in the digestive tracts of duodenal ulcer patients.

To take the test, you swallow a special form of urea, a natural compound, that has been mixed with heavy, nonradioactive carbon. If *H. pylori* is present, it

A Closer Look at Heart Health

It looks like a scene from *Star Trek*: A fully clothed woman on a table is passed through the center of a big metal doughnut. Invisible rays go through her chest. Moments later, doctors can examine a 3-D image of her heart.

Sounds futuristic, but this test, called ultrafast computed tomography (CT), has the potential to spare you the risks and discomforts of angiography, the current gold standard for seeing inside the heart and its arteries. Angiography involves taking pictures of the inside of blood vessels, to determine how clogged they may be. The procedure is usually called for when an exercise stress test reveals potential heart problems. The trouble is that the tools used in angiography can knock bits of artery buildup into the blood, raising the risk of heart attack and stroke. Also, drugs used in the process can leave your head aching.

Ultrafast CT, a new way to potentially rule out the need for angiography, has just passed its first nationwide test with flying colors. Of 427 people with known blockages, ultrafast CT was able to detect 95 percent of the blockages.

Aside from its noninvasive bonus, ultrafast CT may be the inside look of choice because it's the most sensible way yet to spot calcium, a component of arterial plaque (unrelated to calcium intake). Calcium is a very reliable indicator of plaque, explains study author Bruce H. Brundage, M.D., chief of cardiology at Harbor–University of California, Los Angeles, Medical Center in Torrance, California. "Whenever there is detectable calcium in coronary arteries, there is always atherosclerosis; and when you don't see calcium, there is virtually no chance of any significant atherosclerosis." Calcium builds over many years, says Dr. Brundage, so plaque in people under age 45 may not contain enough calcium to be reliably detected.

will feed on the urea and release the carbon. When you breathe into a test bag, the amount of heavy carbon in your breath tells your doctor how much *H. pylori* you have in your digestive system. A positive test for *H. pylori* can confirm a diagnosis of duodenal ulcer.

Glucose check. Many diabetes patients must prick their fingers several times a day to get blood samples for glucose monitoring. But soon there may be a painless alternative to this prickly problem.

One kind of monitor that's being tested uses infrared light to check glucose levels in the blood. When your finger is passed through an infrared beam, circulating blood acts like a prism, dispersing the light into a spectrum. The monitor, which could be available for home use, would simply read the spectrum to determine how much glucose is present.

part three

Day-to-Day Strategies for Peak Health

3

the Hormone Connection

If you were channel-surfing late one night and came across a wonder substance that could energize your sex life, keep your skin youthful, sharpen your memory, strengthen your bones, protect your heart, increase your pain tolerance, and toughen your natural immunity, would you laugh it off as just another bogus cure-all?

If so, Mother Nature would have the last giggle since estrogen—a woman's most powerful hormone—may do all that and more.

"Estrogen is important to women's health beginning at puberty and ever after," says Geoffrey Redmond, M.D., director of the Women's Hormone Center in Cleveland and author of *The Good News about Women's Hormones.*

Sure, most women think of estrogen as the hormone responsible for their menstrual blahs or their premenstrual (PMS) mood swings. And scientific studies seem to show that exposure to your body's natural estrogen can contribute to breast, endometrial, and possibly ovarian cancer. But in fighting heart disease, which kills more women than all those cancers combined, estrogen is a powerful ally. Among its 400 amazing functions, it boosts high-density lipoprotein (HDL), or "good" cholesterol, which helps keep arteries healthy.

What else does estrogen do?

- ❖ *Blesses your heart.* Beyond improving your cholesterol profile, estrogen protects the lining of your blood vessel walls and keeps your blood vessels open so blood flows smoothly, says Dr. Redmond.
- ❖ *Makes strong bones.* Estrogen slows down bone loss while the body naturally replaces it, which helps to prevent osteoporosis, Dr. Redmond says.
- ❖ *Keeps your sex life lively.* It also plays a key role in fostering sexual arousal by preparing brain receptors for activation by testosterone, produced in small amounts by the ovaries.
- ❖ *Enhances your memory.* By boosting production of the enzyme required to make the neurotransmitter acetylcholine, estrogen can help you remember things. It also forges new communication paths between nerve cells.
- ❖ *Sweetens your sleep.* A lullaby hormone, estrogen, when taken over a six-month period, soothes sleep disturbances and gives you a good night's rest by regulating sleep centers in the brain.

20

Head-to-Toe
Pain Relief

R ub it," Mama says when her bambino falls down and goes bump. It's a common mom command. Like "Stand up straight" or "Eat your veg-gies," it's one of those mom-isms that has turned out to be medically correct.

The way rubbing works tells us a lot about the way pain—and pain relief—travel through our bodies, according to Margaret A. Caudill, M.D., Ph.D., co-director of the Arnold Pain Center at Deaconess Hospital in Boston, assistant clinical professor of medicine at Harvard Medical School, and author of *Managing Pain before It Manages You.*

Say you bang your shin on a low coffee table. Three different kinds of fibers, all serving various functions, come into play.

First, pain receptors on your skin yelp the news to sensory nerves rich in A-delta fibers that pick up the message. The yelp speeds along the nerve highway at the equivalent of 40 miles per hour and swerves into your spinal cord, which rockets the pain message to other nerves or to your brain. Right after that sharp flash, you feel another kind of pain—a low, aching, dull throb. That little number is made up of a power brigade of signals that tread along the nerve high-way of C fibers at a more placid 3 miles per hour.

But suppose you rub your shin as soon as you hit it. The rub sets off touch fibers—the A-betas. "Those fibers race at 200 miles an hour to the spinal cord and, theoretically, compete with the pain message," says Dr. Caudill. You'll know those touch fibers won the race when the rub soothes away the pain.

Don't Let Fat Hurt Your Head

New research suggests that if you cut back on fat, you may cut back on headaches, too. When 54 women and men with regular migraines spent a month following a low-fat eating plan, their headaches were less frequent, less intense, shorter in duration, and they needed fewer medications than when they ate their regular fare, according to a California study. When they started adding the fat back in, headaches haunted them again.

Researchers think that fat encourages blood platelets to congregate and damage each other. This prompts the release of the brain chemical serotonin into the bloodstream. This temporary high level of serotonin is then quickly metabolized and excreted, leaving a low serotonin level. With a stingy amount of serotonin, blood vessels are known to widen—and that's when migraine pain begins, says study leader Zuzana Bic, M.D., Dr.P.H., a researcher in the preventive-care program at Loma Linda University School of Public Health in California.

This study found that cutting back to an ultra-low 20 grams of fat a day (about 10 percent of calories from fat) relieved migraines in people who had previously been eating super high fat diets—80 to 120 grams of fat per day. Dr. Bic recommends that people who get migraines should try to limit their dietary fat intake to 10 percent of calories by replacing fatty foods with fruits, vegetables, beans, and grains.

The Essential Chemistry of Pain

Believe it or not, pain is useful. Pain warns you to take your hand off the stove burner, to take care of your back, or to find out why your head aches. Often what makes you hurt also starts to cure you. Those pain messages provoke production of a chemical that sounds like an old sitcom—bradykinin.

This powerful chemical unleashes a torrent of inflammatory chemicals, such as histamines and prostaglandins. They heal but they also hurt. Once you've been warned, and pain has your attention, your body's phenomenal pharmacy starts to kick in. Scientists have discovered that every one of us can make at least eight natural morphinelike opiates, all stronger than the opium from any poppy plant in China. In fact, narcotics such as morphine and codeine work by mimicking our inborn opiate action.

Relief without Drugs

Massage may be the most ancient and natural pain reliever of them all. Even in 2598 B.C., massage was known—and mentioned in a Chinese tome, *The Yellow Emperor's Classic of Internal Medicine*. "Everyone is capable of doing massage on herself or others," says Joan Johnson, author of *The Healing Art of Sports Massage* and director of Sports Massage of the Rockies in Boulder, Colorado. Here are a few of her self-massage pain-relief techniques.

Play lower-back tennis. To loosen a stiff back, lie on the floor with your knees bent, your feet apart, and your hands on your chest. Then position a tennis ball directly under the area of your back that you want to massage, but be careful not to put it directly under your spine or under your lower back, near your kidneys. Rest as much of your body weight on the ball as you can without feeling uncomfortable. Roll your back in a small circle around the tennis ball, then reposition the ball on other areas of your back for more self-massage. Massage each spot for a minute or two.

Be nice to your neck. To massage a stiff neck, stand up straight and reach your right hand over your right shoulder and around to the back of your neck. Press four fingers firmly into the area of your neck directly below your skull, about an inch above the big knob that you can feel on your backbone. The points you want to massage, midway between the bottom of your skull and the top of your shoulder blade, are part of the trapezius muscle.

Hold your fingers at the starting point for a few seconds, then slowly tilt your head to the left, while you drag your fingers down closer to your shoulder. Repeat on your left side using your left hand.

Rock your shoulders. To banish shoulder tension, stand up straight, reach your right arm across your chest, and press the fingertips of your right hand into the muscle at the top of your left shoulder. Rock your fingertips backward and forward to massage the muscle. Then repeat using your left fingertips on your right shoulder. Continue to massage for several minutes.

Press Your Pressure Points into Service

Western medicine is slowly accepting the hallowed pain-relief methods of the Chinese: acupuncture and its at-home variation, acupressure. Both forms rely on stimulating any of the body's 361 acupoints, which lie along 14 lines of energy that the Chinese call meridians. In Eastern therapy, pressure at any of these points restores the proper circulation of the body energy called *chi* (pronounced chee), says Patrick J. LaRiccia, M.D., who has a private practice in alternative medicine at the Presbyterian Medical Center and who is director of the Acupuncture Pain Clinic at the Hospital of the University of Pennsylvania, both in Philadelphia.

"The Western theory is that acupressure releases endorphins, the body's own painkillers," says Dr. LaRiccia. Researchers have found that many acupoints correspond to neuron motor points, where large nerves meet muscle or bone. And meridians may be what scientists now call nerve pathways. In any case, numerous studies have found that the venerable practice helps 56 to 85 percent of people with chronic pain. Here are some ways to find relief.

Soothe heel pain. If your heels ache after too much standing or walking, David Nickel, a doctor of oriental medicine, licensed acupuncturist, and author of *Acupressure for Athletes*, recommends this exercise. Sit down on a rug or mat with your legs comfortably open, and move the foot that hurts close to your body—but not uncomfortably close. Grasp that foot with both hands. Your fingers should be on the top of your foot and your two thumbs on the bottom—over the end of the heel bone that's closest to the center of your foot. Position one thumb over the other for more pressure, then press for 5 seconds and release for 5 seconds. Continue for up to a minute, using Dr. Nickel's breathing technique at the same time: Exhale through your mouth as you press, inhale through your nose as you release.

Rework runner's knee. Sit down on a chair with your legs bent at the knees. If your right knee hurts, use the thumb and forefinger of your left hand to pinch the base of your kneecap. Your thumb and finger should be about $2^{1}/_{2}$ inches apart. Alternately apply and release pressure for 5 seconds each, for up to a minute. Use Dr. Nickel's breathing technique at the same time.

Ice your ivories. The acupoint for tooth pain is on your hand, in the "web" of skin between your thumb and index finger. With your right thumb, feel along the web of your left hand until you're pressing an area near the bone. That's the point the Chinese call *Ho-ku*. At that point, press the area for 5-second intervals, using Dr. Nickel's breathing technique at the same time: Exhale through your mouth as you press, inhale through your nose as you release.

Cue the Relaxation Response

If you have chronic pain, your lifestyle may be contributing to your suffering. Relaxation and sleep could be the keys to relief. "Many women who suffer from some kind of chronic pain just push through daily living until the pain tips them over the edge," says Dr. Caudill. "But there are basic, commonsense things to do—relaxation techniques, taking time for bubble baths, maintaining friendships, and keeping up your social network."

Sleep problems can make pain problems worse, adds Dr. Caudill. She recommends a period of unwinding before you go to bed. One method to help release tension is the relaxation response that was described by Dr. Caudill's colleague, Herbert Benson, M.D., at Harvard Medical School in the early 1970s. Here's how to do it. Sit or lie down in a comfortable position, relax all your muscles, and breathe slowly and deeply. Focus on a phrase or a word, and re-peat it in your mind each time you exhale. If your mind wanders, gently guide it back to your word.

Don't pay attention to thoughts that intrude; just let them passively float through your mind. Practice the relaxation response for 20 minutes once a day or for 10 minutes twice a day, advises Dr. Caudill. If there are some days when you don't have 10 consecutive minutes to yourself, here's a quick relaxer from Dr. Caudill. Take a moment to tense all your muscles at once, then take a deep breath and slowly breathe out, letting all the tension go.

Anatomy of a Headache

Tension headaches bother about 90 percent of all the people in the world, says Alan Rapoport, M.D., assistant clinical professor of neurology at Yale University School of Medicine, co-director of the New England Center for Headache in Stamford, Connecticut, and co-author of *Headache Relief for Women*. The term *tension headache* refers to tense muscles in the head and neck, but it might just as well mean tension from stress—a common headache trigger. Beyond that, many people feel the ache of migraines, cluster headaches, and head pain from allergies or sinus problems.

Migraine headaches are vascular headaches—that is, they involve your blood vessels. First, those blood vessels constrict, which can make you supersensitive to sound and light. Then the blood vessels dilate, producing pain.

The tendency to get migraines is inherited, so if you get them, it's likely that someone else in your family gets them, too. For some women the trigger that sets off the headaches can be biological, such as hormonal swings that accompany the menstrual cycle. Other possible migraine triggers include food, alcohol, and stress. In addition, some people get migraines in response to drops in barometric pressure. Migraine and tension headaches can be hard to tell apart, and some experts believe the two types are part of a continuum, with no clear boundary between them, says Dr. Caudill. Cluster headaches, which are uncommon in women, feel like a sharp, piercing, throbbing, burning pain that bores into one side of your head or around or behind your eyes.

Kitchen Remedies

For people who get headaches, there are specific foods that can cause pain. Migraine triggers such as red wine and chocolate are infamous. But studies show that some foods do the opposite—they actually increase your pain tolerance, says Dr. Caudill. Here's how to sort through the good and the bad.

Talk turkey. Foods, such as turkey and milk, that contain the essential amino acid tryptophan are terrific. Tryptophan is a precursor to the pain-squashing brain chemical serotonin, and it has been used to treat premenstrual problems, depression, and drug and alcohol cravings.

A diet rich in tryptophan, high in complex carbohydrates, and low in proteins may increase pain tolerance, says Dr. Caudill. She recommends tryptophan-rich edibles such as turkey and other lean meats, fish, and low-fat or nonfat milk.

Skip the alcohol. If you get frequent headaches or muscle pain, try eliminating alcohol from your diet and see if you feel better. If alcohol seems to trigger headaches at some times and not at others, try limiting your intake to one glass of dry white wine at a time, suggests Dr. Rapoport.

Beware tyramine, nitrites, and monosodium glutamate. Other possible triggers are foods that contain tyramine, such as aged cheeses, fresh bread, pickled or fermented foods, liver, red wines, yogurt, figs, and bananas. Or you might have to watch out for foods that contain nitrites, chemicals that preserve processed meats such as bologna, salami, pepperoni, bacon, ham, and hot dogs. Other foods that some people have to avoid include nuts, peanut butter, onions, sour cream, and avocados. Still other women react badly to monosodium glutamate (MSG).

Check your cup. Caffeine and products containing aspartame—such as NutraSweet, which is often found in diet soft drinks—trigger migraines in some women. If you suspect a link with your own head pain, try going without caffeine or diet drinks for a week or longer to see if you find relief.

Natural Cold Remedies for Women Who Don't Have Time to Be Sick

Becky Hieter, a 37-year-old mother of two from Ames, Iowa, is no stranger to sore throats, colds, flu, and other infections that frequently plague kids and their busy mothers.

When infection strikes, however, Hieter doesn't turn to over-the-counter medicines like antihistamines. Instead, she relies primarily on herbs, vitamins, and other natural remedies known for their infection-fighting powers. "I swear by echinacea and vitamin C," says Hieter.

Over-the-counter drugs like antihistamines and prescription drugs like antibiotics can help treat and ease cold symptoms and more serious, cold-related sinus infections and sore throats. But they can also cause unpleasant side effects. Antibiotics, for instance, can cause rashes and diarrhea. Yet alternative treatments such as vitamin and mineral therapy, herbal medicine, and homeopathy can get equally good results without the side effects, says Keith DeOrio, M.D., a homeopathic physician in private practice in Santa Monica, California.

Here's the rundown on what works and why.

The Natural Route to Fast Cold Relief

Getting a chill can stress your immunity and give a cold virus free reign. But you don't just get colds when it's cold outside. Anyone who's ever had a miser-

Marital Stress Linked to Colds and Lowered Immunity in Women

Marital bickering can lead to more than emotionally unhealthy relationships. Conflict between spouses can lower a woman's immunity—making her more susceptible to colds and other illnesses, a study has found.

At Ohio State University 90 newlywed couples were asked to discuss a topic that was a source of conflict while investigators monitored physiological changes. Not only did the women's blood pressures soar higher than the men's but they also experienced a greater surge in stress hormones and a decline in white blood cell count, indicating a lowered immune response. Even more worrisome for women, the researchers duplicated their findings with older couples. "Young female newlyweds may experience no serious health consequences," says Janice Kiecolt-Glaser, Ph.D., professor and director of the division of health psychology in the department of psychiatry at Ohio State University in Columbus and lead investigator for the study. "But for older women hostile and chronic conflict might mean the difference between sickness and health."

The reason for this disparity between the sexes isn't yet understood, but the researchers theorize that women pick up more of their partners' emotional signals than men do and are more sensitive to negative interactions.

How can women protect their physical—and emotional—health during conflict? Learn the techniques of fair fighting, suggests Dr. Kiecolt-Glaser—no name-calling, use "I" language, speak in a calm voice, and offer solutions, not blame. The less hostile and negative your disputes, the less you'll stress your immune system.

HEALTH FLASH

able summer cold can attest to that. Colds deserve their name, though, because they stop you cold. When you get struck by a common cold, aches, a stuffy or runny nose, coughing, sneezing, and a sore throat, you can end up feeling out of sorts for seven days or more.

More than 100 different viruses cause colds. Cold medicines treat symptoms only, and many leave you drowsy or fog your thinking. Here are some nondrug approaches to ease the misery of a cold.

Sink it with zinc. Taking a zinc supplement as soon as you sniff that first sniffle is an effective way to sideline a cold, says Sherif Mossad, M.D., clinical doctor in the department of infectious diseases at the Cleveland Clinic in Ohio. "The key is to start taking zinc within 24 hours of your first cold symptoms."

To study the effectiveness of zinc, Dr. Mossad prescribed zinc gluconate lozenges for 50 of a group of 100 employees of the Cleveland Clinic who had early cold symptoms. The other 50 took a mock lookalike drug. The employees who received the zinc gluconate (most of whom were women) took 13.3 milligrams every 2 hours during waking hours for as long as they had the symptoms. Among those who took zinc, most symptoms lasted about $4^1/_2$ days, compared to about $7^1/_2$ days for the 50 people not taking zinc. And, in fact, many people find sucking on zinc lozenges to be an effective way to fight off colds. You can buy zinc lozenges at health food stores and drugstores. Follow the package directions for dosages.

Zinc may help to prevent the attachment of common cold germs to the inside of the nose, says Dr. Mossad. He recommends that you take a daily dose of up to 150 milligrams of zinc gluconate when you start to feel a cold coming on. Talk to your doctor before taking supplements higher than 15 milligrams for more than a few days.

Stock up on C. Another effective standby in the battle against the common cold is vitamin C, says Andrea Sullivan, Ph.D., a naturopathic and homeopathic physician in Washington, D.C., and author of *Naturopathic Medicine for African-Americans*. "Take extra vitamin C when you're under stress or in the winter—both of these conditions leave you more susceptible to a cold. I recommend taking 1,000 milligrams of vitamin C three times a day when you have a cold, to help shorten the duration." Large amounts of vitamin C may cause diarrhea in some people, so cut back if you start experiencing problems.

Pick up some echinacea. The herb echinacea is a natural cold killer, says Dr. Sullivan. "It stimulates the immune system, specifically the white blood cells, to fight infection." Most of the time, echinacea is taken in liquid form—no more than 20 drops in water, juice, or tea three times a day when you start feeling the symptoms of a cold. Or take two capsules three times a day, says Dr. Sullivan. Echinacea is available in health food stores and some drugstores.

Try taking echinacea before long airplane trips in order to prevent colds, recommends Adriane Fugh-Berman, M.D., former head of field investigations for the Office of Alternative Medicine at the National Institutes of Health in Bethesda, Maryland. Because the air in planes is drier and continually recirculated, you're exposed to more viruses, and you're more vulnerable, she explains. "A lot of people pick up viruses on airplanes. So I suggest that you take echinacea the day before and the day of your trip."

Whip up a batch of pesto. Because it's a potent antibiotic and antiviral herb, crushed or mashed garlic can help prevent colds and reduce symptoms, says Dr. Fugh-Berman. As an alternative to garlic-laden food, she suggests enteric-coated garlic capsules, available at most health food stores. Typically, garlic is taken in 300-milligram dosages three times a day, for as long as cold symptoms last. Or you can take a half-clove of the real thing three times a day.

Hurry to homeopathy. Homeopathy offers a variety of cold remedies, depending on your particular symptoms, says Linda Johnston, M.D., diplomate in homeopathic therapeutics, founder of the Academy of Classical Homeopathy in Van Nuys, California, and author of *Everyday Miracles: Homeopathy in Action.* For example, if your left ear aches, the left side of your throat hurts, and you feel worse at night, you might benefit from taking 200C of lachesis, a homeopathic remedy that, among other effects, fights infections, explains Dr. Johnston. (The notation 200C refers to the remedy's potency, which is indicated on the label.) See the package directions for exact dosages. For other cold symptoms, select homeopathic remedies based on the descriptions noted on the packages. These remedies are available in health food stores.

Needle that cold. Acupuncture can cut short a cold's stay, notes Joseph S. Acquah, a licensed acupuncturist and doctor of oriental medicine in Los Angeles. "Acupuncture stimulation of the lung, colon, and liver meridians—energy channels in the body—enhances the body's innate healing ability to clear phlegm from the nose and lungs, eliminate excess waste through the colon, and detoxify the liver. All of these effects will help to relieve the common cold," he says.

Breathing Easy

Whether due to a cold or allergies, the stuffy, clogged-up discomfort of congested nasal passages is still a major pain in the...head.

Over-the-counter nasal sprays and decongestants can help, but sprays shouldn't be used for longer than three days, nor should decongestants be used for more than seven. Overuse can result in a rebound effect—that is, your nose gets stuffed up all over again. And some people find that over-the-counter drugs tend to make them jumpy.

Before nasal congestion drains all of your patience, try these safe, nondrug remedies.

Spice up your menu. Eating any kind of spicy food can temporarily help loosen congestion by thinning out mucus and making your nose run, says Dr. Fugh-Berman. Eating ground red pepper or chili peppers such as jalapeños can increase secretions in your nose and throat, she notes. Or add some hot-pepper sauce (like Tabasco) to soup, salad, or pasta sauce. If you can't stomach spicy foods, try taking two ground-red-pepper capsules four times a day. The capsules are available in health food stores.

Unclog the cause. Spending about 5 minutes in a hot shower allows steam to loosen mucus-clogged sinuses, says Irene von Estorff, M.D., assistant professor of rehabilitation medicine at New York Hospital–Cornell University Medical College in New York City. You can also try putting a towel over your head and leaning over a pot of steaming water that has been removed from the heat.

Rub on an aromatic oil. The essential oils camphor (from camphor trees), menthol (derived from peppermint), and eucalyptus (from eucalyptus trees) are natural decongestants, says Dr. Fugh-Berman. When mixed with neutral oil, such as grapeseed or corn oil, and applied to the skin, these three oils cause a cooling sensation that seems to enhance their decongestant properties. Put some on your neck, under your nose, on your temples, or anywhere that you can smell it. Essential oils should never be applied straight because they can irritate your skin.

Many commercial rubs contain those three essential oils, notes Dr. Fugh-Berman. You can also make your own rub by adding a couple of drops of camphor, menthol, or eucalyptus to a handful of corn oil, and rubbing it on your chest and neck, she says.

Quieting a Cough

Coughs have a knack for perversity. They'll happen during your best friend's wedding, in the middle of a boring speech, and at 3:00 A.M. with sleep nowhere in sight.

No matter how hard you fight back a cough, that hacking, choking sound has to come out eventually. That's because coughing is a natural reflex—many times it's your body's way of trying to get rid of mucus in your lungs.

If you've been coughing for more than two weeks and it doesn't seem to go away, or if you're coughing up colored phlegm (anything other than clear or white), see your doctor. Otherwise, try nature's cures for silencing your cough.

Try nature's cough drops. Cough drops containing eucalyptus or horehound take the edge off your hack, says Dr. Fugh-Berman. Found in drugstores and health food stores, these lozenges help to thin the excretions of bronchial mucus that can make you cough.

Mind your vitamins. Drink plenty of juices made from vitamin-packed vegetables like carrots and beets, and greens like kale or collards, suggests Dr. Sullivan. These juices (which you can either buy in a health food store or prepare at home in a juicer) help you fight germs that cause coughs, thanks to generous amounts of immune-boosting nutrients like vitamins A and C, she says. A deficiency of vitamin A damages the natural protective mucous membrane barrier of the respiratory tract, leaving your throat and lungs vulnerable to bacteria and viruses. Vitamin C boosts immunity by enabling white blood cells to fight infection.

"Drink one glass of vegetable juice a couple of times a day," advises Dr. Sul-

The Uncommonly Annoying Cold

It's bad enough that you end up looking like Rudolph the Red-Nosed Reindeer and sounding like Elmer Fudd. Why does the common cold also have to be so, well, common? Chances are, this year you'll be struck by cold viruses—and succumb to humanity's most prevalent sickness—at least twice and as many as four times.

Since colds are transmitted by hand-to-face contact, one of the best ways to prevent them is to wash your hands frequently. Try not to touch things that you know someone with a cold has touched, says Anthony J. Yonkers, M.D., professor and chairman of the department of otolaryngology–head and neck surgery at the University of Nebraska Medical Center in Omaha. "Everyone worries about people sneezing around them in the office because they think that they'll breathe in germs and get infected," he says. "But if you touch the doorknob that they just touched, and then put your hand to your eye or nose, it's much more likely that you'll be infected."

livan. "If you make your own juice in a blender, add a little water to dilute the vegetables."

Fighting the Flu with Herbs

The flu bug is the most sadistic of germs. When it's at its worst, you'll feel body chills that make you pile on the wool blankets, while at the same time, you're coping with a fever. Add to those miseries a headache, achy joints, and a general feeling that you'll never get out of bed again, and it all spells misery.

So what can you do about this highly contagious respiratory infection? If you drink plenty of fluids, get plenty of rest, and take acetaminophen to help relieve muscle and joint pains and to reduce fever, you should be better in about a week. But if you'd like to rid yourself of the flu a few days earlier—and who wouldn't?—try these tactics.

Grab some echinacea. If you're just starting to feel that tired-all-over general malaise of the flu, try that old standby echinacea. This immune-boosting herb could shorten a flu virus's stay, says Dr. Fugh-Berman. Take two capsules three or four times a day, or take 20 to 40 drops (40 drops equals about one dropperful) of tincture in a beverage three or four times a day, she says.

"It's very important to take echinacea every few hours instead of just once a day, because it doesn't stay in your system for very long," adds Dr. Fugh-Berman. Continue to take echinacea until you feel better, but no longer. If used long-term (for more than a few weeks), echinacea loses its effectiveness, she notes.

Unclogging Stuffed-Up Sinuses

If you have a cold or have allergies, your sinuses may clog up with mucus. Tiny openings in the sinuses are obstructed, so mucus can't drain. With nowhere to go, fluids build up, causing pressure and pain. Worse, bacteria can set up camp in the pools of mucus and infect your sinuses, causing fever, headaches, and facial pain.

If you have a fever, which is a key indicator of infection, see your doctor. If you have pain but no fever, however, you can take the following steps to help drain your sinuses, says Dr. Fugh-Berman.

Sleep with a vaporizer. You can relieve stuffy sinuses as you sleep at night by putting a few drops of eucalyptus, camphor, or menthol essential oil into a steam humidifier set up by your bed, Dr. Fugh-Berman says.

Clear your head with yoga. A legs-against-the-wall yoga pose can help clear your sinuses, says Larry Payne, Ph.D., director of the Samata Yoga Center in Los Angeles and chairman of the International Association of Yoga Therapists.

Lie on your back with your buttocks pushed against the base of the wall. Raise your legs and hold them against the wall for 7 to 15 minutes, says Dr. Payne. "This changes blood flow within the body and changes the flow of your body's lymphatic fluids—the fluids that flow from the space between the body cells into the bloodstream. For the first few minutes of this pose, pressure in your sinuses will increase. But after awhile, the mucus in your sinuses will start to loosen."

One caution: If you have high blood pressure, glaucoma, or if you are at risk for stroke, you should not do this exercise, notes Dr. Payne.

Soothing a Sore Throat

A sore, inflamed throat can be a symptom of an allergy, a viral infection like a cold, or a bacterial infection such as streptococcus (strep throat).

For some people, strep infection can lead to rheumatic fever, a more serious condition that can damage your heart or kidneys. So if you have a sore throat that's not clearly the result of an allergy or cold, you should see a doctor, says Dr. DeOrio. Strep throat calls for different treatment than sore throats due to a cold or allergies. Should your doctor determine that you have strep throat and need antibiotics or other medication, you can still use alternative remedies in addition to your medication, says Dr. DeOrio.

Here's what nature has to offer.

Pick the right homeopathic remedy. For sore throats, Dr. DeOrio often recommends three homeopathic remedies: belladonna, mercurius sol (merc. sol), or lachesis. "These remedies will work no matter what's causing the sore throat. But be sure to match the symptoms to the remedy."

❖ If pain and redness are worse on the right side of your throat or if you have difficulty swallowing and your tonsils appear enlarged, a 30C-potency dose of belladonna three or four times daily is the homeopathic remedy for you, he says. See the package directions for dosage information.

❖ If you have raw, burning pain extending from the middle of your throat to your ears, bad breath, and both swelling and white or yellow discharge in the back of your throat, the ticket may be mercurius sol at 30C potency three or four times a day. The package directions provide dosage instructions.

❖ If your throat feels constricted, looks red and burns, and if the pain is stronger on the left side and extends to your ear, take a dose of lachesis at 30C potency three or four times daily. Determine the correct dosage according to the directions on the package. Continue the remedy until your symptoms subside, typically two to four days, but no longer, says Dr. De-Orio. If you continue to take homeopathic treatments, the symptoms can return.

Rescue Your Joints from Discomfort— Without Drugs

I f you thought the last words on osteoarthritis were "Pop painkillers and suffer," you haven't been talking to the right sources. Cutting-edge researchers who study arthritis relief say they're more and more convinced that how you eat can really make a difference.

If you're among the nearly 25 million American women with osteoarthritis, then you know, or can feel, that the normally tough, resilient padding (called cartilage) that cushions bones inside joints has begun to deteriorate, sometimes wearing away entirely.

In healthy joints cartilage reduces friction and absorbs shock as you move about. But when poorly padded bones rub together, pain strikes. Joints affected most by osteoarthritis seem to be hands, hips, and knees—usually resulting in the most disabling form of the illness. Sometimes inflammation and swelling accompany the pain. Another common consequence is stiffness and loss of mobility, as women with osteoarthritis avoid activity in an attempt to avoid the hurt.

Unburden Aching Joints

There's growing confidence among osteoarthritis experts about the most effective dietary strategy to soothe your joints: If you're beyond a healthy weight

Borage Oil May Relieve Arthritis Pain and Swelling

Research suggesting that a component of borage-seed oil, called gamma linolenic acid, may offer arthritis relief is bolstered by a study from the University of Massachusetts Medical Center in Worcester.

Researchers followed 56 women and men with arthritis for six months, while they took either 2.8 grams a day of gamma linolenic acid or a placebo made from sunflower oil, along with their regular prescription arthritis medications. The results were provocative. Those taking the gamma linolenic acid were more than six times more likely to have significant improvements in swelling, joint tenderness, stiffness, and pain. Symptoms in the other group remained the same or worsened.

For the second 6-month period, everyone got the gamma linolenic acid capsules, and all showed improvement. In fact, those receiving this special fatty acid for the entire 12 months saw progressive improvement. By the end, symptoms were reduced by more than 50 percent in half the gamma linolenic takers. Seven people even opted to reduce the amount of painkillers they were taking, as a result.

While it might appear that gamma linolenic acid could someday become a substitute for painkillers to soothe arthritis, it's important to note that it is not fast acting, says lead investigator Robert Zurier, M.D., professor of medicine and director of rheumatology at the University of Massachusetts Medical Center. In this study it took 6 to 12 weeks to see improvement. Researchers think that gamma linolenic acid may work by changing the balance of substances in the body that affect inflammation. Three months after the study's end, however, swelling and joint pain returned, indicating that the oil would have to be continued to suppress symptoms.

These doses were very large, Dr. Zurier cautions, and gamma linolenic acid use is not approved for arthritis, or any disease, in this country. "Patients can certainly discuss this with their doctors, but no one should take these doses without medical supervision," he advises.

HEALTH FLASH

(as many women with osteoarthritis are), try losing a few pounds, especially through a combination of diet and exercise.

Consider what happened to 48 overweight, postmenopausal women with knee osteoarthritis who participated in a diet-and-exercise trial at the University of Maryland School of Medicine in Baltimore. After six months of walking on treadmills three times a week (for up to 45 minutes per session) and following a reduced-calorie, low-fat diet, the women lost an average of $15^1/_2$ pounds each.

And here's the key payoff: They had much less knee pain. Using a reliable measure called the WOMAC pain score, 40 percent of the women reported only half as much pain. A third of the women experienced 50 percent improvements in functions such as walking up stairs and getting in and out of cars. And compared to the beginning of the study, on average, the women walked 12 percent farther on a 6-minute walking test.

Here's more good news: there's evidence that losing just a little bit of weight may be enough to relieve pain. In a study at Bowman Gray School of Medicine of Wake Forest University in Winston-Salem, North Carolina, women over age 60 with knee osteoarthritis lost an average of 19 pounds over six months with a combination of diet and exercise. Again, pain declined, performance improved. "But some people who lost only 10 pounds experienced as much improvement in pain and disability as those who lost much more," says study researcher Walter Ettinger, M.D., professor of internal medicine and public health science.

Why does losing just a few pounds seem to help so much? Marc Hochberg, M.D., head of the division of rheumatology and clinical immunology at the University of Maryland School of Medicine and leader of the University of Maryland study, explains it this way. When you walk, your knee absorbs a force equal to about three times your body weight with each step. So losing even 10 pounds actually relieves each knee of an approximately 30-pound load with every stride.

Can losing weight help in more ways than reducing pressure on the joints? Maybe. "It's well-known that being overweight raises the risk of getting osteoarthritis in the first place. But why do obese women get more osteoarthritis of the hands—areas that wouldn't be stressed from being overweight?" asks researcher David Felson, M.D., associate professor of medicine and public health at Boston University School of Medicine. "Perhaps," he suggests, "obesity in itself exerts some metabolic influence on bone and cartilage."

The bottom line is that if you're overweight and have osteoarthritis, lose at least 10 pounds. It's critical that you both exercise and cut calories to lose weight, Dr. Hochberg stresses. "Studies show the combo is more effective for losing weight. Plus, we know that sticking with exercise helps keep weight off for the long haul." (Before starting an exercise program, check with your doctor to find out how much exercise is safe for you.)

If you weigh 175 pounds and you walk on a treadmill at a very easygoing 2 miles per hour for $^1/_2$ hour three times a week, you will burn approximately 360 calories.

Where's the C?

Look for the richest sources of vitamin C in the produce aisle—and among the juices—in your local supermarket. Here is how they measure up.

Food	Vitamin C (mg.)
1 guava	165
1 sweet red pepper	141
1 cup fresh-squeezed orange juice	124
1 cup cranberry juice cocktail	108
1 cup orange juice from concentrate	97
1 cup chopped papaya	87
1 cup strawberries	85
1 cup grapefruit juice from concentrate	83
1 cup raw broccoli florets	82
1 kiwifruit	75
1 orange	70
1 cup cantaloupe cubes	68
1 green pepper	66
1 cup Del Monte Gold pineapple chunks	60
1 mango	57
1 cup raw cauliflower florets	46
1/2 grapefruit	41

On the diet front, cut back just 150 calories a day (for a total calorie reduction of 1,050 a week). With this combination, you should be 10 pounds lighter in six months.

The Vitamin Connection

For a decade researchers have kept track of 640 residents of Framingham, Massachusetts, who have osteoarthritis, including recording what they've eaten. Turns out that those getting the most vitamin C had a threefold reduction in osteoarthritis progression—meaning they lost less knee cartilage over time—compared with those getting the least vitamin C.

"Vitamin C may help because it plays a role in making collagen, a material necessary for repairing cartilage," says Tim McAlindon, M.D., assistant professor of medicine at Boston University School of Medicine and lead researcher of the study. He notes that people getting the middle range of vitamin C daily (about 150 to 175 milligrams—an amount easy to get through food) had the same reduced risk of osteoarthritis progression as those taking the most vitamin C (430 to 500 milligrams). His conclusion is that just in case vitamin C is simply a marker for fruits and vegetables rich in other healing compounds, it's best to stick with foods high in vitamin C, rather than relying on a supplement.

The bottom line is that you should eat at least five servings of fruits and vegetables daily, making sure to include rich sources of vitamin C, such as citrus fruits, red peppers, and strawberries. If you live east of the Mississippi, look for an unexpected source of vitamin C in specially bred fresh pineapples called Del Monte Gold. One cup of Del Monte Gold pineapple (about two slices) has 60 milligrams of vitamin C, compared with 15 milligrams for regular pineapple. A delicious bonus is that Del Monte Gold pineapple tastes extrasweet, too.

Another finding from the Framingham study offers one more potential clue to slowing osteoarthritis with diet: getting at least 360 international units (IU) of vitamin D a day. People with vitamin D intakes lower than this level were about three times more likely to have progression of knee osteoarthritis.

How might vitamin D help slow this painful condition? It's known to play a role in keeping bones healthy. Once osteoarthritis breaks down cartilage in a joint, the underlying bone is subjected to greater stress, notes Dr. McAlindon. Low levels of vitamin D may impair the ability of the bone to respond to this increased wear and tear.

One way to ensure that you consume enough vitamin D per day is to look for a multivitamin with 400 IU, equal to 100 percent of the Daily Value (DV). The only other substantial dietary source of vitamin D is milk. One cup of any type of milk has 100 IU (25 percent of the DV); 1/3 cup of nonfat dry milk has 100 IU. Some breakfast cereals are fortified with 40 IU per serving (10 percent of the DV). Experts recommend getting no more than 600 IU of vitamin D on a regular basis.

23

Home Remedies for Tortured Feet

During a lifetime of trekking upstairs and down, indoors and out, over hill and down dale, a woman treads the equivalent of four times around the Earth. Given that your feet get that kind of workout, a little respect for your hardworking tootsies seems in order. Yet in practice, women are more likely to squish their feet into poorly fitted shoes than to care for them.

Take a look at your shoes right now. Eighty-eight percent of women wear shoes that are one or two sizes too narrow, the Women's Shoewear Council of the American Orthopaedic Foot and Ankle Society found. "The fashion shoe is a slowly deforming device," notes S. W. Balkin, D.P.M., attending assistant professor of podiatry in the department of orthopedics at Los Angeles County–University of Southern California Medical Center. Over a lifetime of wearing high heels and tight shoes, each set of five toes assumes the triangular shape of pointed toeboxes. "It's analogous to foot binding," Dr. Balkin says.

And women pay dearly for fashion. Ninety percent of the surgery for common foot problems such as bunions and hammertoes is done on women, notes Carol Frey, M.D., director of the Orthopedic Hospital of Los Angeles Foot and Ankle Clinic and a researcher on the Women's Shoewear Council.

Women are also much more likely than men to suffer from neuroma, an inflammation and thickening of the nerves between the toes. In fact, more than 90 percent of people with neuroma are women. "The modern fashion shoe is to blame, not weight, work, or heredity," says Dr. Balkin. "The sad fact is that these conditions are nearly 100 percent preventable, yet once they have gotten severe enough, they require a lifetime of care or surgery."

Simple, Surprising Solutions for Heel Pain

Inexpensive over-the-counter heel pads and simple stretches can be at least as effective as costly custom-made heel supports for the initial treatment of heel pain, according to a two-year study of this most common of foot ailments.

When researchers at 10 medical centers asked 168 women and 82 men with heel pain to try out various pain-relief measures for eight weeks, the investigators were surprised to learn that an easy stretching routine eased the ache just as effectively as custom-fitted shoe inserts that cost about $120. Even without stretching, almost 9 out of 10 people also felt better wearing inexpensive, off-the-shelf inserts that cost as little as about $6.50, compared to 7 in 10 who wore the custom pads.

Here's an easy stretch for heel pain: Stand with the balls of your feet on a curb or stair and gently lower your heels. "Hold the stretch for 30 seconds and repeat once every hour during the day," says Jane Pontious, D.P.M., associate professor of surgery at the Pennsylvania College of Podiatric Medicine in Philadelphia.

Stretching can be helpful in relieving pain, but, Dr. Pontious adds, "you also need to find out why you're having heel pain." For women, the reasons are many. You may have excessive pronation, in which the arch of your foot rolls inward as you walk. In addition, excess weight puts extra pressure on the heel. A job that involves standing and walking on hard surfaces for long periods of time can also cause problems, as can poorly fitted shoes and high heels.

"If you're not wearing appropriate shoes and getting good shock absorption, a drugstore heel pad is not a bad idea initially," Dr. Pontious says. "But if the condition persists and the pain is not relieved, you should see a podiatrist."

Many women over age 65 have worn pointy-toed pumps for much of their lives, and their feet pay the price: These women have 3½ times more corns and calluses and 13 times more bunions than men.

If the Shoe Doesn't Fit...

"My feet are killing me" is a common expression—but it's usually the shoes that are doing the damage, especially for women. Orthopedic experts estimate that ill-fitting shoes provoke 75 percent of our foot problems, including blisters, bunions, corns and calluses, hammertoes, neuromas, and plantar fasciitis. Here's how they happen.

Blisters. Usually a temporary problem, blisters are caused by rubbing between your toes or between your foot and shoe.

Bunions. A bunion is a bony growth that forms on the joint at the base of your big toe. An inflammation begins on the side of the toe joint, and gradually the metatarsal bone moves outward, as your big toe starts to move inward. That lumpy side growth of bone, combined with the dislocation of the joint, creates the problem.

Corns and calluses. These are created at the parts of your foot where an ill-fitting shoe rubs too much. They're thickened nubs or clumps of dead skin cells, more protection than a problem when they start, but they become painful when they get too big. Corns are smaller and usually form on top of a toe or in between toes. Calluses are bigger and usually form on the bottom of your foot. They can be caused by shoes that have inadequate padding under your feet.

Hammertoes. When a pointed shoe squeezes your toes, your middle toe may get forced upward, resulting in a hammertoe.

Neuromas. If you wear high heels, the foot position pressures your toes into the toebox of the shoe. If the toebox is pointed and tight, a bone at the base of each toe (usually at the base of the third and fourth toes) sometimes rubs. It's the rubbing action that eventually inflames and thickens the nerve between the toes, causing a neuroma. Irritated neuromas cause burning and cramping.

Plantar fasciitis. In terms of body parts, "the heels are the first things to hit the ground," says William Case, physical therapist and president of Case Physical Therapy in Houston. And heel pain most often comes from an inflammation of the plantar fascia, the main ligament that stretches across the bottom of the foot from heel to toe.

When you overuse your foot or pronate (turn your foot inward when you walk), you may irritate and inflame the ligament. If you do that often enough, a bony growth called a heel spur sometimes develops at the point of injury.

Pain from an inflamed ligament or a heel spur feels worst in the morning and diminishes as the day goes on. But the correct shoe insert can cure most heel pain, according to David Alper, D.P.M., visiting professor of podiatry at Northeastern University in Boston.

Sole-Soothing Strategies

There are ways to assuage almost any foot complaint. Here's what foot care specialists recommend.

Stretch your tootsies. "In a way, hammertoes are part of being human," says Melanie Sanders, M.D., chairman of the Women's Shoewear Council and an orthopedist in Indianapolis. "To walk upright, you roll across your foot from heel to toe. That pushes your toes upward, pulling the normal padding upward with them. High heels worsen that tendency," she says. "But you can counterbalance that movement that you do all day long."

Dr. Sanders suggests stretching your toes. First, sit down on a low stool or on a pillow on the floor and place one foot flat on the floor. Then, "put your finger right where the hair on your toes tends to grow and push each toe down firmly so that you feel the stretch on top of your foot. Hold it down for 30 seconds. Do each toe. Then go back and do them again. You can do it while you're watching the news. It takes 4 to 5 minutes," Dr. Sanders says. "Do it daily if your feet are bothering you," she suggests. "For maintenance you just need to do it two or three times a week."

Splint at night. After a day under pressure from shoes, bunions often ache. If you have a bunion that's acting up, try using a foot care product called a night splint. It works while you sleep. You can get a night splint from an orthopedist or podiatrist, according to Dr. Sanders.

A night splint is a small apparatus with a plastic piece that fits the big toe. An elastic strap pulls the big toe into a straighter, more normal position. "The new position helps relieve the pressure and takes the strain off the area around the bunion," she says.

Scrutinize your seams. Athletic shoes are generally good for your feet. But women who have bunions should double-check the construction of their crosstrainers or aerobic shoes, according to Dr. Sanders. "Some sneakers have a little fashion seam that goes right across the top of a bunion." Because the seam doesn't stretch, you get an area of high pressure over the bunion.

Collapse a blister carefully. Blisters are formed when you break in a new pair of shoes or when you do too much walking in the wrong shoes. A blister can make you miserable. You probably won't want to walk or work out very much until the blister heals.

In the meantime, though, "you don't need to wait for it to get big. You can drain it as soon as you see it," says Rodney S. W. Basler, M.D., assistant professor of internal medicine at the University of Nebraska College of Medicine and a dermatologist at the University of Nebraska Medical Center, both in Omaha. Sterilize a needle with the flame of a match and let cool, or sterilize it with rubbing alcohol. Then pierce the blister at its edge. Press it to drain as much fluid as you can, but don't remove the blister's protective skin. "Drain it every 12 hours," says Dr. Basler. "That seems to bring about the fastest healing."

Lift with a cup. To relieve heel pain, you can get a heel cup that goes under the back of your foot to relieve some of the pressure on the ligament. Or find a foam insole that cushions your entire foot. These products are available in drugstores and some shoe stores.

Flex your leather. Before you toss out a too-tight shoe, try using a shoe stretcher, suggests Dr. Sanders. It's a device that you can buy in a full-service shoe store or a shoe repair shop starting at around $11. The stretcher looks like the front part of a shoe tree. Some have round, ball-like attachments that allow you to stretch specific sites—where the shoe presses against a bunion or corn, for instance.

You can use the shoe stretcher alone or maximize its effectiveness with a liquid lubricant available at the shoe repair shop or a drugstore. It works best on leather shoes because they have greater give than most vinyl and are less likely to be damaged by the product. (In fact, some experts say that you shouldn't use the product on vinyl at all, because you'll ruin the shoes—despite what the product label says.) Apply the shoe-stretching liquid to the inside of your shoe. Then position the shoe stretcher, and gently tighten it to press against the inside of the shoe. Let the shoe stretch overnight or longer.

Finding the Perfect Shoe

Despite the bonanza of comfortable athletic shoes—and even some comfortable pumps—it's still all too easy to stray into Sore Foot Gulch. Here are some pointers to keep you safe from painful shoes.

Go round. Whether you buy a flat or a heel, look for shoes with a rounded toebox instead of a deforming pointed toebox. There's a simple test to see whether a shoe is rounded enough. Hold the bottom of the left shoe against the sole of your right foot. Then hold the bottom of the right shoe against the sole of your left foot. If either shoe fails to cover your foot's sole, the shoes are undersize. Pick a larger size or another style and test again.

Strap your heel. In order to get a shoe wide enough for your foot, you may have to buy one with a little too much heel room. "Your heels don't spread with age the way the balls of your feet do," says Dr. Sanders. Try a shoe with an adjustable heel strap. That way, you can get one with ample toe room, then cinch in the strap to prevent slippage.

Add a pad. If you have a favorite pump with the right size toebox, but it's a little too loose on your heel, try a heel pad, suggests Dr. Sanders. It has done the trick for many of her patients, she says.

Remeasure as you age. Once you have reached adulthood, your feet don't grow, but they do change. By the time you're in your thirties, changes in the ligaments that join the bones in the soles of your feet and raise your arches allow your feet to collapse. Your feet begin to spread, or "splay."

"That spread is often responsible for an increase in shoe size of one to two sizes during your lifetime," says James McGuire, D.P.M., director of physical therapy and instructor in the department of orthopedics at the Foot and Ankle Institute of Pennsylvania College of Podiatric Medicine in Philadelphia. In general, your feet are likely to increase in size during and after a pregnancy because of the body's response to increasing demands. In addition, there's a hormone called relaxin that causes the ligaments to relax in the last month of pregnancy—and as the ligaments in your feet relax, your feet may get larger. Exercise can also make a difference. "Aggressive exercise may make your foot meatier and bigger," Dr. McGuire says.

To monitor your changing feet, measure them every three years, suggests Dr. Sanders.

Staying Pain-Free

If you don't want to turn into one of the 43.1 million Americans with feet that hurt, here are some basic all-purpose guidelines to follow.

Don running shoes. You don't have to run to wear running shoes. Many experts tout them as the best all-around shoes for foot support because the heels are so thick and stable. Even if your workplace forbids sneakers on the job, you can do what many businesswomen do—wear them to and from work and at home and play.

Date your sneakers. As the padding in your athletic shoes ages and wears down, your feet start to do double duty in the shock-absorption department. Worn-out shoes sneak up on you. They get old before you know it, and your once-comfortable athletic sneakers may cause real foot problems.

You can keep track of your own athletic shoes, though. Just note the date that you buy each new pair. If you run 25 miles or more a week, replace them every 2^1/$_2$ to 3 months, says Gary M. Gordon, D.P.M., director of the running and walking clinic at the Joseph Torg Center for Sports Medicine at Allegheny University Hospitals, Center City, in Philadelphia. If you take three or more aerobics classes a week, you're wearing out the padding at about the same rate. So you should also replace those sneakers every 2 to 3 months. With a lighter aerobics schedule, replace them every 4 to 6 months.

24

Secrets for Deeper, More Refreshing Sleep

We're a nation of sleep-deprived people. Our sleep debt is so large that Congress established the National Center on Sleep Disorders Research, which is part of the National Institutes of Health based in Bethesda, Maryland, after a three-year federal commission reported that as many as one-third of us toss and turn with insomnia at least once a year.

Forty million Americans have specific sleep disorders, like insomnia, a condition in which we're unable to sleep night after night, or apnea, in which we stop breathing for short periods in our sleep. An additional 20 million to 30 million people have occasional problems falling asleep, staying asleep, or staying on a consistent sleep schedule.

And perhaps no one is more sleep-deprived than women. We juggle family life and work life. And as we age, hormonal changes can make a good night's sleep harder to achieve.

But there's another deficit. Many of those who sleep well don't always sleep enough. On any given day, about one-quarter of us are drowsy and yawning. When you total up all the combined deficits, "well over one-third of us don't get adequate sleep," says Michael Stevenson, Ph.D., clinical director of the North Valley Sleep Disorders Center in Mission Hills, California.

Our brains as well as our bodies need sleep, says Philip Smith, M.D., medical director of the Johns Hopkins University Sleep Disorders Center in Baltimore. "Sleep deprivation makes us moody and irritable and limits our ability to concentrate, make judgments, and perform mental tasks."

Making Friends with Your Pillow

Since we know that we need sleep for mental and physical energy, how do we let ourselves get so tired? "The two answers are that we don't allow ourselves enough time to sleep or we're too tense to fall asleep," says Rosalind Cartwright, Ph.D., director of the Sleep Disorder Service and Research Center at Rush–Presbyterian–St. Luke's Medical Center in Chicago.

Researchers have noted that more women than men are likely to have insomnia. There is evidence that an estimated 40 percent of all women over 40 are fighting insomnia. "The menstrual cycle, pregnancy, and hormone changes at menopause are all reasons that women have many more insomnia complaints than men," says Dr. Stevenson. "And, even in this day and age, women are still the ones who get up with little kids in the middle of the night. That's very disturbing to sleep."

If sleep eludes you so constantly that you can't do what you have to during the day, a visit to your doctor is mandatory, says Tedd Mitchell, M.D., medical director of the Cooper Wellness Program at the Cooper Aerobics Center in Dallas. Insomnia could be a symptom of something else, such as depression. Yet if your sleeplessness is annoying but not debilitating, changes in schedule, exercise, diet, and even eating habits can make you better friends with your pillow.

Get Ready, Get Set, Snooze

While sleep shortages can get to be a habit, some habits are meant to be broken. "You have to court sleep," advises Dr. Cartwright. "Often, people can't sleep because they're too wound up. They rush around all day. They try to work until the last minute. Then they want to fall asleep quickly, and they can't do it. You have to be ready for sleep." To get ready, here are some top methods for attracting the sandman.

Get into hot water. "Take a hot bath. This is the best way I know to court sleep," says Dr. Cartwright. "It sounds so strange, in this day and age when people take morning showers, that people look at me in shock when I mention it. But once they try it, they adore it."

As with many sleep rituals and routines, timing is important. "Take a bath 2 hours before bedtime so that you have $1^1/_2$ hours to do quiet things when you come out," says Dr. Cartwright. "Use bath oil—it floats on the surface of the water and helps the water retain heat. Relax in the tub for 20 to 30 minutes. That relaxes your muscles, too. When you come out, you'll be as limp as a noodle."

Catch a silly flick. After your bath, have a little quiet time before you climb into bed. "Do something mindless—nothing to wind you up, something to wind you down," says Dr. Cartwright. She suggests old Marx Brothers comedies if you like to laugh to release tension. "But don't watch any murder mysteries," she warns. "And don't watch a gory newscast. You want dumb movies."

Stir up some sleepy pudding. Go to bed hungry, and you won't sleep. Go to bed full, and you won't sleep either, say sleep specialists. A good snack, on the other hand, can promote the production of serotonin, "the brain's own sedative and relaxant," says Phyllis Herman, a nutrition specialist certified by the American College of Nutrition and contributor to the *Encyclopedia of Sleep and Dreaming*.

Eat some food containing the amino acid tryptophan, which triggers the serotonin-production process. Milk products, tuna, and turkey are all good choices, says Dr. Cartwright.

One swift but soothing snack to summon sleep is instant pudding, says Peter Hauri, Ph.D., co-director of the Sleep Disorders Center and director of its insomnia program at the Mayo Clinic in Rochester, Minnesota, and author of *No More Sleepless Nights*. Choose the sugar-free variety and make it with skim milk to keep fat and calories down.

Make it vanilla. The smelling and feeling centers in our brains are directly connected, says Alan R. Hirsch, M.D., neurological director of the Smell and Taste Treatment and Research Foundation in Chicago. And certain scents can fill us with feelings of calmness and well-being—such as lilacs in spring or the smell of freshly baked apple pie.

Dr. Hirsch has been studying certain scents in detail, and he's found that some smells can lure sleep by lowering anxiety. Among the best soothers are the scents of lavender, green apple, and vanilla. "Since 90 percent of taste is really smell, one way to obtain the scent in a very concentrated way is to eat the food with the appealing smell," he suggests. So make vanilla pudding. Or slice bananas into nonfat vanilla yogurt. It's two sedative effects in one—the tryptophan in the milk and the calming taste, plus smell, of the vanilla.

Shift Your Thoughts into Slow Gear

You know the pattern. You turn out the light, and today's tiny traumas start replaying themselves in the dark. Or you run through tomorrow's lines for the presentation you're giving at work. You worry whether Junior will get into the college of his choice. You worry about your folks in Virginia. And when you can't sleep, you worry about not sleeping. "We bring yesterday and tomorrow into tonight," says Wilse B. Webb, Ph.D., professor emeritus of psychology at the University of Florida in Gainesville. "The greatest obstacle to getting to sleep is that we keep thinking."

Happily, sleep experts have some techniques to settle or sidetrack our thinking brains.

Keep a worry diary. If you're a worrywart, here's one way to defuse that prickly pastime. Two hours before bedtime, make two columns in a worry diary, Dr. Cartwright suggests. "On the left-hand side of one page, write down what you're worried about," she says. "On the right-hand side, write down what you're going to do about it. Then close the book, put it away, and say, 'Well, I took care of that.' Finish the day."

Count cats. If counting sheep is too corny for you, then count cats or dogs or crickets. But even if you have to resort to the old standby, sheep, as Dr. Webb does, it works. Here's why, he says. "It's a task to do. But it's a task that you want

Reset Your Sleep Clock

As we get older, sleep tends to come in fragments. We spend less time in the deep-sleep stages that refresh mind and body. Patchy sleep patterns are the reason that women in their forties, fifties, and beyond begin finding themselves waking up when it's still dark outside and wanting to fall asleep when it's still light, says Donald L. Bliwise, Ph.D., director of the Emory Clinic Sleep Disorders Center at Emory University School of Medicine in Atlanta. But there are ways to reset your body's sleep clock.

Welcome the dusk. Check the time of the sunset in the newspaper or on the TV news, and time a 20- to 30-minute walk that ends right before the sun's last rays fade away. "Exercise literally reverses the sleep problems that we tend to associate with old age," says Tedd Mitchell, M.D., medical director of the Cooper Wellness Program at the Cooper Aerobics Center in Dallas. Along with the exercise, you get the fading daylight to help reset your body's sleep/wake cycle.

Turn up the lights. Use your brightest lamps to light your evening activities. It's an informal light therapy that will prompt you to stay awake until bedtime, says David N. Neubauer, M.D., associate director of the Johns Hopkins University Sleep Disorders Center in Baltimore. And it helps to reset your body clock so that you don't drowse away the evening in dim light. When you go to bed—and turn off the lights—you're ready.

to give up. The counting distracts you from thinking about things. It interferes with whatever is interfering with your sleep."

Hide the ticktock. Alarm clocks can be, well, alarming to poor sleepers. You tend to keep checking the time—and that only tells you how well you're not sleeping. "The more aware you are of what time it is, the harder it is to fall asleep," says Dr. Hauri.

You need a clock without a cord so that you can stash it under the bed or in a closet. Or "set the alarm and hide it in the top dresser drawer," Dr. Hauri suggests. (Don't forget to first test the alarm in its hiding place to make sure that you will hear it in the morning.)

When Sleep Won't Come

Writer F. Scott Fitzgerald called 3:00 A.M. the "real dark night of the soul." It's when you run out of crickets to count. Dr. Hauri once had a patient who counted 5,865 sheep before she called it a night on that technique. So here's what to do when all the numbers in the animal kingdom fail you.

Stop trying. "Trying to sleep keeps you awake," says Dr. Hauri. "Ninety percent of people with insomnia spend too much time in bed trying to sleep." Instead, read or watch TV until you feel drowsy. Fight sleep, then turn out the light when you no longer can stay awake. But never turn out the light and try to sleep, he says.

Stay calm. Panic turns insomnia from a one-night visitor into a houseguest who just won't leave. "People with insomnia almost develop performance anxiety," says Timothy Roehrs, Ph.D., director of research at the Sleep Disorders and Research Center of Henry Ford Hospital in Detroit. They turn out the light, and then the pressure to sleep banishes sleep. "They need relief from the idea that they have to sleep. Sleep is a natural process, and it will happen."

If it doesn't happen fast enough some nights, Dr. Hauri says not to worry. "You can function quite well after one night of poor sleep, even if you don't think you can. Don't sweat it. Hang in there. Pass the night by reading."

Drift off with lavender. The scent of lavender oil is known to have a light sedative effect. A study by British researchers found that lavender oil was more effective than tranquilizers at helping nursing home residents get a restful night's sleep. In that study essence of lavender oil was introduced into the air with an odor diffuser. But there's another way, if you don't have a diffuser: "You can use a few drops of lavender oil on a handkerchief that you keep on your pillow," Dr. Hirsch says.

The 11 Habits of Highly Effective Sleepers

The things you do or don't do—as well as the things you eat or drink—can add up to shut-eye problems before you realize it. Exercise, caffeine, alcohol, and cigarettes all jiggle your sleep systems. Here is what you can do about them.

Schedule those zzzs. Go to bed at the same time every night—and get up at the same time every morning, say sleep therapists. "You can train the body to go to sleep at a particular time," says Dr. Cartwright. "But if you screw around with that time—2 hours later here, 2 hours earlier there—your body doesn't know when to go to sleep. The more regular the pattern, the more solid the sleep."

Even if you do wind up blowing your bedtime, don't change the setting on your alarm. You can handle an occasional midnight fling. Just don't sleep in, sleep specialists agree.

Sleeping through the bright light of morning jars your body clock even more than lying awake in the darkness. So if you really must steal an hour, take one from night, not day. Otherwise, you'll find yourself going to bed later and later and wanting to snooze the morning away, says Dr. Mitchell.

Move for a better snooze. "Exercise is absolutely the best thing you can do for good sleep," says Dr. Mitchell. "Exercise actually burns off adrenaline, the biochemical that keeps us ready for fight-or-flight and that ups our anxiety level."

A study done at Duke University Medical Center in Durham, North Carolina, supports Dr. Mitchell's assertion. Researchers there looked at 24 men to compare their sleep patterns. Half of those men were sedentary types. The other half were fit walkers, joggers, and swimmers who had exercised vigorously at least three times a week for a year or more. During the study, both groups either exercised for 40 minutes or did no exercise.

It took the sedentary group an average of 27 minutes to fall asleep—but it took the active men an average of only 12 minutes. The inactive men also spent more time awake during the night. And the fit group slept better even on the days when they didn't exercise. So aim for at least a four-day-a-week exercise program. Twenty to 30 aerobic minutes is a good target to shoot for, most experts say.

Check the medicine cabinet. Most poor sleepers know that too much caffeine will disturb sleep. You probably know some of the things that are loaded with caffeine, such as coffee, tea, and cola.

But caffeine is also added to many of the drugs we use, both over-the-counter and prescription ones. Check product labels or prescription package inserts to find out whether caffeine is one ingredient. Other ingredients in drugs can also disturb sleep, says Dr. Mitchell. Watch out for nasal decongestants that contain ephedrine, pseudoephedrine (Actifed, Tylenol, Sudafed), or phenylpropanolamine (Dimetapp); and for bronchodilators—drugs that open up the air passages of the lungs—containing theophylline (such as Quibron or Theophylline) or beta agonists (such as albuterol, found in Proventil or Ventolin).

Antidepressants, weight-reduction drugs (such as phentermine, found in products like Adipex-P or Fastin), thyroid replacement therapy, and methylphenidate (Ritalin), a drug used to treat hyperactivity in children, can also cause sleepless nights.

If you're unsure whether a medicine you're taking could upset your sleep, ask your pharmacist or doctor, Dr. Hauri advises. Even the very drugs given to induce sleep can ultimately disturb it, which is one reason to avoid any kind of sleeping pills, if possible.

Skip the drink. Sure, a glass of wine at bedtime makes you sleepy. But you'll probably pay for it later when you wake up at 1:00 A.M. That's how alcohol works. First it's a depressant; then 3 to 5 hours after you stop drinking, it leaves the body in withdrawal, and you become more alert. In other words, it wakes you up.

Alcohol has a worse effect on sleep than caffeine does, according to Merrill Mitler, Ph.D., director of research for sleep medicine at the Scripps Clinic and Research Foundation in La Jolla, California. "Alcohol is a terrible sleep disrupter—particularly in people over the age of 30."

Calculate Your Sleep Quota

Maybe you're tired because you've cut corners on sleep time and now you can't make up for lost snoozing. You go to bed late, and you get up too early. But how much sleep do you need, anyway?

"Sleep is highly malleable," says Peter Hauri, Ph.D., co-director of the Sleep Disorders Center and director of its insomnia program at the Mayo Clinic in Rochester, Minnesota, and author of *No More Sleepless Nights*. "Everybody needs a different amount. There's no use talking about averages."

The range of sleep needs is wide, experts say, from 4 hours up to 10. While most of us do need at least 8 hours or so, we often make do with about an hour less than we need. "You've slept enough if you're not tired during the day and if you can watch TV at night or go out to a movie without falling asleep," says Dr. Hauri.

Falling asleep at the drop of a hat does not mean that you're a good sleeper. It means that you're sleep-deprived. And many sleep experts say that use of an alarm clock is proof of that deprivation. A well-rested person wakes up naturally, without the need for that jolt.

If you're tired of being tired, you can figure out how much sleep you need. Start by systematically adding a small amount of sleep to your schedule. "Go to bed $^1/_2$ hour earlier each night for a week. Then, if you're waking up spontaneously and maintaining your alertness throughout the day, that extra $^1/_2$ hour is what you need," says Timothy Roehrs, Ph.D., director of research at the Sleep Disorders and Research Center of Henry Ford Hospital in Detroit.

Add the sleep at the beginning of the night, not in the morning, he suggests. That way, you won't throw off your natural body-clock rhythms. If you're still waking to the alarm clock and falling asleep in your armchair, add another $^1/_2$ hour in the same manner.

Most sleep experts caution against drinking anything more than a glass of wine or beer early in the evening. Some experts caution against any at all for the poor sleeper. It's an individual thing, says Dr. Hauri. Know your limits. If you sleep poorly after a glass of wine, consider that before you decide to indulge.

Bag the butts. Here's one more reason not to smoke. The average smoker snoozes 30 minutes less than a nonsmoker, according to a series on sleep that was published by the *British Medical Journal*. That's because nicotine is a stimulant. It raises your blood pressure, works your heart faster, and speeds up your brain waves. And heavy smokers sometimes wake up during the night craving a cigarette.

Sleep soundly with your spouse. Admittedly, this isn't always easy. If snoring keeps you awake, offer the offender a wedge-shaped pillow. Frequently, just the change of pillow puts an end to snoring problems. If your spouse's tossing and turning bothers you, invest in a king-size bed or twin beds. Or you can "sleep separately but be united during the day," advises Dr. Hauri.

Quiet restless legs. One strange but not-so-uncommon medical condition, restless legs, can cause sleep problems. If you or your spouse has this problem, be sure to tell your doctor. Sometimes it can be treated with small doses of the prescription medicine L-dopa, a drug used to treat Parkinson's disease, says Dr. Hirsch.

Customize the temperature. Too warm is just as bad as too cold. If you like it warm while your partner likes it cool—or vice versa—get an electric blanket with separate heating controls, one for each side. Or let the chilly party have an additional blanket on just that side of the bed.

Darken the room. Biologically, "you really need not to have light at night," says Dr. Cartwright. To block light, use a sleeping mask. But make sure that you try it before you buy it to see if the band holding it to your head is comfortable and if it fits well.

Good-quality lined drapes will keep the light out of your room. So before you buy your next set of drapes, first ask about their room-darkening capacity. Pull-down shades come in room-darkening versions, too. Just make sure that the tube they come in has the words "room darkening" on it.

Hush noise. If you choose lined drapes to darken your bedroom, the extra thickness of the lining will also help to absorb noise. Wall-to-wall carpeting serves the same purpose. You can also try putting a damper on obnoxious sound—from traffic to snoring spouses—with silicone or foam earplugs.

Fans or air conditioners can be used to mask noise, says Dr. Mitchell. Or, try white noise. Get it by setting your radio dial to the hum at the end of the radio band or by buying a white noise generator, available at electronics stores or bedding stores.

Find the optimal position. If you have a bad back, sleep on your side with or without a pillow between your knees. If you get heartburn, sleep with your head elevated. You can do that by placing 6-inch blocks under the head of your bed. Or, if you sleep with someone, you can elevate yourself by using a wedge-shaped pillow.

If you snore, sleeping on your side or stomach may help you. Snoring occurs because the muscles in your throat naturally relax during sleep. When you're on your back, this fleshy tissue partially blocks your airway and vibrates, says Dr. Roehrs. Other contributing factors for snoring are alcohol and sleep deprivation.

Feeling sleepy already? With this bag of sleeping tricks, you'll soon find yourself refreshed and ready to greet the dawn with new energy.

part four

Maximum Nutrition for Busy Women

the Hormone Connection

Think of it as new cuisine for a new stage of life. Even before menopause arrives, it's time to start building a new food pyramid that will energize and protect you through this new phase of life, says JoAnn Hattner, R.D., a clinical dietitian and nutritionist at the Stanford University Medical Center and a spokesperson for the American Dietetic Association.

Your body's need for calories and some nutrients, such as iron, will decline at this time, as your menstrual bleeding stops. Yet your need for other nutrients will be greater in order to boost protection against heart disease, cancer, and osteoporosis. For example, you've probably already guessed that it's time to start proudly wearing your milk mustache again (or diving into other rich sources of calcium) to combat the dramatic bone loss that accompanies the drop-off in estrogen levels at menopause. Calcium-rich foods include broccoli, shellfish, almonds, canned salmon with the bones as well as fortified orange juice. At menopause, aim for 1,500 milligrams a day, says Hattner. Your other dietary needs are also fluctuating, she notes. Here's how she suggests meeting them.

Enjoy soy. Soybeans, soy milk, and tofu contain natural plant estrogens called isoflavones that may combat menopause symptoms, lower your cholesterol, and work with calcium to fight osteoporosis.

Stress vitamin E. Find this good-for-your-heart nutrient in vegetable oil, wheat germ, green leafy vegetables, and whole grains.

Boost your veggies and fruits. Eat seven to nine servings of fruits and vegetables daily. The antioxidants in a plant-based diet protect you against cardiovascular disease and cancers of the colon and breast.

Pour a bowl of cereal. A high-fiber diet will protect you against colon cancer and also helps prevent constipation, an aggravating complaint of many menopausal women. Get 25 to 30 grams a day by starting off with a high-fiber cereal, eating your seven to nine servings of fruits and vegetables a day, and choosing whole-grain breads. Then munch on some pumpkin seeds, which have 4 grams of fiber per ounce) for an afternoon snack.

Iron out your iron needs. If you experience heavy menstrual bleeding as you approach menopause, you may need more iron. Iron-rich sources are liver, red meat, shellfish, nuts, and enriched grain products as well as cream of wheat or other iron-enriched cereal products, dried fruits, dried beans and peas, and even molasses.

Does Your Diet Pass the Nutrition Challenge?

I f only you could open wide, say "ah"...and get your diet checked! "The next time you come in," your doctor might say as he peered down your throat, "I want to see more carrots and not so many caramels down there!"

Then there's reality. More than half the time, diet—and by diet, we mean your daily food choices, *not* a weight-loss plan—isn't even mentioned by doctors in their examining rooms, according to a recent survey.

That's too bad. Sooner or later a careless diet puts out the welcome mat for heart attacks, stroke, cancer, diabetes...even blindness. A healthy diet, on the other hand, helps give all kinds of illnesses the slip. The optimum diet checkup is a complete diet analysis with a registered dietitian (R.D.). Ask your doctor to send you for a consultation with an R.D. Or make an appointment with one yourself. The American Dietetic Association's hotline is (800) 366-1655. (Note: Most health insurance doesn't cover R.D. counseling.)

Holly McCord, R.D., a dietitian and nutrition editor for *Prevention* magazine, designed this nutrition quiz. It should help you see where your diet may be off track so that you can make healthy course corrections. The way you answer each question generally reveals a whole pattern of dietary habits.

Your answers also uncover whether you're really trying to maintain the best diet or you just think you are. Even when we have the best intentions, we can fall short without realizing it. Just use what you learn as inspiration to make better choices in the future.

Open Up Some Canned Goodness

Don't assume that you're settling for second best every time you reach for a canned good for the sake of convenience. A University of Illinois analysis points out that canned fruits and vegetables often pack as much vitamin A or C as their fresh or frozen counterparts.

Intrigued? Grab the can opener—here are some surprising examples.

❖ Most canned carrots have the same amount of vitamin A as fresh, cooked carrots—more than 300 percent of the Daily Value (DV), the amount most adults need every day, per $1/2$ cup.

❖ A $1/2$ cup of canned pumpkin has over 250 percent of the DV for vitamin A—more than 10 times the vitamin A of fresh pumpkin that's been cooked and mashed.

❖ Canned pineapple has 20 percent of the DV for vitamin C per $1/2$ cup—just as much as if the fruit were fresh.

In fact, with canned pineapple on hand, you can sip a vitamin C–packed piña colada smoothie whenever the mood strikes. (We're thinking Sunday afternoon...you lounging on the patio with the paper...) For a 12-ounce shake: Open and partially thaw a frozen 8-ounce can of crushed pineapple packed in juice. In a blender or food processor, combine the pineapple with juice, $1/2$ cup plain nonfat yogurt, and $1/4$ teaspoon imitation coconut extract. Per serving: 200 calories, 24 milligrams vitamin C (40 percent of the DV), 200 milligrams calcium (20 percent of the DV), 2 grams fiber.

HEALTH FLASH

The Quiz

Add up your yes answers to the following questions to determine your personal Healthy Eating Score.

1. Do you usually leave a restaurant with doggie bag in hand?
   Yes___ No___

2. Does your breakfast cereal have at least 5 grams of fiber per serving? (If you don't know, if you don't eat cereal, or if your cereal box has cobwebs, answer no.)
   Yes___ No___

3. Have you taken a calcium supplement in the last 24 hours?

Yes___ No___

4. If you got an invitation to a "Come as You Were at Your Senior Prom" party, could you knock 'em dead in the same dress you wore back then?

Yes___ No___

5. Do you do most of your eating before the six o'clock news comes on?

Yes___ No___

6. Do you know exactly how many servings of fruits and how many servings of vegetables you ate yesterday?

Yes___ No___

7. Have you taken a multivitamin/mineral supplement in the last 24 hours?

Yes___ No___

8. If you buy your favorite fat-free or low-fat cookies, chips, frozen yogurt, or ice cream to eat all by yourself, will there still be any left a week later?

Yes___ No___

9. Can you recite the number of grams of fat you're allowed to eat in one day without blowing your fat budget?

Yes___ No___

10. Do most of your meals and snacks come from your own kitchen as opposed to a restaurant, drive-up window, deli, food court, convenience store, or vending machine?

Yes___ No___

Your Healthy Eating Score (total number of yes answers): ___
What does your number mean? Here's the key.

9 to 10: Absolutely fabulous! Your body thanks you for feeding it so well.

6 to 8: Very impressive. A score this high means that you're trying hard and experiencing success. But why not try to shore up the few weak spots you do have?

3 to 5: It's a start. You do some things right, but there's still plenty of room for improvement.

0 to 2: Careless eating alert! It's time to make some changes in your diet.

A Closer Look at Your Eating Patterns

Now, let's see what your answer to each question, whether yes or no, reveals about the state of your nutritional health. If you're ready to transform each no to a yes, you'll find doable tips to get you started on your healthiest diet ever.

Question 1: Do You Practice Portion Control?

Are you a doggie bagger? If you said yes, congratulations. You're practicing the powerful secret of portion control. If you said no, chances are you're getting stuffed to the gills every time you eat in a restaurant. If that happens often, it's a problem.

We all love eating out. But most restaurant entrées could feed Bluto, Mrs. Bluto, and the four little Blutos. Confirmed doggie baggers, however, simply eat half or less of their full entrées and take the rest home in doggie bags. They avoid a huge hit of calories and fat (plus they have a microwave treat ready for later).

You know what else doggie bags say about you? If you keep portion sizes sane in restaurants, where people feel entitled to splurge, you most likely keep portion sizes sensible at home, too. Eating sensible quantities, at home and away, may be the surest way to keep weight in the healthy zone. Here's a better strategy for huge restaurant portions.

Make that doggie bag automatic. When you order, ask the waiter to serve only half of your entrée on your plate. Ask him to bring the other half in a take-home container at the end of the meal. What you don't see won't tempt you. (This works just as well with a humongous sandwich in a deli as with a filet mignon in a five-star palace.)

Or make it superfluous. Many restaurants already offer half-portions. Or they will let you split an entrée with a companion (ask the waiter to serve it on two plates). Or you can order an appetizer instead of an entrée.

Note: If you do this, change your answer for Question 1 to a yes.

Question 2: Are Your Mornings High-Fiber?

Does your cereal have at least 5 grams of fiber? A yes here says three good things about your diet. First, it says you eat breakfast. Studies show that breakfast eating gives you a lead in folic acid, calcium, vitamin A, vitamin C, iron, and fiber that breakfast-skippers never make up the rest of the day. Also, breakfast-eaters are less apt to be obese—maybe because they don't set themselves up to overeat later in the day out of hunger.

Second, if you know the grams of fiber you get from your cereal, that means you read food labels. In other words, you practice one of the healthy-eater's basic survival skills—checking what's in your food. Third, those 5-plus grams of fiber suggest that you're aware that more fiber may mean less colon cancer,

What a Difference a Dab Makes

Which is better for your heart, butter or margarine? One study indicates that the smarter choice for your heart is margarine—even if you eat a low-fat diet.

In New Zealand researchers gave 49 women and men with high cholesterol a diet with 26 percent calories from fat. Some of the people used about 1 tablespoon of butter per day, while others used the same amount of margarine. Both spreads contain fatty acids that raise blood cholesterol—butter has saturated fats, while margarine has trans-fatty acids. Researchers have debated which is better, or worse, for your heart.

After six weeks, both diets reduced total cholesterol and low-density lipoproteins (LDLs), the so-called "bad" cholesterol, a bit. No surprise there; a low-fat diet usually does improve cholesterol levels. But the margarine diet dropped cholesterol more. In fact, LDL dropped 10 percent more. It looks like a little margarine beats butter, even on a low-fat diet. Or better yet, use reduced-fat or fat-free spreads and sprays.

breast cancer, heart disease, and diverticular disease. We need a minimum of 25 grams of fiber daily. A fiber-rich breakfast cereal speeds you toward your goal. Get additional fiber with these techniques.

Say "later" to cereal. "Allergic" to breakfast? Then eat cereal later—for morning break or dinner or a satisfying bedtime snack. And check the label to get a brand with 5 grams of fiber or more per serving.

Build an on-the-go-wich. No time to eat before you dash to work? Buy whole-grain bread with 3 grams of fiber per slice. Make a sandwich from two slices spread with diet margarine and low-sugar jam. Eat it when you get to your desk or while you ride the bus or train to work.

Have beans every day. Every ½ cup provides 5 grams of fiber or more. In the summertime, what's a picnic without baked beans or three-bean salad?

Question 3: Are You Getting Enough Calcium?

Do you take a regular calcium supplement? If you said no, then you need a game plan to get the three to four servings of calcium-rich foods that you need every day (each serving providing at least 300 milligrams of calcium). Otherwise, your bones will pay for the days that your calcium intake is low.

If you said yes, you do take a calcium supplement, you're giving your bones a smart nutritional safety net. (But don't stop trying to get as much calcium as you possibly can from calcium-rich foods like milk.)

Protect your bones these easy ways.

Add a supplement. Many American women manage only a single glass of milk or a cup of yogurt each day. If that describes you and you're under the age of 50, a supplement with 500 milligrams of elemental calcium should bring your intake up to the recommended 1,000 milligrams. If you're 50 or over, you'll need two 500-milligram supplements, taken separately, to get you up to the recommended 1,500 milligrams.

Remember D. Make sure you get 400 international units (IU) a day of vitamin D to ensure calcium absorption. Your best bet is a multivitamin/mineral supplement with 400 IU of vitamin D. (Forget about supplements that contain only vitamin D; they make it too easy to get too much, which can be harmful.) Other sources include milk and some fortified breakfast cereals.

Pick up a bar. Look for a supplement in a bar—a Calcium Almond Blitz bar. Found in health food stores, these are yummy, 150-calorie treats with 1,200 milligrams of calcium and 2 grams of fat.

Question 4: What's Your Weight History?

Can you still wear your prom dress? Aside from the stir you'll create, what's so good about a yes to this question? Assuming you were a healthy weight in high school or college, the closer you stay to that weight as the years go by, the better your health. For 16 years a huge study followed U.S. nurses between 30 and 55 years of age. Those who stayed the slimmest over the years had the lowest risk of death from all causes, including heart disease and cancer.

If you've added some pounds over the years, take heart. The same study showed that losing weight also lowers risks of heart disease and cancer.

Check your BMI. To decide whether your weight is putting you at risk, find your body mass index (BMI). First, divide your weight (in pounds) by your height (in inches) squared. Multiply the resulting number by 705. (Or see "Calculate Your Body Mass Index" on page 219.) The answer, your BMI, will usually be between 19 and 30. Experts say a BMI over 25 is likely to increase risks to your health.

Work toward a healthy weight. If your BMI is over 25, pay special attention to the slimming tips in Questions 1, 2, 5, 6, 8, 9, and 10.

Question 5: Is Night Bingeing Your Style?

Do you eat the bulk of your calories before six o'clock? That makes you unusual. A study of American women's diets showed that the average woman eats almost half her daily calories at dinner and later.

Since evening snacks tend to be chips and cookies instead of fruits and vegetables, it's not surprising that the same study found women who eat more food after 5:00 P.M. get less vitamin C and vitamin B_6, less folic acid, and more fat. Weight-control experts theorize that saving most calories for later in the day may contribute to obesity by setting us up to binge. We feel entitled to a reward for starving ourselves during the daytime.

With these meal-scheduling ideas, even the busiest woman can eat at optimal times for weight control and better nutrition.

Think mini-meals. Spread out your food in mini-meals throughout the day. Eat cereal, milk, and fruit for breakfast; a bagel and juice for midmorning break; a salad and sandwich for lunch; soup for a midafternoon pick-me-up; pasta with vegetables for dinner; and a yogurt-and-fruit parfait for a bedtime treat.

Munch on nutritious fare. If you must nosh after dinner, chuck the empty-calorie stuff. A bean dip with baked tortilla chips provides fiber, folic acid, and magnesium. A baked potato with fat-free sour cream offers fiber, vitamin C, and potassium. Blend cantaloupe cubes with orange juice for a vitamin C, beta-carotene, and potassium smoothie.

Question 6: Do You Fit In Five a Day?

Do you count your fruits and veggies? Every day, we need a minimum of two servings of fruits and three servings of vegetables. Experts think this super-important strategy can cut our risk of cancer in half. How do you make sure you get five a day? It's simple. You count.

Not sure what counts as a serving? Use the following easy system.

Add up the tennis balls. A tennis-ball-size, or $1/2$ cup, portion of cooked vegetables, raw vegetables, or cut-up fruit each counts as one serving. Most pieces of whole fruit count as one serving, too. (Be reasonable. A tiny tangerine may count as a half-serving, a huge apple as $1^1/2$.)

The exceptions: For one serving of raw, leafy greens, you need two tennis balls. And for dried fruit, count a golf ball as one serving.

Question 7: What's Your Supplement IQ?

Do you take a regular multivitamin/mineral supplement? Of course, you should aim for the most nutritious food choices possible. But for insurance, cover potential shortfalls in your diet with a multivitamin/mineral supplement with close to 100 percent of the Daily Value (DV), the amount an average adult needs, for most vitamins and minerals.

In fact, the Centers for Disease Control and Prevention urges doctors to recommend to their patients multivitamin/mineral supplements that include the DV of 400 micrograms of folic acid. Studies show that getting 400 micrograms of folic acid daily prevents women from giving birth to babies with certain birth defects. Experts also suspect that diets high in folic acid help prevent heart disease in both women and men. You can get 400 micrograms from diet alone, but only if you're very determined.

Here's a supplement strategy that works.

Go for 100 percent. Get yourself a multi with close to 100 percent of the DV for most vitamins and minerals. Exception: Men and postmenopausal women should look for a multi with less iron (0 to 50 percent of the DV). After menopause, women need less iron because menstruation—and the loss of iron-rich blood—has ceased.

Get a separate calcium supplement. Don't count on a single-dose multi to cover your needs for calcium—they simply don't contain enough.

Don't adopt a junk-food diet. Taking supplements simply fills in the gaps—the best nutrition, including thousands of protective ingredients that researchers are only beginning to understand, are found only in good food.

Question 8: Are You a Fat-Free Fanatic?

Can you handle fat-free chips and sweets without bingeing? If you said yes, that's sensational. You're avoiding one of today's biggest mega-calorie temptations. Plenty of women who wouldn't dream of eating one serving of a high-fat snack or sweet can't resist scarfing a whole pack of fat-fat cookies, a whole box of low-fat crackers, a whole bag of fat-free chips, or a whole half-gallon of low-fat ice cream at one go. Eating like that, at up to 2,500 calories a pop, is an express train to obesity. Here are practical tips for handling the new fat-free treats.

Face the calories. After you take a reduced-fat treat home, take a minute to multiply the calories per serving by the servings per container. Many cookies and snacks run about 900 calories a box or bag. That means you add a quarter-pound of extra weight for every box you finish. If you know the consequences, it's harder to binge.

Create single servings. Buy snack-size resealable plastic bags. Divide snacks like cookies or chips into individual portions.

Go for pops. Switch from containers of yogurt or ice cream to fat-free ice pops. When one pop is gone, don't go for seconds.

Question 9: Have You Counted Your Fat Grams Lately?

Do you follow a fat-gram budget? A yes here is very important. It says you take low-fat eating—one of our major weapons against heart disease, cancer, and obesity—seriously enough. You would think that we should be able to go low-fat simply by choosing low-fat foods and low-fat cooking methods. Adding up grams of fat in everything we eat shouldn't be necessary...in theory. In the real world diets are complicated. It's helpful to check once in a while to make sure that you're truly keeping your fat intake low enough—not just hoping that you are. To do that, you need a fat budget. Here's how to figure out the best one for you.

1. Pick a weight that would be healthy for you. This may be your current weight or what you'd like to weigh someday.
2. Multiply this healthy weight by 12 if you're inactive, by 15 if you're active (you get 30 minutes to 1 hour of aerobic exercise three times a week), or

by 18 if you're very active. This gives you the level of calories you need to sustain yourself at a healthy weight.

3. Using the chart below, find the number of grams of fat that corresponds to your calorie level. By limiting fat to this amount, you'll keep calories from fat to 25 percent or less of your total calories, the healthy level many health experts recommend.

Calories	Fat (g.)
1,200	33
1,400	38
1,600	44
1,800	50
2,000	55
2,200	61
2,500	69
2,800	77

Question 10: Are You an At-Home Eater?

Do most of your meals and snacks come from your own kitchen? If you said yes, you're avoiding one of the worst threats to a healthy diet: eating out. Outside the house we face a gauntlet of Titanic Burgers at the drive-up window and Triple Chocolate Torpedo Cake at the diner.

Several years ago, nutritionists compared the healthiness of several different eating patterns. They found that women who got about half their food in restaurants (and another 10 percent from drive-up windows and cafeterias) consumed the fattiest diets. Women who got about a third of their food from fast-food drive-ups consumed the most calories. The healthiest diets were eaten by women who prepared about 70 percent of their meals at home. Out of many different groups, these women ate the diets lowest in fat and highest in fiber, folic acid, and vitamin C.

If your lifestyle dictates that you eat your meals away from home, the following tips can help you make healthier choices.

Order extra fruit and veggies. In restaurants make sure you order a side dish or two of vegetables. Order fruit as an appetizer, salad, or dessert. This helps to boost fiber, vitamins, and minerals.

Think small. At the drive-up window request the smallest burger they have, plain. Add ketchup and mustard, but skip the cheese and special sauce. Then stop at the nearest convenience store to buy some fresh fruit and a $\frac{1}{2}$ pint of nonfat milk to complete your meal.

Bring your own. Make your purse or briefcase a healthy "vending machine" that dispenses cans of low-sodium tomato juice, mini boxes of raisins, packs of whole-grain crackers...even Calcium Almond Blitz bars.

Don't Let Your Body Run Dry

I t was worse than feeling fuzzy. Robin, 42, was hazy and disoriented—as if the television and her husband's voice were a million miles away. For no reason she could imagine, she felt weaker than watered-down lemonade, and she wondered if she was going to be sick to her stomach.

That morning, she'd been fine. She took her usual 4-mile walk before the temperature had a chance to soar into the 100s, like it threatened to. She made it to her tooth-pulling appointment on time. Picked up the painkillers on the way home. And went downhill from there. When she tried to get out of bed the next morning, she hardly had the strength to roll over.

This funny feeling of weakness overcame Liz, 55, too. It was the third Olympic event she'd attended in three days. When she applauded the sprinters, she felt kind of surreal, like someone else's hands were doing the clapping. She's not the swooning type, but she started to feel dizzy. Cramps started clenching at her legs. She felt queasy and figured she should get up, but she hardly had the energy.

Robin and Liz, who asked us not to use their last names, are fit, smart, and healthy. What knocked them limp in the first round was something that they thought could never happen to them: dehydration. Fortunately, Robin's spouse and Liz's buddies recognized the fatigue, dizziness, cramps, and nausea as the danger signs of dehydration, and they got some water for their companions. If it's left untreated, however, dehydration can send body temperatures dangerously skyward. Dehydration can also create life-threatening heart-rhythm disturbances.

Cancer Protection from Your Faucet

HEALTH FLASH

Here's one more reason to sip a cool, clear glass of water today: A study suggests that water may lower women's risk of colon cancer.

Researchers at the Fred Hutchinson Cancer Research Center in Seattle examined data gathered from diet questionnaires completed by more than 400 middle-aged women and men with a history of colon cancer. When they compared the answers with those of a group of cancer-free people, they discovered a water link.

Among women who drank more than five glasses of plain water a day, there were fewer cases of colon cancer. In fact, their risk was about half of what it was for women who drank fewer than two glasses a day. The connection was less clear for men.

Scientists aren't sure exactly how water might provide this apparent benefit, but they offer several possibilities. Increased water intake could help prevent constipation and speed up the works in general. That might reduce the contact with, and concentrations of, carcinogens in the colon.

All the more reason to pour more water. Aim for at least eight 8-ounce glasses a day. Drink it with every meal and rehydrate in the midmorning and midafternoon. Keep a fresh pitcher in the fridge and a filled water bottle close by.

Dehydration: As Common in the Suburbs as in the Sahara

Like most Americans, Robin and Liz thought that dehydration was something that happened only to Olympic athletes, the elderly, and to sojourners lost in the desert. True, some people—those with diabetes or those on diuretics—are more likely to get dehydrated than others. But you can be perfectly healthy and still run dry. In fact, in some regards the less of an Olympian you are, the more likely you are to run dry. People who are more fit have a greater percentage of water in their blood. The water acts as a reserve to allow for extra sweating when needed.

What takes most healthy folks from "it won't happen to me" to "it did happen to me" is pretty obvious. Either you don't drink enough water or you lose too much. What's not so obvious is that it's often a combination of factors ganging up on you that dries you out.

For instance: The steam-bath temperatures alone weren't enough to leave healthy folks like Robin and Liz dry. In Robin's case, a sweaty walk plus not drinking water because of her tooth extraction equaled trouble. For Liz, two days of extra sweating, plus cheering for the hopefuls, plus a little holding back on fluids (bathroom lines, you know) added up to a visit to the first-aid station.

Part of the dehydration problem is that most people's fluid stores aren't terribly well stocked in the first place. People care for their lawns' water needs better than they care for their own bodies' needs. Experts suspect that few people actually drink the recommended eight 8-ounce glasses of water in a day. Which may leave less room for error when any dehydrating events come along.

Drink Up: Heeding Nature's Call

Most of the time, the thirst mechanism keeps a normal person from teetering close to the rim of dehydration. The hypothalamus in the brain notices when the blood has an increase in sugar or salt—a sign that the water level is getting too low. It sends out an all-points bulletin to the thirst mechanism, which in turn sends that person running to the water cooler.

As you age, however, the mechanism becomes a little less sensitive. The kidneys lose some function, too, and may let more water go through than they used to, leaving less for your body to use. Not only do you miss Mother Nature's call to drink something, but the amount that you need to drink may be even more than you realize.

Even when the thirst mechanism is intact, people don't always heed it. "I've seen athletes suffer because they're preoccupied with the event that they're competing in, they're some distance from water, or they're just unwilling to stop training or interrupt competition to rehydrate," says Lawrence E. Armstrong, Ph.D., an exercise and environmental physiology professor at the University of Connecticut in Storrs.

Symptoms such as dizziness kick in when you've lost as little as 4 to 7 percent of your body weight in water (although some older or less-fit folks may feel them sooner). Smaller losses, from 2 to 4 percent, probably won't send you to the hospital, but they may affect the way you do a day's work. One small study of bicyclists saw performance dip at water losses as little as 1.8 percent. That kind of water loss could happen in as little as an hour or two of walking in the heat.

What's so dangerous about this drought condition in your body is that it first draws the water it needs from your bloodstream. With less blood (and more-concentrated, "sludgy" blood, at that), the heart has to work harder to pump blood to the points it sees as most important: the heart, head, and kidneys.

So starts the downward cascade. "Your body also redirects blood from the places where it doesn't need to go," says Paul D. Thompson, M.D., director of preventive cardiology at the University of Pittsburgh Medical Center. One of the places that the body kind of gives up on is the skin. And that's a major problem because the skin is your radiator. Blood carries heat away from the engine—your muscles—and delivers it to your skin, where it dissipates. But if blood is diverted away from your skin, you can't get heat away from the engine, and everything breaks down. In extreme situations muscle breaks down and releases the potassium that can cause an irregular heartbeat.

But all of these problems can be stopped before they start by paying attention to both sides of the equation. You have to know how to meet your body's daily quota for H_2O (not always so easy), and you have to be able to deal with those sneaky situations that can zap amazing amounts of water right out of you.

The Well-Watered Body

You don't have to feel like you've swallowed the Gulf of Mexico in order to be well-watered. Just get a grip on how small the requirement really is. Your daily requirement is 64 ounces. That's only the amount in three 20-ounce soda bottles, plus one good drink from the water fountain. (Experts estimate an ounce per slurp, so four sips should do it.) Most tall drinking glasses hold at least 12 ounces. Five refills and you're done.

If you don't feel like keeping score of how many refills you've had, fill a pitcher with all the water you need in a day, keep it in your refrigerator, and always refill your glass from that. Some people make water drinking pleasurable for themselves by drinking it out of Grandma's crystal or from another cup they like.

If you'll be out all day in hot weather, fill a plastic bottle with water and tuck it in the freezer the night before. Cool water all day doesn't only feel great on your tongue, it also gets absorbed into the body faster than water at air temperature does.

Embellish the water with lemon slices if taste is your barrier. Buy flavored seltzer water if you like a bubbly treat or try adding flavor to plain seltzer with cranberry juice, peach nectar, or whatever kind of juice you like. Juices and flavored waters count ounce-for-ounce toward your daily water totals. Milk is 90 percent water, so you can count most of it toward your daily total.

The only things you can't count one-for-one toward your totals are beverages containing caffeine and alcohol, as these compounds are diuretics. Count 3 cups of coffee as only 2 cups of fluid. Alcohol doesn't even count at all. It can actually suppress an antidiuretic hormone in your body. So for every alcoholic drink you have, whether it's wine, beer, or liquor, have an extra glass of water.

You can also help the fluid cause a little by putting smart choices on your plate. A juicy slice of watermelon (92 percent water) can help your hydration along better than a handful of pretzels can (5 percent water). But you really

Filling Your Water Deficit

Eight 8-ounce glasses of water is the daily requirement for your basic desk jockey. But if you're going to be doing anything else, your requirement goes up. How much it goes up depends on your weight, your gender, the outdoor temperature and humidity, how fit you are, and how intensely you're working.

But based on a 135-pound woman who walks for 30 minutes every day, here's about how much extra water she needs in these basic situations.

Activity	Extra Glasses Needed (8 oz.)
Flight from New York to Los Angeles, 5 hours of flying time	4–5
Sitting at an afternoon baseball game, air temperature 90°F, for 3 hours	$2^1/_2$–5
Swimming in a pool, water temperature 68°F, for 1 hour	$^1/_2$–2
Walking indoors on a treadmill, air temperature 72°F, for 1 hour	$1^1/_2$–$2^1/_2$
Walking outdoors, air temperature 90°F, for 1 hour	2–$3^1/_2$
Hiking in rolling hills, air temperature 70°F, for 4 hours	10–14
Hiking in rolling hills, air temperature 90°F, for 4 hours	13–16
Running at 6 miles per hour, air temperature 90°F, for 1 hour	5
Playing tennis, air temperature 70°F, for 1 hour	2–10
Sleeping late, for $2^1/_2$ hours	$^1/_2$

can't expect to get more than 35 percent of your daily requirement of water from various food sources. After all, it's easier to drink 16 ounces of water than it is to eat a pound of watermelon or 20 pounds of pretzels.

If you've lost count of the glasses of water you've had, you can also tell that you're well-hydrated when your urine is pale yellow or clear. Most well-watered folks also visit the restroom once every 2 to 3 hours.

Compensate for Sweat

The 64-ounce recommendation is all well and good when you're sitting at your desk all day. "But that reasonable guideline goes to pieces really fast when you become active," says E. Wayne Askew, Ph.D., director of the division of foods and nutrition at the University of Utah in Salt Lake City. Dr. Askew's research with Army personnel at the U.S. Army Research Institute of Environmental Medicine in Natick, Massachusetts, helped keep Desert Storm troops hydrated. And he knows this: The more you move around, the more water you require. If you're doing a 3-hour marathon, for instance, the amount of water lost from your body can rise from the recommended 64 ounces to about 104 ounces. That's 13 of those 8-ounce glasses.

And whatever you're doing, water loss increases if you're in a warm environment. Case in point: Hoover Dam builders were "dropping like flies" from dehydration until their sleeping quarters were air-conditioned, says Dr. Thompson. That saved those workers from sweating profusely for at least a portion of the day.

The clearest way to know how much water to replace when you exercise is to weigh yourself before and after your workout, says Phillip B. Sparling, Ed.D., professor of exercise physiology at Georgia Institute of Technology in Atlanta and a member of the Heat Stress Task Force for the 1996 Olympic Games. Replace every pound you've lost by drinking 16 ounces of fluid.

Better yet, hydrate before you go to the gym. Drink 8 to 16 ounces at least an hour before you head off to exercise. While exercising at 50 to 70 percent of your maximum heart rate, you need 20 to 40 ounces ($2^1/_2$ to 5 glasses) per hour, which is 4 to 8 ounces every 15 minutes.

If you are on medications, consult with your doctor on your water needs. Being on diuretics, for instance, doesn't always mean that you need more water. Some people with congestive heart failure may actually be harmed by dousing themselves with too much extra water. Other dry-prone people, such as diabetics, should just be sure to take regular water breaks.

Forget about Salt Pills

When you sweat, you lose sodium as well as water. Sodium is important because it helps maintain the right balance of fluid between the blood and cells of muscles and organs. Sodium is so important to body functions, in fact, that the body learns to hold onto it.

In the first few days of exercise in a hot climate, you lose more sodium than you'll lose when you're acclimated to the heat, 8 to 10 days later. Nonetheless, first hot day or last, you don't need to fill up with extra sodium. Despite what anyone's told you, salt pills are "a terrible idea," says Felicia Busch, R.D., spokesperson for the American Dietetic Association and registered dietitian in St. Paul, Minnesota.

Too much sodium can accelerate dehydration. Your body needs more water to get rid of the extra sodium. Plus, says Dr. Thompson, "You don't need salt pills because your body is extremely good at holding onto sodium, so it can regulate itself as long as you're not on medication," he says.

Do You Need a Sports Drink?

Water is your best after-sport choice, unless you've been going really long or really strong. Intense exercise, that is, working at 70 percent or more of your maximum heart rate for more than an hour, depletes your carbohydrate stores, which sports drinks can partially replenish. The rest can be replaced by increasing your intake of carbohydrates over the next 24 hours. If carbohydrate stores are left bare, the result will feel like fatigue.

These stores also get sold out during long-term exercise. So if you're likely to be hiking for 2 to 4 hours or more, sports drinks might be smart. Your daily lunchtime walk, however, should require only water afterward. A study by Dr. Armstrong suggests that 90 minutes of walking at 36 percent of maximum heart rate didn't deplete carbohydrate stores in the muscle.

That said, sports drinks do have a place in keeping you from dying of thirst. Their best asset is that the sugar and salt in them help their water content get absorbed into the intestines, and thus the rest of the body, faster than plain water does. This makes them good candidates for rehydrating the person who's started to feel dizzy, nauseous, crampy, or fatigued.

Would sugared sodas work just as well? Not really. Sports drinks are about 8 percent carbohydrates. When carbohydrate concentrations get very high—as they are in sodas and fruit juices—gastric emptying actually slows down. This means that it takes longer for the fluid to get to the parts of your body that need it.

But if you like the taste of sports drinks, serve 'em up as you like 'em. Staying away from drought damage simply means water as you like it. And if you do stay well-watered, you'll at least be treating yourself better than you treat your lawn.

Supplemental Insurance, from A to Zinc

Nobody's perfect. You aim for a superhealthy diet, but on occasion you work right through lunch...or grab fast food before the movie...or indulge in frozen chocolate yogurt instead of dinner. It happens.

And even when you try your best, you may come up a little short on nutrition. In one study when registered dietitians planned some daily menus, they found it was tough to get recommended levels of every essential mineral and vitamin in less than 2,200 calories. That's why a multivitamin/mineral supplement makes sense.

But which one? Walk down the vitamin aisle of any drugstore, and you'll see that it's a supplement jungle out there. Gazillions of vitamin and mineral products loom at you from the shelves. So how do you find the best one without a Ph.D. in nutrition and a spare weekend? Help is here.

To help you select a multivitamin/mineral supplement, nutrition pros offer this "Test for the Best"—a quick checklist that lets you evaluate multivitamins in no time. Plus, you'll find out which two vitamins and one mineral that nutrition experts suggest you take as single supplements—and why.

If you already take a multi, get it out and see if it makes the grade. If it flunks, you'll know exactly how to find a new one that rates A-plus.

Test for the Best

Picking a great complete multivitamin is easy—we've whittled down more than 25 essential vitamins and minerals to only nine key nutrients that you

Coming soon to a supermarket near you...white bread, pasta, and rice—now fortified with folate. Getting enough—400 micrograms a day—is so important for women of childbearing age that the federal government has now decided to require that folate, or folic acid, as the supplement is called, be added to certain grain foods. By law, white rice and all foods that are made from refined flour or cornmeal and that are enriched with B vitamins and iron must also be enriched with folate by January 1998.

Why is folate so crucial? Studies prove that supplements of 400 micrograms of folic acid help prevent neural-tube birth defects such as spina bifida. These defects occur in developing fetuses before most women know that they are pregnant, so getting enough folate prior to conception is important. Also, diets low in folate are linked to heart disease. And our diets are low: American women typically get about 195 micrograms a day, half of what we need.

How much folic acid will enriched foods deliver? An average slice of white bread, half a hamburger roll, or a small dinner roll: about 40 micrograms. A $1/2$-cup serving of white pasta, noodles, or rice: about 60 micrograms. Whole-wheat products and brown rice will not be enriched with folic acid, but they're still worth eating for the fiber and for minerals such as magnesium and zinc that are lost when white flour and rice are refined.

need to zero in on. Why these nine? They're the ones that experts said were most likely to be lacking in American diets...and to be present in multis in amounts likely to be effective.

Don't be fooled just because a product calls itself a multi or says it's complete. If you check, you may be surprised to find that some multis contain vitamins only, or have just a few vitamins and minerals. But the more of the following nine nutrients a multi contains in levels close to experts' recommendations, the more complete it is.

Iron

This should be the first item you check for when choosing a multi, since the amount you need differs depending on your age and gender. Find a multi with the iron level you want before you check for other nutrients.

How much do you need? Premenopausal women should look for up to 18 milligrams, which is 100 percent of the Daily Value (DV). Menopausal women should look for 0 to 9 milligrams, 0 to 50 percent of the DV.

One note of caution about iron. Premenopausal women lose iron each month through menstrual bleeding, and they may need the help of a supplement to replace it. But women not having periods lose little iron normally. And since some research indicates that excess iron raises the risks of heart disease and colon cancer, many experts now advise menopausal women to look for supplements with no or low iron. Also, check your breakfast cereal; some cereals are heavily fortified with iron. Take that into account when you select a multi.

Be aware that unless you're diagnosed with iron-deficiency anemia, there's no reason to take levels above 100 percent of the DV. In fact, for women with a genetic condition called hemochromatosis, iron overload can actually be toxic.

Vitamin A/Beta-carotene

How much do you need? Look for a multi with 5,000 international units (IU), which is 100 percent of the DV. In most multivitamins, the vitamin A is a mix of preformed vitamin A and beta-carotene, a substance that is converted into vitamin A in the body. Not all multis tell you how much of the supplement comes from each. But even if a multi is all preformed vitamin A or all beta-carotene, 5,000 IU is considered a very safe level of either one.

Don't take preformed vitamin A supplements of more than 10,000 IU because more than 15,000 IU can be toxic. Pregnant women should not take more than 5,000 IU because too much vitamin A can cause birth defects.

It may also be possible to get too much beta-carotene. Studies show that people with diets high in beta-carotene have lower risks of heart disease and cancer. But in two studies of long-term smokers, those taking high-dose beta-carotene supplements (25 milligrams or more) developed more lung cancer. Until we know more, a reasonable limit of beta-carotene from supplements (not food) is 6 milligrams.

Vitamin D

How much do you need? Look for 400 IU (100 percent of the DV).

Our bodies can manufacture vitamin D from the action of sunlight on the skin, but experts believe that many people, especially the elderly and those who routinely use sunblock, may not be exposed to enough sun.

Don't get more than 600 IU of vitamin D a day from supplements plus fortified foods on a regular basis. Be sure to count the vitamin D that you get from milk (100 IU per 8 ounce glass of milk or per $\frac{1}{3}$ cup nonfat milk powder) or fortified breakfast cereal (amounts vary).

Vitamin B$_6$

How much do you need? Look for 2 milligrams (100 percent of the DV). American women's diets appear to be routinely low in B$_6$, and for some women, oral contraceptives may increase the need for supplements. Low intakes are linked to higher levels of heart attack risk and poorer immune functioning.

Don't overdo B$_6$ (or any other vitamin or mineral, for that matter). Megadoses of 100 milligrams are associated with reversible nerve damage, and problems have been seen at intakes of 50 milligrams. Reports of high doses of vitamin B$_6$ relieving carpal tunnel syndrome or premenstrual syndrome have not been confirmed by research.

Folic Acid

How much do you need? Look for 400 micrograms, which is 100 percent of the DV. This amount may be listed as 0.4 milligram, which is the same as 400 micrograms. Higher amounts of folic acid can be toxic.

Studies prove that women taking supplements with 400 micrograms of folic acid prior to becoming pregnant and in the first weeks of pregnancy reduce their risks of giving birth to babies with serious brain and spine defects. There's a strong indication that all people who have higher intakes of folic acid may reduce their risks of heart disease and colon cancer.

It's difficult to get 400 micrograms of folate (the form of folic acid that is found naturally in food) in your diet unless you choose several rich food sources every day. Most Americans' diets fall short. The U.S. Public Health Service, therefore, has urged doctors to tell patients about the benefits of supplements containing 400 micrograms of folic acid.

Magnesium

How much do you need? Look for 100 milligrams, 25 percent of the DV. That's the most you'll find in any single-dose multi because more would make a too-big-to-swallow pill. In a divided-dose multi, look for up to 400 milligrams, 100 percent of the DV, in the daily total.

This mineral has been tentatively linked to protection from diabetes, osteoporosis, atherosclerosis, hypertension, and migraine headaches, but Americans routinely get far less than 100 percent of the DV through food.

Excess magnesium can lead to diarrhea, as more than 400 milligrams can be toxic. People with abnormal kidney function should not supplement magne-

A Label Readers Guide to Supplements

Supplement labels include a lot of useful information—and some that's useless. Here's what you really need to know.

❖ *Expiration date.* Be sure to look for one. Don't buy a bottle containing more tablets than you can use before the product expires.

❖ *Ability to dissolve.* The letters USP (for the nongovernmental United States Pharmacopeia) on the label mean that the supplement should dissolve inside you. If you don't see USP, experts say stay with a major brand or major store brand. Is there a simple home test of dissolvability? For multis, experts say the answer is no.

❖ *Ability to be absorbed.* Experts say that there's no convincing evidence that the chemical form of supplements—such as minerals in "chelated" or "colloidal" form—makes much difference. One exception is if you want to get the most iron, look for ferrous fumarate or ferrous sulfate.

❖ *Natural versus synthetic.* It makes no difference which you choose. More expensive doesn't necessarily mean more effective.

❖ *Timed-release multis.* These are intended to keep blood levels of nutrients even over time. The trouble is that nutrients may not be fully released before the supplement leaves your digestive system, so you could miss out on important nutrients. Try divided-dose multis, which are two or more capsules taken at different times of the day.

sium without a doctor's supervision because magnesium overload could lead to nausea, vomiting, breathing problems, and even comas.

Zinc

How much do you need? Look for 15 milligrams, 100 percent of the DV.

Surveys show that this may be the mineral most lacking in Americans' diets. Zinc is necessary for a strong immune system and proper wound healing.

Don't take supplements with more than 15 milligrams a day on a regular basis. Too much zinc—in one study, 50 to 75 milligrams a day—can backfire and lower heart-helping high-density lipoprotein (HDL) cholesterol.

Copper

How much do you need? Look for 2 milligrams, 100 percent of the DV.

Here's another mineral that runs low in the average diet. Copper plays a role in bone and heart health, blood sugar regulation, and iron use. Do not take more than 10 milligrams of copper a day, as it can be toxic at that amount.

If your supplement contains zinc, make sure that it has copper, too. Elevating zinc intake without taking in enough copper can suppress copper absorption.

Chromium

How much do you need? Look for 50 to 200 micrograms, a safe and adequate range set by the National Research Council. Research indicates that it may be difficult to get even the minimum amount of the chromium that we need from food. This important mineral helps the body handle blood sugar. Does extra chromium help with weight loss or building muscle? Most studies so far don't bear this out.

Supplement labels may not include a percentage of the DV for chromium. Instead, they may have an asterisk (*) that indicates "Daily Value not established." That was the case until 1996, when the Food and Drug Administration (FDA) set a DV for chromium of 120 micrograms. It may take time for the labels on some brands of supplements to catch up. Do not take chromium at levels above 200 micrograms a day, as it can be toxic.

Extras

What if other vitamins and minerals are present in a multi? Consider them nice to have, but not necessary. For information on calcium and vitamins C and E, see below. For most of the others, it's preferable if levels stay in the 100-percent-of-the-DV-or-lower range. (Exception: People over the age of 60 may want to take extra vitamin B_{12}—from 200 percent to 500 percent of the DV, or 1,200 to 3,000 milligrams—to make up for problems some have in absorbing vitamin B_{12} from food.)

Important Single Supplements

Wondering why we omitted three superimportant nutrients—vitamin C, vitamin E, and calcium—from the list of nutrients to look for in a multi? Because we think there's good reason to consider taking each one as a single supplement in amounts you won't find in the standard single-dose multi.

Calcium

How much do you need? Depending on the calcium in your diet, consider single supplements containing about 500 to 1,000 milligrams of this crucial bone protector. It surprises many women that single-dose multis are never "complete" with 100 percent of the DV for calcium (1,000 milligrams). In fact, that would be impossible—all that calcium would make a single tablet too big to swallow.

Some single-dose multis do have about 200 milligrams of calcium. But since surveys show that many people's diets lag well behind recommended levels, a separate calcium supplement is worth considering. For more information on calcium, a vital supplement for women, see chapter 28.

Vitamin C

How much do you need? Consider taking 200 to 500 milligrams of this antioxidant vitamin as a single supplement. (Antioxidants protect body tissues from breaking down, offering protection from heart disease, cancer, and other major health problems.) Otherwise, make sure that your multi has at least 60 milligrams, 100 percent of the DV.

A study last year at the National Institutes of Health (NIH) in Bethesda, Maryland, found that we need 200 milligrams of vitamin C to keep blood cells at 85 percent saturation with the vitamin. For 95 percent saturation, we need 400 to 500 milligrams.

People with diets high in vitamin C have lower rates of cancer and heart disease. Although we are far from having proof, some studies hint that vitamin C supplements may help lower the risk of cataracts as well as help those with diabetes.

Look for vitamin C supplements in 100-, 250-, or 500-milligram tablets. Or find chewable tablets (to protect tooth enamel, chew only one a day) or effervescent tablets or powder that dissolve in water. You may find 100 milligrams or more of vitamin C in some multis. Should you get a natural or a synthetic supplement? The truth is, your body doesn't know the difference between vitamin C from rose hips or from a laboratory.

Don't gulp all your C at one sitting. The best way to take it is to divide your dose in two; take half in the morning, half at night. The reason for this is that after 12 hours, your body returns to presaturation levels, no matter what amount of vitamin C you've taken.

Can you get 200 to 500 milligrams from food? It's possible if you eat a lot of vitamin C–rich fruits and vegetables. An 8-ounce glass of orange juice from concentrate, for example, has 100 milligrams. A cup of fresh strawberries has 85 milligrams. A 1/2 cup of cooked broccoli has 40 milligrams.

Although 1,000 milligrams of vitamin C yielded 100 percent saturation of blood cells in the NIH study, some research (but not all) suggests that taking that much vitamin C may increase the risk of kidney stones. The vitamin becomes toxic if more than 1,200 milligrams are taken per day.

Vitamin E

How much do you need? Consider taking 100 to 400 IU of this antioxidant vitamin. Most multis supply only about 30 IU (100 percent of the DV), much less than the levels that some research indicates may fight illness, especially heart disease. If you don't take extra vitamin E, make sure that your multi has at least 30 IU.

Among the best indicators that extra E may help fight heart disease is a British study of more than 2,000 men and women with narrowed coronary arteries. Participants took either 400 IU of vitamin E, 800 IU, or a placebo. After 18 months, all of the vitamin E recipients, regardless of dose, lowered their chances of having a nonfatal heart attack by 75 percent. Other research suggests (but doesn't prove) that extra E might reduce the risks of cataracts and some cancers and might help people with diabetes.

Look for vitamin E supplements in 100-, 200-, or 400-IU capsules. It's also available in chewable or liquid form. Though natural vitamin E is more active in the body than synthetic vitamin E, the difference in potency is taken into account in the IU. That means that 100 IU of synthetic vitamin E are as potent as 100 IU of natural vitamin E. Most research, by the way, uses synthetic vitamin E. To find out which type your supplement has, read the list of ingredients. Natural vitamin E is d-alpha-tocopherol; synthetic is dl-alpha-tocopherol.

Can you get 100 to 400 IU of vitamin E from food? You'd need 2 cups of corn oil, one of the best sources, to get 100 IU. But it's best to take E with a meal that contains at least a little fat, to help with absorption.

If you're on blood-thinning medication or if you're at risk for uncontrolled bleeding, talk with your doctor before taking vitamin E at these levels because it may interfere with blood clotting if you have a cut or wound. Vitamin E can be toxic for anyone who takes more than 600 IU per day.

Customize Your Calcium

Confused about calcium supplements? It's no wonder. At a midsize drugstore in Washington, D.C., 25 different calcium products line the shelves. And at a health food store there are 31 more—each somehow different from the others.

The number of different products isn't the only cause for consternation. Just read the fine print on the labels—what's not there is the information that you really need most: the form of the calcium and how much usable calcium is in each tablet.

Women ask a lot of questions about calcium. Do certain calcium supplements get absorbed better? Should supplements have extras like vitamin D? Will they make you constipated? Can you take too much? Getting good answers is crucial because getting enough calcium is vital for building and preserving strong bones. So we've compiled a guide to steer you successfully through the maze.

Do You Need a Supplement?

Frankly, unless you love milk, reaching recommended levels of calcium through diet alone takes careful planning. It can be done, but too often it isn't. According to government figures, the average calcium intake of almost all Amer-

Over-come the Calcium Follies

What do tofu, dried figs, and kale have in common? A mistaken identity as top calcium sources. The truth is, these superhealthy foods do not deliver big-time calcium in amounts that women would eat every day. But they show up all the time, right next to milk, on lists of high-calcium foods. Holly McCord, R.D., a dietitian and nutrition editor for *Prevention* magazine, took a whole gang of the worst offenders and computed how much you'd actually have to eat to get the same amount of calcium found in just one 8-ounce glass of milk. (Keep in mind that you need more than three times this much calcium every day.)

- ❖ Firm tofu. For many brands, you'd need a quart.
- ❖ Cooked kale. Are you up for 3 cups?
- ❖ Almonds. One whole cup would do you. The problem is, that would contain almost as much fat as a whole stick of margarine.
- ❖ Dried figs. You'd need 11 figs...but don't "fig out" too much. Eleven dried figs tally up 525 calories—more than a hot-fudge sundae.
- ❖ Frozen yogurt or ice cream. No calorie bargain here. You'd need $^3/_4$ pint of most brands. Even if you go nonfat, that's 300 to 500 calories.
- ❖ Canned salmon (if you eat the bones). Picture yourself eating almost a whole $7^1/_2$-ounce can.
- ❖ Cooked broccoli. Dish out 3 cups. Even for broccoli-lovers, that's a stretch.
- ❖ Brown sugar. You'd need more than $1^1/_2$ cups. Think of the calories.

For your bones' sake, take McCord's advice. Focus on the foods that *Prevention* calls Calcium Champs. To be a Calcium Champ, a food must be easy to eat every day and must deliver 300 milligrams of calcium or more per realistic serving. Calcium Champs are nonfat or low-fat milk, many nonfat or low-fat yogurts and cheeses, and calcium-enriched orange juice and soy milk. Get three to four servings of Champs every day, and you'll automatically hit that important calcium target.

HEALTH FLASH

ican adults—both men and women—fails to meet standards for healthy bones set by the National Institutes of Health (NIH) in Bethesda, Maryland. Women over the age of 50 average less than half the calcium that they need.

That's why many health experts recommend considering a calcium supplement. Research proves that calcium supplements can decrease the risks of bone loss and fractures due to osteoporosis and that getting too little calcium increases the risks. High-calcium diets are also linked to lower risks of heart disease, high blood pressure, and colon cancer.

We'd never suggest a calcium supplement in place of calcium-rich foods. The ideal approach always is meeting nutrient needs with a super diet. But in the real world, "some people are either unwilling or unable—often because of low-calorie diets—to eat enough high-calcium foods. For them, a supplement makes sense," says Barbara Levine, R.D., Ph.D., director of the Calcium Information Center in New York City. Moreover, medications prescribed to treat osteoporosis, such as hormone-replacement therapy (HRT), alendronate, and nasal calcitonin, were designed in conjunction with calcium supplements.

A recent review of research with HRT and nasal calcitonin found that simultaneously taking calcium supplements with these medications nearly tripled their bone-preserving effects.

Which One Is Best?

Once you've started looking for a calcium supplement, here's what you need to know about what's out there. First, here's a list of the most common types of supplements found in stores, along with what percentage of each is actually calcium.

Supplement	Calcium (%)
Calcium carbonate	40
Dicalcium phosphate	38
Bonemeal	31
Oyster shell	28
Dolomite	22
Calcium citrate	21
Calcium lactate	13
Calcium gluconate	9

Notice that calcium carbonate is 40 percent calcium, the highest proportion in any type of supplement. That means that supplements made from calcium carbonate deliver the most calcium per tablet, so you'll have fewer pills to swallow or tablets to chew. It also makes calcium carbonate supplements the least expensive, as a rule. It's for this reason that top osteoporosis specialist Robert Heaney, M.D., professor of medicine at Creighton University in Omaha, Nebraska, recommends trying calcium carbonate first, if you need a supplement.

Unfortunately, not all supplement labels make it easy to determine the source of the calcium, especially because there's no standard format. You may have to search. Some labels tell the source of calcium in big print on the front, others in tiny print on the back (sometimes under "Ingredients" or "Source").

What about the Extras?

You'll find that some supplements offer calcium alone. But many others offer combinations of calcium and other nutrients. Some combinations include vitamin D, a vitamin that helps you absorb calcium (though you don't need to take it simultaneously). Others may contain the minerals magnesium, zinc, copper, and/or manganese, all linked, in some research, to bone health.

Do you need the extras? If you take a complete multivitamin/mineral supplement, skip them. But make sure that your multi has 400 international units (IU) of vitamin D, 100 percent of the Daily Value (DV); 100 milligrams of magnesium, 25 percent of the DV; and 15 milligrams of zinc, 100 percent of the DV, all of which are lacking in many diets. If you don't take a multi, look for a calcium supplement that provides some vitamin D, magnesium, and zinc.

Beyond Pills

Do you have trouble swallowing pills? Besides tablets and capsules meant to be swallowed whole, supplements come as chewable tablets and as liquids.

You'll find chewable calcium carbonate tablets (such as Tums or Rolaids, also used as antacids for heartburn) and calcium citrate chewables. Flavors include peppermint, spearmint, fruit flavors, and malted milk. Chew them well (don't swallow them whole), and try to drink some water with them.

Try supplements in the forms of powders or tablets meant to be dissolved in water. Or try syrup or liquid in a bottle. Citrical Liquitab is a calcium citrate effervescent tablet that dissolves in cold water into a pleasant, bubbly, citrus-flavored drink.

With Meals or in Between?

You may wonder how much of the calcium you take is actually absorbed into your body and whether some forms of calcium are better absorbed than others. Amazingly, top calcium pros, including Dr. Heaney and Bess Dawson-Hughes, M.D., chief of the Calcium and Bone Mineral Metabolism Lab at Tufts University in Boston, say that there's little difference in absorption among sources of calcium as long as supplements are taken with food. So if you time your supplements to coincide with meals, the main thing to look for is whichever supplement supplies the most calcium for the least money—and that's often calcium carbonate.

Studies indicate that if supplements are taken on an empty stomach, calcium citrate is the best absorbed. This is especially true for people over the age of 60, though Dr. Heaney's research suggests that it applies to younger people, too.

The Easy Way to Calculate Your Calcium Needs

First, find your daily requirement, set by the National Institutes of Health in Bethesda, Maryland.

❖ Women up to 24 years old: 1,500 milligrams of calcium.
❖ Women 25 to 49 years old: 1,000 milligrams of calcium.
❖ Women 50 years and older: 1,500 milligrams of calcium.
❖ Women who are pregnant or nursing: 1,200 to 1,500 milligrams of calcium.

Using this number, there are two ways to tell whether and how much to supplement. There's a general rule-of-thumb recommendation used by some doctors (based on surveys of average calcium intakes): If your daily requirement is 1,000 milligrams, supplement with 500 milligrams; if your daily requirement is 1,500 milligrams, supplement with 1,000 milligrams.

To determine specific needs based on your diet, do the following:

1. Count up your daily servings of Calcium Champs—the foods that you eat every day that supply substantial calcium. The Calcium Champs that are most likely to be eaten daily (in single-serving amounts) are 8 ounces (1 cup) of nonfat or 1 percent milk, 8 ounces of nonfat or low-fat yogurt, 8 ounces of calcium-fortified orange juice, 8 ounces of nonfat or low-fat calcium-fortified soy or rice milk, two 1-ounce slices of nonfat or reduced-fat cheese.
2. After you've determined your daily servings, count 300 milligrams of calcium for each serving of Champs (or check the product labels—calcium contents can vary among brands).
3. To this number, add an estimated calcium total for all the other foods you eat throughout the day—generally, 200 milligrams.
4. If you take a multivitamin/mineral supplement, add to your total the milligrams of calcium contained in that. (Don't assume that a multi will cover your needs. Most multis have too little calcium to make up average shortfalls.)
5. Subtract the total of steps 2, 3, and 4 from your daily requirement. Anything higher than zero represents how many milligrams of calcium you are falling short of in a day. Always try to boost calcium with extra servings of Calcium Champs. But do make up any remaining needs with a supplement.

Note: One type of supplement often taken between meals is chewable calcium carbonate tablets. According to Dr. Heaney, however, even these are best absorbed if used at mealtime.

With food or between meals, for best absorption, don't take more than about 500 milligrams of calcium at one time, say experts.

Before a supplement can be absorbed, it has to dissolve. With chewables (especially if taken with enough fluid) and liquid supplements, dissolving is assured. As for capsules and tablets that you swallow whole, experts say most have improved since the 1980s, when tests showed that some weren't breaking apart in the body.

To increase the odds that a product will dissolve, look for the letters USP, standing for United States Pharmacopeia, a nongovernmental organization that has set quality standards for how well a calcium supplement dissolves. Or look for a major brand or major store brand, a possible predictor of quality control. To check how well your supplement dissolves, place a calcium supplement in white vinegar. Stir every 5 minutes for 30 minutes. By then, the supplement should be 75 percent dissolved.

Deciphering Label Lingo

It seems outrageous, but some labels on packages of calcium supplements make it difficult to find the most basic information, such as how much usable calcium you're getting per tablet. The following steps should help you decipher any label.

Step 1: Determine the milligrams of usable calcium. Ideally, but not often, the label will specifically say how much "elemental calcium" there is in the product. If it does, that's great. The elemental calcium is the same as usable calcium.

If the supplement's label doesn't use the words "elemental calcium," you can look for the milligrams of "calcium." But be very careful that you do not mistake calcium carbonate, calcium citrate, or anything else for just plain calcium. Otherwise, you can mistakenly think that a supplement has much more usable calcium than it really does.

Step 2: Determine how many tablets, capsules, wafers, or teaspoons you need to take to get the amount of usable calcium listed on the label. (Don't assume that you only need one tablet for this amount; we've seen up to six required.) Again, be careful; label format is anything but standardized.

More Answers to Calcium Questions

What about other concerns that women have about calcium supplements, the bone builders in bottles? Read on for answers.

Will calcium supplements make me constipated? Some women report symptoms of constipation, bloating, or gas when they take calcium carbonate sup-

Get Extra Calcium after Bed Rest

When you're back on your feet after a week or more of bed rest, top calcium pro Robert Heaney, M.D., professor of medicine at Creighton University in Omaha, Nebraska, recommends boosting your calcium intake to 2,000 milligrams a day for a period about seven times as long as the time you spent in bed.

Why? During bed rest, you lose bone. Fortunately, once you're up and putting weight on your skeleton, your body starts to put lost bone back. But only, says Dr. Heaney, if you provide it with the building material it needs—extra calcium. So, make calcium supplements and high-calcium foods part of every post-illness regimen, he advises.

But don't take this large quantity of calcium for any longer than the time that Dr. Heaney suggests. It can interfere with absorption of other key minerals and could lead to additional health problems.

plements. Research fails to verify that calcium carbonate actually causes these symptoms, according to Dr. Dawson-Hughes, but she suggests that you switch to a different type of calcium supplement if you experience these side effects.

What about lead content? A 1993 study found that "natural" supplements made from oyster shells, dolomite (a natural mineral containing both calcium and magnesium), and especially bonemeal contained levels of lead that greatly exceeded the lead in a quantity of milk supplying an equal amount of calcium. At present, most experts consider these levels unwise only for children. Nevertheless, for adults who want to keep lead intake as low as possible, a non-"natural" calcium supplement is the best choice, especially since no advantage to taking "natural" calcium supplements has been demonstrated.

Be aware that sometimes oyster shell calcium is identified only as "natural" calcium carbonate, and the words "oyster shell" do not appear on the label. If a calcium carbonate product doesn't say "natural" or "oyster shell," however, it has been made from limestone refined in a laboratory. Refined calcium carbonate products have low levels of lead similar to milk.

Can I get too much calcium? According to the NIH, a regular calcium intake of up to 2,000 milligrams per day is safe. But there's no reason to supplement with more than 1,500 milligrams unless your doctor prescribes it, says Dr. Heaney. Going overboard could make it difficult for your body to eliminate calcium it doesn't need. Calcium can also be toxic if you take more than 2,000 milligrams per day.

I don't have any need for an antacid—my stomach is fine. Will it hurt to take calcium in the form of antacid calcium carbonate chewable tablets? No. They're no different from any other form of calcium carbonate supplements.

Is bedtime a good time for me to take a calcium supplement? Yes, because this may help keep blood levels of calcium high enough overnight to stop calcium from being pulled out of bones.

What foods or drugs don't mix with calcium supplements? The only food that seems to impair calcium absorption significantly is wheat bran. Avoid taking a supplement with ultrahigh-wheat-bran cereals. If other foods impair calcium absorption, the effect is so insignificant that you don't need to worry.

Ideally, take calcium supplements separately from multis because the absorption of iron and zinc can be impaired. Calcium supplements also impair the absorption of certain drugs, such as the antibiotic tetracycline. When you have a prescription filled, ask the pharmacist about the effects of calcium.

Do calcium supplements increase the risk of kidney stones? Diets high in calcium from food appear to be linked in studies to lower risks of kidney stones. But at least one major study suggests that calcium supplements taken between meals are linked to a higher risk. If you're being treated for kidney stones and simply can't get the calcium you need from your diet, check with your doctor. She may give the okay to supplements taken with meals, based on urine tests for calcium and oxalate, a substance that, at high levels, promotes the formation of kidney stones.

29

Chocolate Milk Shakes for Menopause

W hen I was younger, I suspected that older women were exaggerating how miserable hot flashes make you feel. Not anymore."

"The first few times, I kept checking. Wasn't anybody else in the office burning up except me?"

"If it happens in bed, I have to tear all my covers off immediately or I go crazy!"

If you identify with these tales of discomfort, chances are you're in the throes of hot flashes and night sweats, like these women. About 75 percent of American women endure fiery episodes of "internal combustion," along with sleep disturbances and mood swings, as menopause closes in. In some cases these symptoms can begin years before, and continue for years beyond, women's last periods.

Until now, the only antidote to hot flashes has been hormone-replacement therapy (HRT), medications prescribed to replace the estrogen and other hormones that our bodies start making less of. But this may change. Researchers at two leading American universities are serving up something else in hopes of relieving hot flashes: foods made from the simple soybean. These foods range from delicious stir-fries to puddings to, yes, thick-and-creamy chocolate milk shakes.

The Asian Connection

The trail of evidence linking soy with a hot-flash-free menopause starts in Asia. There, women in the menopausal years rarely, it seems, suffer hot flashes or sleep disturbances. In fact, there isn't even a word for hot flash in the Japanese language.

Among the first to suggest that diet may be the reason that Asian women don't experience the unpleasant menopausal symptoms that plague their American counterparts was Sherwood Gorbach, M.D., professor of medicine and community health at Tufts University School of Medicine in Boston. For 2,000 years, foods made from the soybean—including tofu, tempeh, and roasted soybeans—have been diet staples in Asia, he explains. And we now know that soybeans contain special compounds, called isoflavones, that are actually a natural plant form of estrogen. In one day, a typical Asian woman, who eats about

$^1/_4$ pound of soy foods daily, may be getting 30 to 50 milligrams of isoflavones from her food.

Stay Tuned for These Soy Studies

The intriguing fact that isoflavones are a type of estrogen, although 500 to 1,000 times weaker than human estrogen, has led Dr. Gorbach and other researchers to wonder: Could soy foods have a cooling effect on hot flashes similar to the effect produced by estrogen-replacement therapy?

We're beginning to get answers. The first results from a small pilot study at Bowman Gray School of Medicine of Wake Forest University in Winston-Salem, North Carolina, are in, and so far, so good. In the study 43 women who had hot flashes at least once a day tested soy powder (stirred in cereal or juice daily) containing 34 milligrams of isoflavones. (About $^1/_2$ cup of tofu yields a helping of isoflavones equal to the amount used in the study.)

During the six weeks that they took soy, the women's hot flashes became significantly less intense. The hot flashes raged on in women who took a carbohydrate powder with zero isoflavones for six weeks.

Larger studies are currently underway and will yield more information about soy's purported power to soothe hot flashes. Among them are the following two studies:

❖ A study of 240 women over the age of 45 who are experiencing hot flashes or night sweats is being conducted by Gregory L. Burke, M.D., vice-chairman and professor in the department of public-health sciences at Bowman Gray School of Medicine. Every day for two years, the women will drink an 8-ounce soy beverage containing either less than 1 milligram, 34 milligrams, or 50 milligrams of isoflavones, without knowing which level of isoflavones they're receiving. Researchers will track whether isoflavones lower the number of hot flashes and night sweats the women experience as well as other menopausal symptoms (such as anxiety or mood swings).

❖ Sixty women with hot flashes are being followed by two studies at Tufts University, in Dr. Gorbach's department. For three months, these women will eat either two specially designed almond- or chocolate-flavored soy breakfast bars containing 20 milligrams of isoflavones each (for a daily total of 40 milligrams of isoflavones) or two placebo bars without isoflavones. Researchers will track the women's reports of hot flashes and night sweats and their levels of estrogen and other hormones. Although these studies have not been completed, preliminary data suggest that the women receiving isoflavones are getting relief from their symptoms, Dr. Gorbach says.

The Joys of Soy

Why wait for the final word to add soy to your diet? Even if research into soy and hot flashes doesn't pan out, other studies show that soy lowers cholesterol and suggest that it may help prevent breast cancer and osteoporosis. "A serving of soy every day could turn out to be a good bet," says Dr. Gorbach.

If soy isoflavones prove to be hot-flash coolers, researchers say that they will likely recommend consuming in the range of 30 to 50 milligrams per day. Is it okay if you eat soy foods that put you above that amount? Dr. Burke notes that many Asians routinely consume up to 100 milligrams of isoflavones a day. "If there were side effects, I think we'd have seen them by now," he says.

But not soy fast! Pardon the pun, but finding isoflavones isn't as simple as just buying foods with soy in their names. With some soy products, isoflavones are removed when the food is prepared.

If you're wondering about isoflavone capsules that are sold in health food stores, remember this: Just as recent studies seem to show that beta-carotene may not work if taken alone as a supplement, the same may be true for isoflavones. Plus, the possibility of megadosing on isoflavone supplements worries some doctors. One such doctor is soy researcher Kenneth Setchell, Ph.D., director of the clinical mass spectrometry center at Children's Hospital Medical Center in Cincinnati. Isoflavones are weak forms of estrogen, Dr. Setchell emphasizes; in fact, he was one of the first scientists to focus on this. At levels far above the 100 milligrams upper range of Asian diets, we don't know whether isoflavones could be harmful to a woman's body in some way, for example, by possibly encouraging the growth of breast or endometrial cancers.

Your best bet? Get your isoflavones from food instead of pills.

Tastebud-Friendly Soy Foods

It's true: The top sources of isoflavones don't show up on many American shopping lists...yet. "It's hard to convince the average woman to eat soy. Most Americans are not going to rush out and buy tofu or tempeh," says Dr. Setchell.

If this describes you, try some of the new, isoflavone-rich soy products on the market, such as silken tofu that can be whipped into a pudding or added to chocolate soy milk for a thick milk shake. Then there's textured soy protein (TSP), which can take the place of ground beef or turkey in sloppy joes, becoming an all-American comfort food.

Try TSP granules, reconstituted with hot water or broth, as a superhealthy ground beef substitute—high in protein, low in calories, with almost zero fat and substantial fiber. The price is right, too. TSP, sometimes called textured vegetable protein, is sold in health food stores, but our favorite kind, Beef(Not), is sold via mail order.

Where the Isoflavones Aren't

Though these foods may have a place in your diet, you won't find many isoflavones in the following:

❖ Soy sauce
❖ Soybean oil
❖ Foods with a lot of other ingredients besides soy. Examples include canned meal-replacement drinks, soy cheese, soy hot dogs, soy bacon, and tofu yogurt.
❖ Miso, which does have isoflavones; but since each serving is so small (1 teaspoon), you only get about 6 milligrams.
❖ Soy foods made from soy protein concentrate. Examples in this category, such as many vegetarian burgers, may or may not have isoflavones, depending on how they're processed.

Want something more mainstream? Have soy for breakfast with Nutlettes, the only soy ready-to-eat breakfast cereal that we're aware of. This slightly nutty-tasting cereal packs 9 grams of fiber in a $^{1}/_{2}$-cup serving and stays crisp in milk. Add fruit for sweetness. Another breakfast choice could be Take Care High Protein Beverage Powder, available in plain sweetened, chocolate, strawberry, or unsweetened/unflavored versions to mix with water, juice, or milk. Take Care was the soy beverage used for the hot flash study at Bowman Gray. It's a soy food with controlled levels of isoflavones. Normally, levels of isoflavones vary somewhat.

Fancy a roasted soy-butter-and-jelly sandwich? Roasted soy butter is a brand-new product with a peanut butter taste and consistency. It's available in supermarkets as Morningstar Farms Roasted SoyButter or in health food stores as Natural Touch Roasted SoyButter. Roasted soy nuts can be eaten like roasted peanuts. Watch your portions, though, because of the high fat content. You could also use soy milk in instant nonfat pudding or nonfat hot chocolate.

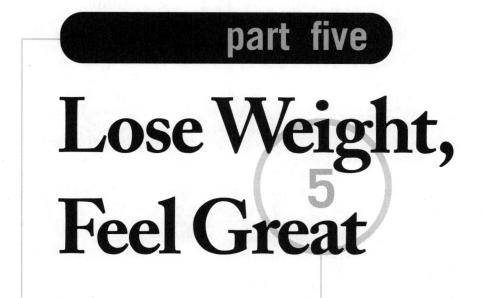

part five

Lose Weight, Feel Great

the Hormone Connection

When a woman's reproductive years end, a drop in levels of the hormone estrogen can trigger changes that reshuffle her weight, her shape, and even the proportions of muscle and body fat that she carries. "Menopause may accelerate weight-gain and body-composition changes," says Eric Poehlman, Ph.D., professor of medicine at the University of Vermont in Burlington. "But I say, fight it."

When Dr. Poehlman and other researchers at the University of Vermont tracked the body compositions of 35 women for six years, they found that those who entered menopause lost 6½ pounds of what the researchers call fat-free mass—that is, muscle, bone, organs, and so forth. "We think that a significant portion of what they lost was muscle mass," says researcher Michael Toth, Ph.D., a physiologist and postdoctoral fellow in the department of medicine at the University of Vermont who worked on the study.

Significantly, the researchers also discovered that the women became less active as they got older—actually burning 230 fewer calories a day by the time they reached menopause. "That could be one of the reasons that they also had more body fat," Dr. Toth says.

"A sedentary lifestyle explains about 80 percent of body fatness," says William Evans, Ph.D., professor of applied physiology and nutrition and director of the Noll Physiological Research Center at Pennsylvania State University in University Park and author of *Biomarkers: The 10 Keys to Prolonging Vitality*. "When a woman is inactive, she loses muscle mass. With less muscle mass, her body burns significantly fewer calories around the clock."

The antidote is to stay active every way that you can. Small steps count, like parking at the far end of the parking lot at the mall, supermarket, or office, and striding to your destination. Like strolling at lunch, playing with the dog, or gardening.

While sculpting a firmer, healthier, more attractive body can require new strategies as women age, "it is absolutely possible to look and feel 20 or even 30 years younger," says Miriam E. Nelson, Ph.D., an exercise physiologist in the human physiology laboratory at the U.S. Department of Agriculture Human Nutrition Research Center on Aging at Tufts University in Boston.

Dr. Nelson believes that middle-age spread is not inevitable—it's not written into our genes, our hormones, or the laws of nature. Firming up, she notes "takes time. It doesn't happen overnight. It takes a commitment. But a woman can look fantastic. She can have that youthful spark. That bounce in her step. That firmness when she walks."

30

What Do You Really Have to Lose?

For Jill Cude, a 42-year-old engineering-company manager from Houston, the weight-loss countdown began one January. "I wanted to lose weight in time for my 20th high school reunion, scheduled for August," she says. "The question was, how much to take off?"

Jill weighed 143 pounds but longed to return to the lithe 122 pounds she had weighed as a high school senior. "But the dietitian who was helping me suggested that we talk about a more appropriate weight—128 pounds, a weight that I could maintain and one that would not make me look emaciated," she recalls. "At first, I wasn't sure that I'd like it."

By August, Jill had shed 15 pounds, reaching her revised but realistic goal. On reunion night, she slipped into a size 6 red, silk pantsuit with rhinestones sparkling at the shoulders, and she discovered that realistic also meant attractive. "My outfit looked fabulous," she recalls. "I got a lot of compliments."

Best of all, Jill has maintained her new weight ever since by following a healthy eating plan and fitting a lot of activity into her day. At 128 pounds, she looks and feels great, and she can maintain her new slim look with a comfortable amount of physical activity and with meals that don't sacrifice nutrition or the foods that she loves.

Balancing Wants, Needs, and Reality

Determining your true weight-loss needs is a balancing act that requires a careful look at your desires, your needs, your lifestyle, and your body's natural

Avoid Dumbed-Down Dieting

You're on a diet. You're trying not to think about food. But you are thinking about food. You're dreading your next encounter with the scale. You're disappointed about your last encounter with the scale. Let's just face it—diets are distracting.

And that is precisely what Michael Green, Ph.D., senior research psychologist at the Institute of Food Research in Reading, England, has shown with a series of studies involving women on self-imposed diets. The same women scored lower on tests of mental tasks when they were dieting than when they weren't. Could their impaired brain functions be caused by nutritional deficiencies from dieting? Dr. Green was able to rule that out when he found that women on diets scored lower whether they had lost any weight or not.

Dr. Green's theory is that the stress of restraining your appetite and anxiety about how much weight you'll lose just plain preoccupies the brain. You're not really dumber, just distracted. The mental skills that suffered in the study were vigilance, immediate free recall, and simple reaction time. In everyday terms that means that, when you're dieting, you might need extra time to balance your checkbook, you might forget to buy milk when you grocery shop, or you might not hit the brakes as fast as usual when the car in front of you comes to a sudden halt.

Where does all this leave us? The healthiest way to lose weight is coincidental weight loss—the kind that just happens by itself when you focus on eating and exercising for super health. We've known that it's better for your body; now we know that it's also better for your mind.

HEALTH FLASH

tendencies, says Shiriki Kumanyika, R.D., Ph.D., professor and head of the department of human nutrition and dietetics at the University of Illinois at Chicago and a member of the advisory committee that established the U.S. government's 1995 Dietary Guidelines for Americans.

"There is no magic number," says Dr. Kumanyika. "A woman cannot pick a goal weight off a chart. She has to factor in her own current weight and weight history, her family's health history, her personal health goals, her eating patterns, and her level of activity. Then, she can pick a weight-reduction target that makes sense."

For women making this highly personal decision often means stepping away from our culture's loud-and-clear message that thinner is better. "Weight is a huge emotional issue for women," says Debbie Then, Ph.D., a psychologist in private practice in Los Angeles. "Women are valued by society for their looks, while men are more often valued for what they do. So women feel much more pressure, from within and from outside, to be thin. As a result, many women never really appreciate their own unique, beautiful bodies."

Why Do You Want to Shed Pounds?

Why? is the simple question that Michael Hamilton, M.D., program and medical director of Duke University Diet and Fitness Center in Durham, North Carolina, asks women who want to lose weight. "The best reason to lose weight is that you feel that your weight is in some way negatively impacting your life," says Dr. Hamilton.

"Excessive weight could be jeopardizing your health. Or it could be interfering with your ability to get up in the morning with the energy to do the things that you want to do. It could be making you feel embarrassed and unwilling to go out socially to the movies or on a hike or to parties," Dr. Hamilton adds.

So ask yourself if your weight interferes with your life—physically, socially, or psychologically. If your answer is yes, consider the reasons. Do you find yourself turning to food to calm stress or to soothe difficult emotions? If so, it may be time to break the emotional-eating cycle. Do you simply feel too big to take part in activities that you enjoy? Or do you know that your weight is a health risk? Then a new eating plan and more physical activity may be all you need, says Dr. Hamilton.

Do you find yourself postponing changes that you would like to make in your life, telling yourself that happiness, new relationships, new interests, or a different job must wait until you've lost weight?

The real barrier may not be your weight at all, says Marcia Hutchinson, Ed.D., a psychologist in the Boston area and author of *Transforming Body Image*.

"I like to ask women, 'Well, what would be different about your life if you were thinner? How would your relationships change? How would the way you project yourself in the world change? How would the way you care about yourself change? How would the way you feel about yourself as a sexual being change?'" Dr. Hutchinson says.

"Getting rid of extra pounds won't change other parts of your life unless you can also make a change in the way you think about yourself," Dr. Hutchinson points out.

Do You Have a Clear Picture of Your Body Right Now?

Often, women approach weight loss by dreaming about the number of pounds they would like to lose, rather than by having a clear picture of how their bodies actually look. If your mental image of your body shape is inaccurate—if, for example, you dislike your hips and thighs because you think that they're huge, when in fact they're only slightly padded—you may set an unattainable weight-loss goal.

"It's important for a woman to have a realistic sense of her body before beginning a weight-loss program," says Yasmin Mossavar-Rahmani, R.D., Ph.D., assistant clinical professor in the department of epidemiology and social medicine at Albert Einstein College of Medicine of Yeshiva University in New York City. "Otherwise, she may diet unnecessarily or try to lose too much weight."

In a study at a Brooklyn hospital, Dr. Mossavar-Rahmani and other researchers asked 150 women hospital employees—from doctors to laundry workers—to estimate their body sizes. When the researchers compared the women's guesses with accurate measurements, they found that half the women had inaccurate perceptions of themselves, believing that their bodies were bigger, or sometimes smaller, than they actually were. The less accurate a woman's self-perception, researchers found, the more likely she was to diet.

Body Mass Index: More Accurate Than a Scale

You can pin down your "real" size with a measurement tool recommended by weight-loss experts: the body mass index (BMI).

Body mass index is a single number based on a scientific formula that compares your height to your weight. The result helps predict whether you are at risk for weight-related health problems. Most likely, your BMI will fall somewhere between 19 and 32. If you're 5 feet, 4 inches tall, for example, and you weigh 122 pounds, your BMI is 21. But if you're 5 feet, 4 inches tall and weigh 157 pounds, your BMI is considerably higher—27. Dr. Hamilton says that the safest range is 20 to 25.

What's your healthiest BMI? The answer depends a great deal on your personal and inherited risk for a variety of health problems, including the following:

Heart disease. If you're at risk for heart disease, a BMI below 22 may be safest, according to Harvard University's ongoing Nurse's Health Study.

Diabetes. Women with BMIs over 28 raise their risks of diabetes, according to the American Diabetes Association.

Calculate Your Body Mass Index

To find your body mass index (BMI), locate your height in the left column. Move across the chart to the right until you hit your approximate weight. Then follow that column down to the corresponding BMI number at the bottom of the chart.

HEIGHT						WEIGHT (lb.)								
4'10"	91	96	100	105	110	115	119	124	129	134	138	143	148	153
4'11"	94	99	104	109	114	119	124	128	133	138	143	148	153	158
5'0"	97	102	107	112	118	123	128	133	138	143	148	153	158	163
5'1"	100	106	111	116	122	127	132	137	143	148	153	158	164	169
5'2"	104	109	115	120	126	131	136	142	147	153	158	164	169	174
5'3"	107	113	118	124	130	135	141	146	152	158	163	169	175	180
5'4"	110	116	122	128	134	140	145	151	157	163	169	174	180	186
5'5"	114	120	126	132	138	144	150	156	162	168	174	180	186	192
5'6"	118	124	130	136	142	148	155	161	167	173	179	186	192	198
5'7"	121	127	134	140	146	153	159	166	172	178	185	191	197	204
5'8"	125	131	138	144	151	158	164	171	177	184	190	197	203	210
5'9"	128	135	142	149	155	162	169	176	182	189	196	203	209	216
5'10"	132	139	146	153	160	167	174	181	188	195	202	207	215	222
5'11"	136	143	150	157	165	172	179	186	193	200	208	215	222	229
6'0"	140	147	154	162	169	177	184	191	199	206	213	221	228	235
BMI	19	20	21	22	23	24	25	26	27	28	29	30	31	32

Breast cancer. If you have a family history of breast cancer, a BMI below 27 may be safer.

Other health conditions. With a BMI above 27, your risks rise for arthritis, gout, and above-normal levels of cholesterol and triglycerides (blood fats that can increase your risk of heart disease).

What if your BMI is outside the ideal range? The good news is that a woman can reduce her health risks if she loses just 10 to 14 pounds—dropping from, say, a BMI of 30 to a BMI of 28.

Tummy Fat versus Hip Fat

Where you're overweight can be just as important as how much you weigh. Women who carry extra fat on their abdomens are at higher risk for weight-related health problems, while fat packed on their hips and thighs poses much less risk (though such fat may be harder to get rid of), says Susan Fried, Ph.D., associate professor of nutritional sciences at Rutgers University in New Brunswick, New Jersey, who studies the links between health and abdominal fat.

Get a clear picture of this fat zone with another measurement tool, the waist/hip ratio. Find yours by measuring your waist at its smallest point and your hips at their widest point. Then divide your waist measurement by your hip measurement. (If your waist is 34 inches and your hips are 42 inches, for example, your waist/hip ratio is 0.8.) For women, waist/hip ratios over 0.8 indicate increased risks of diabetes, heart disease, and high blood pressure, says Dr. Hamilton.

Diet, aerobic exercise, and strength training all help burn that excess fat. And the best way to keep track of your progress is with an old-fashioned tape measure—or your bedroom mirror, Dr. Hamilton adds.

Aim for Easy Weight Maintenance

You may find another important clue to your body's natural, healthy weight range by thinking back over your weight history as an adult—or by looking through the back of your closet for the clothes that once fit, says Dr. Hamilton.

Take a look at your past and think about a weight that has seemed natural for you as an adult. Perhaps you weighed 140 pounds for many years, then suddenly began putting on the pounds. Perhaps your easy-maintenance weight was a bit higher or a bit lower than that. Regardless of the number, it was a weight that seemed to maintain itself, staying nearly the same whether you ate a little more or a little less, or whether you engaged in a little more or a little less physical activity.

"I like to find out what a woman weighed before she started to gain weight in adulthood," Dr. Hamilton says. "I ask if there was a weight that she somehow easily maintained for a period of time. If there was, then that weight is probably a reasonable goal to set."

If you've always been overweight, you may find useful clues in the weights and body sizes of your relatives, he says. "If both parents gained weight at a certain time of life, there is probably a strong genetic tendency for their children to gain weight then as well," Dr. Hamilton notes. "That simply means that you have to be realistic and careful. Genes may influence 30 to 50 percent of your weight, but you can stay in control through a healthy diet and an exercise program."

Putting It All Together: Your Goal Weight

So there you have it: three very good ways to decide on a goal weight. You may want to lose 5 pounds or 45 pounds. You may not want to lose any weight at all; perhaps you simply want to lose body fat and firm up. Whatever your goal is, try these tips, suggested by weight-loss experts, to get started working toward that target.

First, hold the line. If you've been gaining more and more weight, your first step might be simply to stop putting on pounds, says Dr. Kumanyika. "Ninety percent of diets are a failure," she notes. "Your best strategy might be to first understand how to hold the line, and then to evaluate how and whether you can lose weight."

Set a small goal. Losing just 5 to 10 percent of your weight can dramatically improve many weight-related health problems. Small losses of 10 pounds or less can also give you a big boost of self-confidence, says Dr. Hamilton. "And within days of changing your diet, you'll feel more energetic, too."

Break a big goal into small goals. If your goal is a big one, break it down into a series of small victories, suggests Anne Dubner, R.D., a nutrition consultant in Houston and a spokesperson for the American Dietetic Association. "Don't set unrealistic expectations for yourself," she says. "Set your sights on losing 10 pounds or less. Concentrate on that. You'll get good results." Then go to the next goal, and the next.

31

Fill Your Plate and Watch the Pounds Disappear

We all know them—those lucky women who seem naturally, effortlessly slender. Young or old, they walk to work and spend the day with an extra, rosy glow about them. The type who never awakens thinking, "What will I wear today—that fits?"

The fact is, it's not terribly difficult to become one of them. Becoming effortlessly slender doesn't mean clearing your favorite foods from your plate or spending all your free time in the gym. (Those tactics just leave a nasty aftertaste of deprivation.) All you need to do is twist your plate a little more than 90 degrees—we'll tell you more about that in a minute—and fill it up. Then, shift your mind a little bit, too. It's time to get outside and have some fun.

This approach isn't about grand, sweeping changes. It's about easing your way into the good life.

Never Feel Deprived Again

"Avoiding feelings of deprivation is critical to adopting permanent eating changes," says Ronette L. Kolotkin, Ph.D., director of behavioral programs at the Duke University Diet and Fitness Center in Durham, North Carolina. That means making sure that portions look filling, tasty, and visually appealing.

Is Chocolate a Vegetable?

You've heard that red wine may fight heart attacks, thanks partly to substances called antioxidants that protect your cells from damage. Now, chemists at the University of California at Davis reveal that chocolate contains these same antioxidants, called flavonoids. In fact, a 1½-ounce milk-chocolate bar has the same quantity of flavonoids as a 5-ounce glass of cabernet sauvignon.

We regret to report, however, that chocolate will never be a health food, according to researcher Andrew Waterhouse, Ph.D., assistant professor in the department of viticulture and enology at the University of California at Davis. In spite of its flavonoids, chocolate is too high in fat and empty calories to be heart smart. (White chocolate, by the way, has zero flavonoids.)

But Dr. Waterhouse also found flavonoids in cocoa powder (chocolate with most of the fat removed). In fact, a cup of hot chocolate made with 2 tablespoons of cocoa powder has about 75 percent of the flavonoids in a glass of red wine. Make hot chocolate with skim milk, and you get a nice big splash of calcium and vitamin D, almost no fat...and at least a few fightin' flavonoids. Still, the healthiest way to fill up on flavonoids is to eat a lot of fruits and vegetables.

How to fill up that plate without filling out your trousers? A redesign. If you put the average American meal on one of those paper plates with dividers, the largest section—about half the plate—is filled with meat. "Most of the rest is refined starchy food and added fat," says James J. Kenney, R.D., Ph.D., nutrition research specialist at the Pritikin Longevity Center in Santa Monica, California. That design just doesn't fuel the body optimally.

As a result, Americans eat few nutrient-dense vegetables but, as a nation, we do eat some 839 billion fat calories each year. That's about 34 to 36 percent of our calories as fat, a megadose compared with the 15 to 25 percent that we should be eating.

Now, about this redesign. Instead of plopping the meat in that large section at the bottom of the divided plate, move it around about 90 degrees and put it in one of the smaller compartments. When the meat (or chicken or fish) fills no more than one-quarter of the plate, it generally becomes the 3-ounce serving that earns kudos for being very healthy. (It'll be about the size of a deck of playing cards.)

Fill the largest plate compartment with vegetables and put grains in the other space. (Actually, it's great to let the grains spill over a bit into the veggies section.) When you're finished losing weight, you can play with the vegetable and grain proportions, making them about equal. Increasing grains relative to vegetables later for maintenance will increase calories slightly without affecting weight control, says Lori Wiersema, R.D., associate director of the Johns Hopkins Weight Management Center in Baltimore.

"Redesigning your plate to create the right fuel mix automatically slashes fat grams and calories to a healthier level," says Wiersema. As you prepare soups and stews, modify recipes to yield the same proportions of vegetables, grains, and meat. Add to your satisfaction by filling up snack times with a mélange of juicy, fresh fruits. Try kiwifruit, mangoes, papayas, and other fruits that you normally pass by.

Start redesigning your plate by redesigning your grocery cart. Fill the bottom of your cart with fruits, vegetables, and whole-grain foods, then you need just the foldout top basket for meat and added fat products.

Wake Up Your Tastebuds

Skeptical that a plate redesign will satisfy you as much as we say? Here's how to maximize your enjoyment.

Go for less meat, more satisfaction. A great way to enjoy smaller portions of meat, fish, and poultry is to give them intense flavor, says Marilyn C. Majchrzak, R.D., food-development manager at the Canyon Ranch Health Resort in Tucson, Arizona. "While we strongly recommend limiting all fat, especially saturated fat such as butter, using just 1 teaspoon wisely can make a huge difference in feeling satisfied." At Canyon Ranch, culinary experts add fresh crushed herbs to 1 teaspoon of melted butter, using it as a richly flavored sauce for broiled fish.

Don't forget to satisfy your sense of sight, too. Three ounces of chicken doesn't look like paltry poultry when it's sliced and arranged.

"If you have a hard time stopping at 3 ounces of roast beef, double up on roast night, and then go vegetarian the next night. Dietary changes have to work for you," says Wiersema.

Choose flavor-rich fruits and veggies. Summer isn't the only time to reap the rich vegetable harvest. Try winter veggies or dip into the freezer.

"Granted, some things are better fresh, such as summer and winter squash, pea pods, cabbage, tomatoes, and lettuce. But corn, green beans, green peas, carrots, and broccoli are almost as great frozen, when fresh isn't available or convenient," says Jennifer Flora, food-development coordinator at Canyon Ranch.

Don't skip the fresh produce aisle in winter. "All types of citrus, apples, potatoes, root vegetables, and winter squashes are especially abundant and wonderful in February," says Sarah Delea, vice-president of communications for the United Fresh Fruit and Vegetable Association. As the California growing season begins to wind down in late January, grapes from Chile begin to come in, she says, so start looking for those. Also, keep an eye out for strawberries in later February. Bananas are great year-round.

Cook for your tastebuds. Stove-top steaming and microwaving are the best ways to bring frozen vegetables back to life. Cook them with as little water as possible. "When it comes to nutritional goodness, frozen, canned, and fresh vegetables are quite comparable," says Barbara P. Klein, Ph.D., professor of food science and human nutrition at the University of Illinois at Urbana-Champaign.

Focus on great grains. When we say grains, we mean whole grains, not processed-to-the-limit starches. Fortunately, grocery stores are packed with great whole-grain options. Try whole-wheat pasta, brown rice, barley, millet, bulgur, multigrain dinner rolls, and 12-grain bread. Whole grains give you not only more vitamins and minerals but also more fiber, says Wiersema. "That's a big help in making you feel full for longer periods of time, which is another aid in weight loss." One of the tastiest grain options is rice, which comes in an array of varieties, each with its own subtle flavor. Add interest to the grains section of your plate by trying something other than the bland instant rice that Mom used to make. Brown and longer-cooking rices are tasty, substantial, and satisfying.

Brown rice is the best for nutrients and fiber, and it has a chewy texture and excellent nutlike flavor. Parboiled or converted rice is next best because some of the nutrients are retained in the parboiling process, although its fiber content is low. This rice is fluffier than brown rice. By the way, to retain nutrients in any type of rice, never rinse it before cooking.

The size of the kernels determines how the rice cooks up. Long-grain rice produces light, dry grains that separate easily. The shortest grains produce moister kernels that stick together. A short-grain rice called arborio is used to make creamy risottos.

All rices are not the same. The rice called Texmati has a subtle, pecanlike taste. For added flavor in all types of rice, culinary experts at Canyon Ranch suggest tossing an herbal tea bag into the water while the rice cooks. Favorites of spa guests include orange, almond, and ginger herbal teas.

Put cooking time to good use by making a big batch of brown rice and freezing some of it. Cooked rice can be stored for up to seven days in the refrigerator and for six months in the freezer. To reheat, add 2 tablespoons of liquid per cup of cooked rice. Then microwave the rice and liquid for about $1\frac{1}{2}$ minutes, or heat it on the stove top for 4 to 5 minutes.

32

To Slim Down Fast, Walk This Way

Have you heard the call? Sometime in a woman's life, her faithful body starts sending messages. Maybe you tug a sweater off over your head and notice that your shoulders feel creaky. You might pull on your favorite jeans and find them suddenly more snug. Or you reach out one arm to push open a heavy door and find that you need both arms to budge it.

Pay attention. These signals are a major wake-up call. As you age, unexercised joints stiffen up. Unexercised muscles peter out. And when muscles peter out, weight gain speeds up. Better face it: Use-it-or-lose-it time has arrived. "Exercise me," your body is pleading.

The trick is finding the right exercise. You need to work on everything—muscles, joints, heart, and lungs—to stay fit. But who can spend all day at the gym? Plain old walking is always great for your heart and lungs, but it won't do a lot for the joints and muscles in any parts of your body besides your legs. Another consideration is protecting your knees. The ideal physical-activity plan should minimize stress on your knees. And let's throw in the fact that you may be a total newcomer to the exercise scene. Is the situation impossible?

Not on your life. There is one exercise that seems to do it all. It's a special "ultra" form of walking in which your own two feet can carry you to the pinnacle of fitness. You'll be surprised at how much fun it is.

Heel-to-Toe Strolling

If you've never been introduced, may we present heel-to-toe walking? In a nutshell, it's a style of walking that involves your whole body in one great, gliding, heart-pumping, joint-flexing, muscle-working, calorie-burning motion. Heel-to-toe walking delivers everything women need for fitness in one doable exercise.

Never exercised before? Don't worry—you can do this. True, heel-to-toe walking involves a little more than regular walking—like the fun of mastering a new technique—but it gives a whopping return. What are the benefits?

Toning muscles everywhere. A key goal of exercise is stopping the loss of muscle strength and tone that comes with aging. To perform heel-to-toe walking, even regular walkers will be using muscles that they didn't know they had, particularly around their waists, buttocks, hips, thighs, and arms. "Heel-to-toe walking spreads the workload over the whole body and creates real muscular balance," explains Martin Rudow, a former Olympic heel-to-toe coach.

Staying loose. Experts tell us that the way to keep joints flexible is to use them. This is exactly what heel-to-toe walking makes you do—much more so than regular walking. You'll be giving joints in your ankles, feet, hips, and shoulders more action and stretching than they've ever seen.

Built-in knee protection. Knee injuries sideline too many people, even affecting regular walkers. But with the heel-to-toe walking technique, your knee is extended completely when your heel strikes the ground. "That means that the shock is absorbed all the way up your leg and in your hip and trunk, rather than just under your kneecap, as it is when you walk normally," says James Elting, M.D., an orthopedic surgeon and fellow with the American Academy of Sports Physicians.

Calorie crunching. Step right up if you're counting calories. Staying slim is a good health strategy. Studies link gaining weight as we age with poorer health. The good news is that because so many muscles are involved in heel-to-toe walking, you burn more calories than when regular walking at the same speed. If you heel-to-toe walk a 12-minute mile, you even burn more calories than when jogging at the same pace, without the pounding.

Kind to your heart. No question about it, heel-to-toe walking gives your heart and lungs a healthy workout, without the knee trauma that other aerobic exercises can deliver.

Therapy for the spirit. Heel-to-toe walking gives you a sense of mastery and self-esteem as you learn and endlessly perfect your technique. More than any other sport, heel-to-toe walking lets you spot where you need to improve, because you can slow down and observe yourself. "If you tried to do that on a bike, you'd fall over. If you were swimming, you'd sink," says Rudow. Once you get hooked, you'll never be bored.

Ready, Set, Ramble

Actually, racewalking is the official name for heel-to-toe walking. But it's better to stick with heel-to-toe walking, the original name. Why? If you think of it as simply walking really fast and beating somebody in a race, you might miss what a fabulous, fun exercise heel-to-toe walking really is.

Once you get used to it, heel-to-toe walking feels amazingly good—rhythmic and more powerful than regular walking. But it's difficult to learn heel-to-toe walking just by reading about it. Descriptions of the four basics—posture, footwork, hip work, and arm work—can at least get you started. Try out each one at a time (a full-length mirror helps at first) before putting them together.

Then after you've experimented a little, you may want more information.

Heel-to-Toe Beginner's Warmup

To help you get ready for your roadwork, here's a warmup program designed by Elaine Ward, walking coach, author of several fitness and competitive walking books, and managing director of the North American Racewalking Foundation. Especially important is the toe-tapping exercise to strengthen shins, which often turn out to be a beginning heel-to-toe walker's weakest point.

❖ *Walking warmup.* Walk for 5 minutes at an easy pace to warm up your muscles.
❖ *In-place warmup.* Stretch and strengthen for 5 minutes with these exercises.

1. Shoulder roll. Keeping your arms at your sides, roll your shoulders in alternating circles, left and right, as if you were doing the backstroke. Repeat 20 times.
2. Side stretch. Start by facing forward, with your hands resting at your waist. Slowly turn to your left and right, and look behind you. Repeat 20 times.
3. Back stretch. With your knees slightly bent and your pelvis tucked under, lean forward with your head and arms hanging down. Don't push or strain. Let gravity stretch you. Hold for 30 seconds. (If you have osteoporosis, omit this stretch.)
4. Calf stretch. With your arms straight and your hands on a wall, bend your left knee and lean into the wall. Stretch your right leg out in back, pressing your heel into the ground. Count to 20 slowly. Repeat, bending your right knee and stretching your left leg.
5. Toe taps. Stand with one foot in front of the other so that your feet are about walking distance apart. Repeatedly tap the toes of one foot on the ground, bringing your toes up high. Do 12 reps, then change feet. (You can do this exercise anytime, even sitting down.)
6. Foot rockers. Stand with one foot in front of the other so that your feet are about walking distance apart, and rock from heel to toe and back. Repeat 10 times.

Videos are especially helpful. And personal coaching may be available in your area. But, here are the techniques to get you started.

Check your posture. Stand tall, chin up, with your weight slightly forward on the balls of your feet. Lean forward just slightly from the ankles, without bending at the waist. (Check your position in the mirror.) Imagine that your body is a board, and it's starting to tip forward, all in one plane. Avoid swayback by tucking under your buttocks and tucking in your stomach, but don't strain. Keep your shoulders relaxed. This forward lean allows gravity to help you move forward.

Add footwork. Start walking. Try to point your feet straight ahead. Don't force it, but make gentle corrections when you see one of your feet pointing out or in. Land on each heel with your toes and forefoot raised at a 25- to 30-degree angle off the ground. (Landing on your heel this way helps straighten your knee, a critical part of heel-to-toe style, and diverts impact from your knee joint.) Allow yourself to roll forward on your foot, pressing down on the outside portion of the bottom of your foot so that you feel continuous contact with the ground. Push off with your toes.

As you read this, just walk around the house in your bare feet, heel-to-toe walking style, to get the feel of it. You'll notice a distinct push forward when you use this rolling motion, in contrast to your normal, more flat-footed stride. Go slowly and you'll also notice just how strong your toes are and how much motion you can get out of your whole foot. You'll also notice greater use of the muscles in your buttocks than you do in regular walking.

Put some hip into it. First, let's clear the air. If you're afraid to try this technique because you've seen racewalkers who looked like waddling ducks, relax. Hips that waddle from side to side are a result of faulty technique. When you heel-to-toe walk with proper form, you look powerful and graceful, not anything like a duck.

That's not to say that heel-to-toe walkers don't use their hips. They do use them to the max, but in a graceful, natural forward-and-back motion that feels like gliding. (Most regular walkers do not use their hips when they walk. This is more a matter of poor posture, stiffness, and cultural taboo than proper biomechanics.)

To check out the proper hip motion for heel-to-toe walking, before you decide to go public, stand in front of that mirror again and try this exercise suggested by Elaine Ward, walking coach, author of several fitness and competitive walking books, and managing director of the North American Racewalking Foundation. Walk in place by moving your knees forward and back. Stand tall, and let your arms swing naturally at your sides. Begin to let your hips swing, forward and back, with your legs. You'll feel a twisting motion at your waist.

If it's hard to get your hips moving, pretend that you're holding onto a towel and drying off your behind. Notice that the movement of your arms helps your hips move forward and back even farther. Feels good, doesn't it?

When you're walking, this hip movement allows you to keep your back foot on the ground a bit longer, extending your stride behind you and giving power to your push-off. Not to mention toning your waist and massaging your lower back.

Pump your arms. Arm movement complements leg and hip movement and turns heel-to-toe walking into a total-body, integrated movement. When you use your arms properly, you'll feel a delightful sense of rhythm and coordination, plus extra power. Your shoulder joints stay flexible, too.

Bend your arms to at least a right angle; a little more is better according to some coaches. Let them swing like pendulums from your relaxed shoulders. (Let's go back to that mirror.) Cup your hands in a loosely clenched fist as you swing one arm forward and the other backward. Don't hunch up. Your hands should swing no higher in front than the midline of the chest. They should swing straight ahead, not diagonally. As you swing back, your hands should go as far as an imaginary back pocket, but no farther. Your elbows should stay close to your body. Swing your arms in front of the mirror until you feel relaxed and comfortable. Notice how hard it is to keep your hips still? Good. Let them rotate back and forth freely.

This mirror exercise can help you immensely to get the feel of a proper arm swing. And it can also give you confidence that you don't look silly. What does look awkward is punching the air in front of your body or thrusting your arms high in the air. As you swing your arms, concentrate more on the back swing than the forward swing and feel how that helps move you forward.

Hitting Your Stride

Once you hit the pavement to try your new sport, take it slowly to master proper technique, but don't get too obsessed with perfection. "I tell my non-competitive walkers to consider all the tips a smorgasbord," says Jeff Salvage, heel-to-toe-walking coach and United States Track and Field MidAtlantic Racewalk chairman. "Feel free to pick and choose what you like. Any one of them will enhance your technique."

But when you do start to speed up, remember this very important point: Heel-to-toe walkers go faster by taking short, quick steps, not long strides. This is what makes you feel like you're gliding instead of bounding, and it takes the bounce out of your walk, making fast walking easier on your joints.

What's the key to short, quick steps? The quickness and the size of your stride is directly related to your arm swing. If you swing your arms too far out in front, you will be forced to take too long a stride to keep your balance. If you keep your arm swings short and quick, your legs will tend to move in sync, and vice versa.

33

Toss Those Control-Top Panty Hose: Body Toners That Work

You can see a significant difference in your body after just six weeks of body toning with weights, says Rebecca Gorrell, a certified fitness instructor and wellness-education director at Canyon Ranch Health Resort in Tucson, Arizona.

"Body shaping is one of the very few natural ways that you can change the way you look," adds Larry A. Tucker, Ph.D., professor and director of health promotion at Brigham Young University in Provo, Utah.

That is good news—but wait, there's more. Change comes so predictably that it builds self-esteem in addition to better bodies. Researchers at Brigham Young, led by Dr. Tucker, conducted a 12-week study of 60 women with an average age of 42. Half of the women were assigned to exercise by walking; the rest of the women were assigned to a strength-training group. The scientists found that the body images of the walkers improved during the 12 weeks. But they also discovered that the body images of the women who strength-trained improved significantly more. "We saw substantial mental, emotional, and physical changes," says Dr. Tucker.

Exercise Lowers "Bad" Cholesterol

There's a new way that exercise helps women's hearts. In a study of 377 women and men with moderately high levels of low-density lipoproteins (LDLs, the so-called bad cholesterol that raises heart disease risk) and moderately low levels of "good" high-density lipoproteins (HDLs), researchers saw that people who worked out and ate low-fat diets reduced their LDLs further than people who tried to just eat their way to good health. Women who added exercise to smart eating lowered their LDLs twice as much as women who only used low-fat diets.

"This demonstrates that exercise is not just important for managing HDL cholesterol, which is where it has been thought to have a role. Exercise is also very important for controlling LDL cholesterol. Previously, people have focused only on diet to manage LDLs," says Marcia Stefanick, Ph.D., senior research scientist at the Stanford Center for Research and Disease Prevention.

Exercise is thought to influence LDLs by helping women lose abdominal fat. Abdominal fat is a problem, according to one theory, because the blood circulating through it drains right into the liver. The liver, receiving fat-laden blood, manufactures fat molecules like LDLs. But when fat in the abdomen is reduced, the blood-fat mill in your liver might have fewer raw materials with which to create damaging LDLs.

Exercisers in this study worked out for 45 minutes three times a week. Now you have another good reason to add physical activity to your weekly routine.

A Workout for Busy Women

Try a time-efficient total-body-shaping workout for yourself. It takes just 20 minutes two or three times a week. To do the basic body-shapers, you'll need a set of 2-pound dumbbells and a set of 5-pound dumbbells, or one set that allows you to gradually increase the amount of weight that you're lifting.

A set of single-piece dumbbells generally costs under $10. The kind that allows you to add more weight to increase resistance costs about $15 to $30 per set in most sporting goods stores. Or you can fill plastic jugs or bottles with just enough sand or water to make your own 2- and 5-pound weights.

(Remember: Sand is heavier than water, so you won't need as much of it to make your weights.)

For the exercises that are done on the floor, you'll probably want to use an exercise mat or a folded blanket. And a few of the exercises call for an exercise band, which is a strip of flexible rubber that you can buy in most sporting goods stores. Exercises calling for a bench can be done on a padded exercise bench or on a low bench with a cushion.

Before you begin, warm up for 5 to 10 minutes. Walk briskly in place or jog. Extend your arms to the sides and do arm circles. Then, begin the shape-up routine.

Do each exercise 8 to 12 times. (You can start with 8 repetitions and work your way up to 12 as your fitness level increases.) This repetition is called a set. If you cannot complete 8 repetitions, or reps, that means that you're lifting too much weight. If you can do 12 reps without feeling muscle fatigue, you should be lifting more. If you have been doing the routine for several weeks and it feels comfortable, you can begin doing a second set of all the exercises. Progress to heavier weights very gradually, as an exercise starts to feel easy.

Following the basic workout, you'll find exercises that help tone different parts of your body. Start with all of the basic body-shapers, then add or substitute some of the optional toning moves as you progress.

Basic Body-Shapers

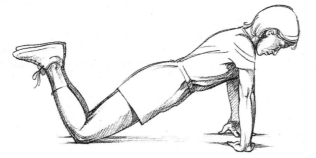

Push-Ups

This helps tone your entire chest, even if you start with a half rather than a full push-up. Kneeling on an exercise mat, lean forward and place your hands shoulder-width apart on the mat. Your fingers should be pointing inward and your elbows outward. When you're in the upright position, your arms and back should be straight, and your knees should touch the floor. Lower your chest to the floor, keeping your upper body rigid. Then push up, straightening your arms, and repeat.

Squats

This exercise tones your thighs and buttocks. Stand with your feet approximately shoulder-width apart and your toes pointed straight ahead or slightly out to the sides. With your feet flat on the floor, lower yourself into the squat position, extending your arms straight ahead as you do so. You're in the right position when your trunk leans forward (up to 45 degrees), your buttocks move back slightly, and your thighs and arms are almost parallel to the floor.

While squatting, look forward at all times and keep the natural curvature in your spine. Do not lower yourself so that your knees extend beyond your feet. Keep your heels flat on the floor to avoid stress on your knees. Then raise yourself to a standing position and repeat.

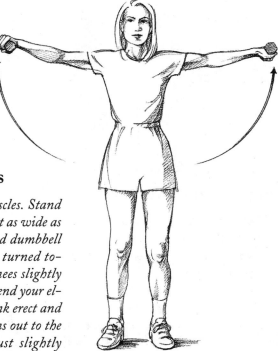

Lateral Shoulder Raises

This tones your shoulder muscles. Stand with your feet spread apart about as wide as your hips. Hold a 2- or 3-pound dumbbell in each hand, with your palms turned toward your thighs. Bend your knees slightly so that they're not locked. Now bend your elbows slightly. Keeping your trunk erect and your elbows bent, raise your arms out to the sides until your elbows are just slightly higher than your shoulders. Lower the dumbbells to your sides and repeat.

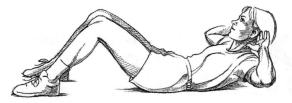

Abdominal Crunches

This exercise tones your upper abdominal muscles. Lie on your back on a mat, with your knees bent and your feet flat on the floor. Place your fingertips behind your ears, with your elbows out as wide as they'll go. Tighten your stomach muscles to curl your trunk, lifting your shoulders until they clear the floor. Keep your elbows out, not in near your ears, so that you lift with your abdominal muscles rather than by straining your neck, arms, and back. Hold the crunch for a few seconds at the top of the lift. Then lower your upper body and repeat.

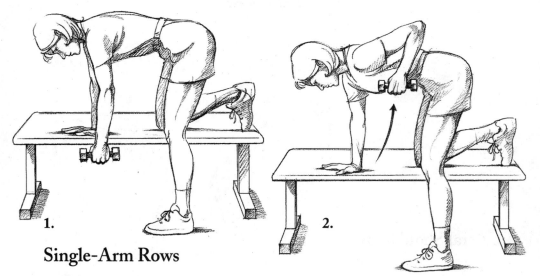

Single-Arm Rows

This exercise tones your shoulder and back muscles.

(1) With your left foot on the floor and your left knee slightly bent, position your right knee on a bench so that your knee is directly under your hip. Lean forward, placing your right hand on the bench, with your back flat and parallel to the floor. Grasp a dumbbell in your left hand, with your arm fully extended downward and your palm facing toward you.

(2) Squeezing your shoulder blades together, pull your left arm up while bending your elbow, until the point of your elbow is a few inches above your back. (The motion is like pulling the cord on a lawn mower.) Return to the starting position and repeat. After you complete 8 to 12 repetitions, switch sides and repeat.

Optional Toning Moves

Here are optional toning exercises that can be added to the total body-shaping workout or substituted for exercises in the workout. In addition, see chapter 34 for more tummy-tightening routines.

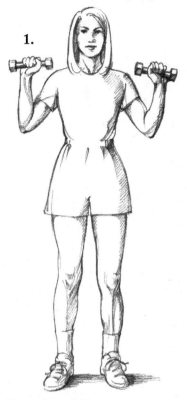

1.

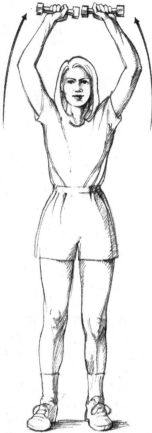

2.

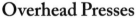

Overhead Presses

A good set of shoulders in a backless sundress is one of summertime's sassiest sights. With toned shoulders, you're virtually assured of a prouder bustline. You can banish round, stooped shoulders with the following exercise. The exercise requires 5-pound dumbbells (to start).

(1) Stand and grip a 5-pound dumbbell in each hand, with your elbows bent so that your arms form Vs at your sides. The dumbbells should be slightly more than shoulder-width apart, and your palms should face forward.

(2) Keeping your back straight, raise your arms and press the dumbbells up over your head so that the heads of the dumbbells touch at the top. Be sure that you don't lean back while you're making this motion. Slowly lower the dumbbells to the starting position, then repeat.

Do two sets of 8 repetitions each. Then slowly increase to three sets of 10 reps each, using 10-pound dumbbells.

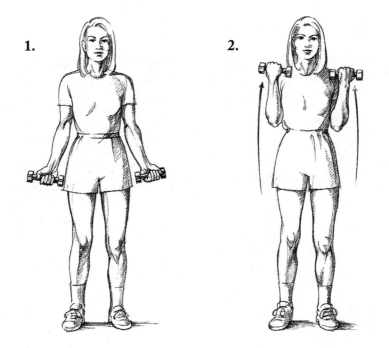

1.

2.

Biceps Curls

Located on your upper arms, your biceps are the muscles that you use to lift boulders, babies, and bowling balls. A sturdy set of biceps will also help you yank heavy bags of cat litter out of the trunk and hoist 5-gallon bottles of water into the house. Just what you always needed, right? To do this exercise you will need 5-pound dumbbells (to start).

(1) Pick up a pair of dumbbells and stand in an upright position, maintaining the normal curvature of your spine. Keep your elbows and upper arms along the sides of your body, and hold the dumbbells with your palms facing up.

(2) Raise the dumbbells toward your shoulders. Don't swing the dumbbells or arch your back. Slowly lower the dumbbells until they're in the starting position.

Do 8 repetitions. Beginners should use 5- to 8-pound dumbbells, and those at an intermediate level should use 10- to 12-pound dumbbells. Do two sets, with a rest of about 30 seconds between sets. Gradually work your way up to 10 to 15 repetitions. Increase the weight when the curls start to feel easy.

Triceps Kickbacks

The muscles along the back of your upper arms are called the triceps. If they become too flabby, though, some people might jokingly call them bat wings. There is good news, however: You can quickly make the backs of your arms shapely with this exercise, using an exercise bench and a 2-pound dumbbell (to start).

(1) Stand with your right side next to a bench and hold a 2-pound dumbbell in your left hand. Bending at your hips, lean forward and place your right hand on the bench. Make sure that your back is flat and parallel to the floor. Keeping your left foot flat on the floor, place your right knee along the edge of the bench as shown, making sure that your knee is directly under your hip. Squeezing your shoulder blades together, pull your left arm up while bending your elbow, until the point of your elbow is a few inches above your back. Pause for a moment.

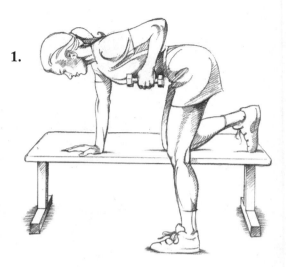

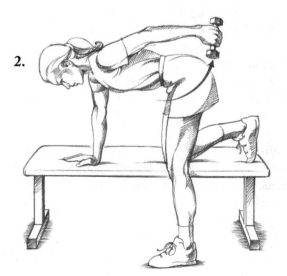

(2) Then move your forearm down, back, and up in an arc, straightening your elbow as much as possible for maximum results. The final position of the dumbbell should be well above the level of your back, but it should get there with lifting, not swinging. Slowly lower your arm to the starting point.

Do one set of 4 repetitions, then repeat with your right arm. Gradually increase the routine to 20 reps per arm using a 5-pound dumbbell. To progress further, work up to three sets: 10 reps per arm with a 5-pound dumbbell for the first set; 8 to 10 reps per arm with an 8-pound dumbbell for the second set; and 15 to 20 reps per arm with a 5-pound dumbbell for the third set.

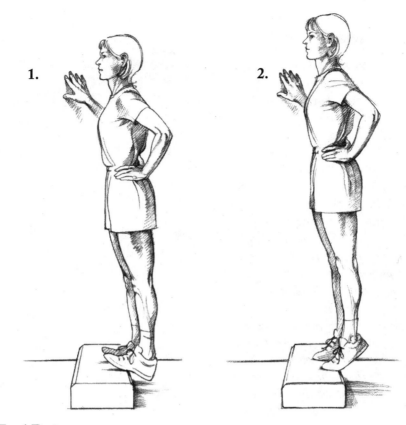

1.

2.

Heel Raises

It's a gargantuan word: gastrocnemii. So fitness folks call the big muscles in the back of the calves the gastrocs for short. If you build and firm both of these babies, they'll make your ankles look slim—even if you have naturally thick anklebones and Achilles tendons. The bottom line is a shapelier leg line. To do this toning move you need an exercise step. Or you can do it on the bottom step of a staircase.

(1) With the balls of your feet on the edge of the step and your heels hanging off the edge, lower yourself as far as you can without tottering backward. Sink until you feel a slight stretch in both your calf muscles and your Achilles tendons.

(2) Then raise your heels as high as you can, while keeping your back and legs straight. Hold this position for a second or two, then return to the starting position and repeat.

Start with one set of 3 to 4 repetitions. Gradually increase the number of reps to 15 to 20. Work your way up to three sets: 10 reps in the first set; 15 reps in the second set, holding an 8- to 10-pound dumbbell in one hand at your side; and 20 to 25 reps in the third set, still holding the dumbbell.

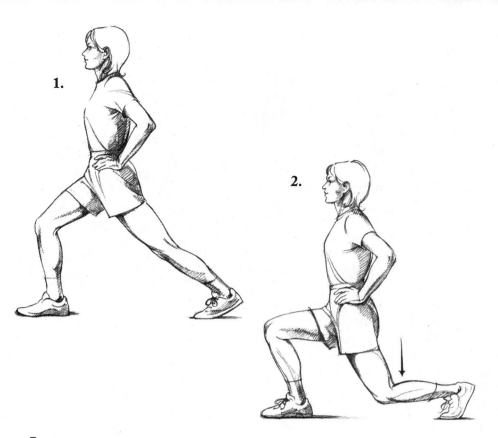

Lunges

Thighs—they're surely the front-runners in the contest for least popular body parts. Make them fit, firm, and fine by working the quadriceps muscles, or quads, on the front of your upper legs.

(1) Stand in a well-balanced position, with your feet slightly more than hip-width apart. Step forward with your right leg, using as long a stride as possible.

(2) Keeping your trunk erect, lower yourself until your hip muscles begin to feel taut.

When you've developed good flexibility in doing this exercise, you should be able to lightly touch the floor with the knee of your rear leg in a relaxed, slightly bent position. Shift your weight backward, and take as many small steps as needed with your right leg to return to a standing position. Repeat with your left leg.

Start with 3 repetitions per leg and work your way up to 20 reps per leg. To progress further, gradually work up to these three sets: 5 to 8 reps per leg for the first set; 10 reps per leg, holding 5-pound dumbbells if you're a beginner or 10-pound dumbbells if you're at an intermediate level, for the second set; and 15 to 20 reps per leg using 5-pound dumbbells for the third set.

Hip Extensions

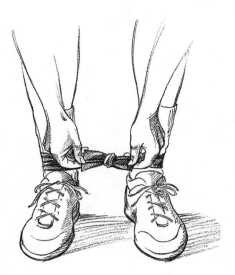

The gluteus maximus is the bulkiest—and, for some of us, the balkiest—muscle in the body. It's the muscle in each buttock; the more we shape the glutes, the less we leave to chance in this area. To do this exercise you will need an exercise mat and an exercise band. To begin, wrap the exercise band very loosely around your ankles and tie the ends into a half-bow (only one end has a loop), as shown in the illustration at right.

(1) Kneeling on a mat, lower yourself until your elbows and forearms rest on the mat and your weight is balanced on your knees and forearms. Slide part of the band down your left foot and latch it over the top of that foot. Extend your right leg straight back so that your toes rest on the floor.

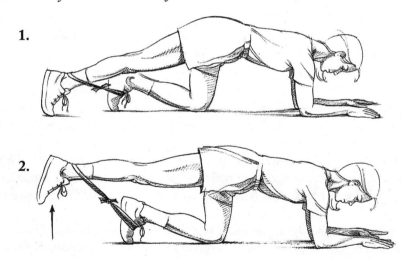

1.

2.

(2) Slowly lift your right leg no higher than your buttocks, and hold it in the raised position for a few seconds, resisting the pressure of the exercise band. Slowly return your right toes to the floor.

Do one set of 8 repetitions with your right leg, then switch to your left leg. Gradually increase the number of sets until you're doing three sets with each leg, switching from your right leg to your left leg for each set. And gradually decrease the length of the band so that it offers you more resistance. To protect and strengthen your back, hold your mid-section in a tight contraction and keep your back straight while you do the exercise.

1.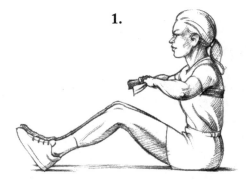

2.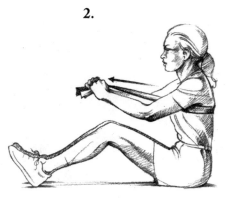

Horizontal Chest Presses

Sorry, you can't increase the actual size of your breasts by body shaping. But you can firm and tone the pectoral muscles that lie beneath them, and that will make your breasts look fuller. Toning your chest muscles will give you a natural breast lift. You will need an exercise band to do these presses.

(1) While either standing or sitting, place an exercise band across your back so that it stretches horizontally across both shoulder blades. Your hands should be positioned near your armpits as they grip the ends of the band, with your palms facing down. Take up the slack until the band feels snug across your back.

(2) Slowly press your hands and arms forward, keeping your palms down. Return to the starting position with a single, fluid motion.

Do one set of 8 chest presses. Gradually increase to three sets of 8 repetitions. And shorten the band to make it more snug so that it offers more resistance.

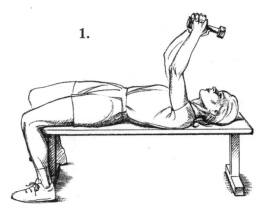

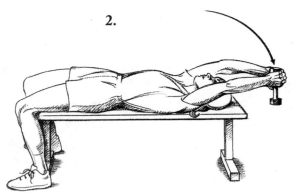

Pullovers

This is another move that firms pectoral muscles. You will need a 5-pound dumb-bell (to start).

(1) Lie on your back on a padded exercise bench, with your head near one end of the bench and your feet flat on the floor, positioned shoulder-width apart. Grasp one end of a 5-pound dumbbell with both hands. Raise it directly overhead, with your arms fully extended. This is your starting position.

(2) Keep your arms relatively straight and lower them backward until the bottom end of the dumbbell reaches a point even with or slightly below the level of your back. Allow your arms to bend just enough to prevent uncomfortable stress on your elbows. Then return the dumbbell to the overhead position. Relax and repeat.

Start with 2 or 3 repetitions. Gradually increase to 15 reps, using a 10-pound dumbbell. To progress beyond that, work up to three sets: 10 reps using a 5-pound dumbbell for the first set; 8 to 10 reps using the heavier dumbbell for the second set; and 15 reps using the heavier dumbbell for the third set.

Cooldown Stretches

When your workout is through, shake your legs and walk around for about 5 minutes. Then, stretch. This elongates your muscles, keeping them flexible and preventing them from tightening up. Do each of these two stretches slowly and deliberately, reaching and bending without bouncing.

Figure-4 Stretches

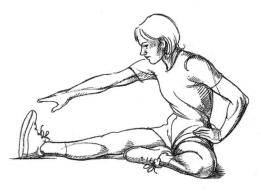

Sit on the floor on a mat, with your right leg straight in front of you and your toes pointing up. Bend your left knee to place your left heel against the inside of your right thigh, close to your crotch. Meanwhile, try to keep your left knee as close to the floor as possible.

Bending from your hips, not from your waist, slowly reach out with your right hand as though trying to touch your right toes or ankle. Don't arch your back; just maintain the natural curvature of your spine. Hold the position for 30 seconds, return to the start position, then reverse leg positions and stretch your left hand toward your left toes for another 30 seconds. Finally, repeat this stretch, starting with your right leg bent and your left leg straight.

Lying Side Stretches

Lie on your back on a mat with your feet together and your arms straight out to the sides. Keeping your left leg fully extended on the floor, slowly lift your right leg in the air, keeping your right knee slightly bent. Then, without bending your left knee, rotate your right hip and stretch your right leg straight across your body. Keep both hands on the floor. Hold this position for 30 seconds, continuing to stretch without bouncing. Return to the start, and repeat the stretch a second time. Then do the same exercise again with your left leg, repeating it twice.

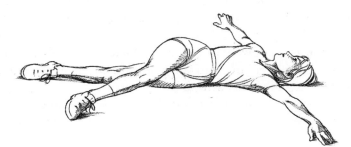

34

Tighten Your Tummy—Fast

What's the usual advice for someone who wants to have a flat belly? Maybe something like "Do a thousand sit-ups and call me when you can't move anymore."

That's no way to live. Not only that but experts say that you can do thousands of sit-ups (or "crunches") a month and still not get the results that you want. The grain of truth in the thousands-of-crunches theory is that the right kind of abdominal exercise can tighten up your abdominal muscles. And tightening your abdominal muscles is an important part of flattening your belly. (The other key ingredients, of course, are a low-fat, moderate-calorie diet; aerobic exercise; and strength training.)

Just doing plain, old sit-ups, though, probably won't help you much in the bulging-tummy department. But the right program of abdominal exercises, done in the right way, can. "Most people learn to do abdominal exercises the wrong way," says Jeffrey Young, M.D., assistant professor of physical medicine and rehabilitation at Northwestern University Medical School in Chicago. "If your form is off, no matter how hard you work and how many repetitions you do, you're not getting the full benefit of the exercise."

So here's a really smart tummy-tightening regimen recommended by our experts—one that you can easily handle even if you haven't done a sit-up since high school.

Isolate Those Abdominal Muscles

The most important part of this program is what goes on in your head during it. Here's what you need to be thinking about to get the most out of your efforts.

"When most people do crunches or other conventional abdominal exercises, they're recruiting at least three muscle groups: the abdominals, the hip flexors, and some of the quadriceps, or thigh muscles," says Peter Francis, Ph.D., director of the biomechanics lab at San Diego State University in California. That means that whatever benefit is being gained from the exercise is being spread out over all three muscle groups, even though the point was to work just the abdominals—abs, for short. But if your abs do all the work, they'll respond quicker by getting stronger and tighter. "Opening up people's awareness of what it is that they're doing allows them to consciously activate the targeted muscles, making the exercise much more effective."

Here's an exercise from Dr. Francis to help you better focus on your abs during any abs workout. While standing, place the thumb of your left hand on the bottom of your rib cage. With your fingers spread wide, place your middle finger of the same hand on the front of your hipbone. Slowly kick your left foot forward, 6 to 12 inches off the floor. That's pure hip flexion. You should notice that the distance between the ribs and pelvis (or between your thumb and middle finger) does not change.

Now for pure abdominal flexion. Shift all your weight to your right foot. Your left foot should be lightly touching the floor. Keeping your left leg loose, contract your abdominal muscles by pulling your rib cage and pelvis toward each other. (Your leg will move a little.) This is kind of like doing a mini-crunch while standing, but nothing above your chest moves. If you're doing it correctly, the distance between your thumb and middle finger should decrease by about ½ inch.

Besides teaching you what true abdominal contraction feels like, this exercise is good to practice almost anywhere for some added toning and tightening. Just remember to exercise both your left and right sides. "It sounds terribly easy," says Dr. Francis. "But if you put electrodes on the abdominals during this simple exercise, you would see bursts of activity in the major abdominal muscles."

In any exercise for abdominal strengthening, you need to make sure that your abs alone are getting the workout. To do that while doing a crunch involves four important steps.

Step 1: Lie on the floor with your knees bent and your feet flat and close to your buttocks, and completely relax your abdominal muscles. (Your lower back will be slightly curved, and your tummy may stick out a bit.) This relaxed stage gives you a baseline during the exercise so that you can better distinguish when your abs are getting all the attention and when they're not.

Step 2: Without moving any other parts of your body, tense your abs by slightly pulling your rib cage toward your pelvis. "This allows you to focus on exactly which muscle you want to use to lift you up," Dr. Francis says. "It's going to take longer to do a sit-up, but what you're really doing is going for quality rather than quantity."

Step 3: Tilt your pelvis so that your lower back stays flat on the floor as you curl and release. This is the secret to belly-tightening crunches. One study found that when people maintained a pelvic tilt, abdominal muscle activity doubled compared with when the pelvis wasn't stabilized. "When you do sit-ups incorrectly, you activate only the upper abdominals," Dr. Young says. "To work the lower abdominals, you have to engage the pelvis."

Hint: To find out if your pelvis is in proper alignment, have a friend try to slide her hand under your back while you do crunches. If she can get it under there, your form is getting sloppy and you should stop. To improve your staying power, practice holding a pelvic tilt while you lift and lower each leg. Remember, you want quality not quantity.

Step 4: Relax your abs and begin again.

Get Off the Fast Track

The best muscle development comes from controlled tension on muscles. Keeping your abdominal exercises slow, instead of popping off the floor, prevents momentum from helping out the abs. "A few slow crunches are far better than 100 fast crunches," says Wayne Westcott, Ph.D., strength training consultant to the YMCA of the United States of America, based in Quincy, Massachusetts.

How slow is slow enough? About 7 seconds for each repetition—3 seconds on the lifting stage, hold for a second, and then 3 seconds on the lowering stage. It's especially important to keep the movement slow on the lowering phase of the exercise. Often people flop back onto the floor when during crunches, and they're missing out on half of the exercise.

Your Personal Tummy-Toning Level

Since this program is designed for all levels of experience, here's how to determine how many crunches you need to do each week. (You'll need a friend or family member to assist you.)

1. Lie on a carpeted floor or an exercise mat, and get in proper crunch position: knees bent, feet flat on the floor, fingertips lightly touching the sides of your head, and elbows out to the sides. The objective is to do as many perfect crunches as possible. Keep them slow—3 seconds to lift your head and shoulders, pause for a second with the abs fully contracted, and then 3 seconds to lower your body.

2. Check for perfect form. This is where your partner comes in. Have her count aloud one-one-thousand, two-one-thousand, three-one-thousand to ensure that you don't cheat. At the same time, she should check to be sure that on each crunch your shoulder blades are coming off the floor about 3 inches—about the width of her hand. As soon as you're unable to do the crunches in perfect form anymore, stop.

3. Do the arithmetic. Start with the number of perfect crunches that you just did. Call this your score. If your score is between:

1 and 5, subtract 1 from your score:	_____.	You are at Level A.
6 and 10, subtract 2 from your score:	_____.	You are at Level B.
11 and 15, subtract 3 from your score:	_____.	You are at Level C.
16 or more, subtract 4 from your score:	_____.	You are at Level D.

This is your number of reps per set; that is, the number of times that you need to repeat the crunch without taking a break. You'll need to do three sets of each crunch described.

4. At the end of each week, retest yourself as described above. This gives you your number of reps per set for the next week. If you haven't advanced to the next level—for instance, if your score was in Level A all week, and it's still in Level A—repeat last week's workout.

If you scored lower than 4, get started by practicing the pelvic tilts described in this chapter for a week. Then take the test again. Once you're able to complete at least four perfect crunches, you're ready to begin the following three-week regimen.

Your 21-Day Smart Abs Workout

Now here's the routine. Do three sets of each of the exercises—the crunch, crunch with a twist, and reverse crunch—using your personal number of repetitions. For best results, work your abdominal muscles five days a week.

The program is broken into weeklong segments to provide progressive resistance—the same way that you increase the amount of weight that you lift when doing body-toning exercises—by changing the positions of your arms and/or legs each week. That way, your abs will be challenged without upping your repetitions to exorbitant numbers.

During Week 1, you will learn the simplest way to do a basic tummy-tightening crunch—with your feet flat on the floor and your arms crossed on your chest. This firms the rectus abdominis, the large muscle across your tummy, running from the lower border of your rib cage to your pubic area. Next, you'll tone the oblique muscles along the sides of your waist by performing a crunch with a twist. Finally, your Week 1 daily workout concludes with a reverse crunch, a move that calls on your abdominal muscles to actually lift your hips slightly off the floor.

Once you've completed Week 1, reassess how many crunches you can do. If you're able to advance to the next level of perfect crunches, you can move on to Week 2. If not, spend a few more days, preferably another week, on Week 1 exercises, then test yourself again.

All along, be sure to follow the directions closely. Stop if you feel strain or pain in any area. When you do the crunch and crunch with a twist, be careful not to yank yourself up by your neck or head. And rest if you need to. Also, be aware that while toning will firm the abdominal muscles, aerobic exercise, such as a walking program, will burn off the coat of fat that covers them.

The Crunch

Lie on the floor and concentrate on pulling your rib cage and pelvis toward each other as you slowly curl your head and shoulders off the floor. Keep your head and neck in line by imagining that you're holding a softball between your chin and your chest. When your hands are by your ears, don't pull on your head.

Do three sets of crunches at least five days a week for best results. Use your personal tummy-toning level to determine how many crunches you should perform in each set.

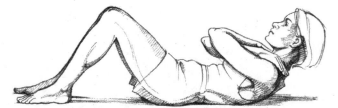

Week 1
Knees bent, feet on floor, arms crossed on chest

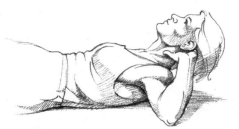

Week 2
Knees bent, feet on floor, fingers behind head

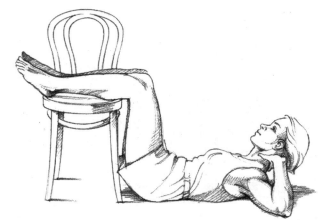

Week 3
Knees bent, legs on chair, fingers behind head

Crunch with a Twist

Lie on the floor and concentrate on pulling your rib cage and pelvis toward each other as you slowly curl your head and shoulders off the floor. Keep your head and neck in line by imagining that you're holding a softball between your chin and your chest. As you curl upward, twist your upper body to the left and concentrate on pulling your right shoulder toward your left knee.

Do three sets of crunches on each side, using your personal tummy-toning level to determine how many crunches you should perform in each set. Perform the crunch with a twist at least five days a week.

Week 1
Knees bent, arms on chest

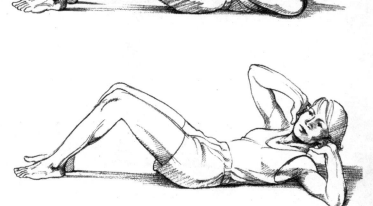

Week 2
Knees bent, fingers behind head

Week 3
Knees bent, legs on chair, fingers behind head

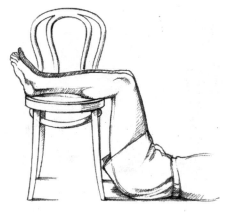

Reverse Crunch

    Contract your abdominals, pressing your back into the floor, so that your hips come 1 to 2 inches off the floor. Hold and then lower.

    Do three sets of crunches at least five days a week for best results. Use your personal tummy-toning level to determine how many crunches you should perform in each set.

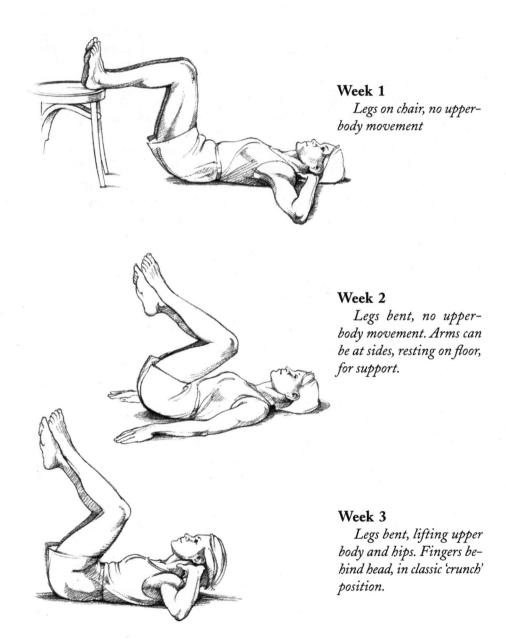

Week 1
    Legs on chair, no upper-body movement

Week 2
    Legs bent, no upper-body movement. Arms can be at sides, resting on floor, for support.

Week 3
    Legs bent, lifting upper body and hips. Fingers behind head, in classic 'crunch' position.

Advanced Abs Workout

Once you are able to do at least 16 perfect crunches, you can graduate to this advanced program. Whether your goal is a washboard stomach or you'd just like some variety in your abs program, here are some challenging variations to keep you motivated.

Extend your upward reach. The farther your arms are away from your trunk, the harder it makes a crunch. "You're changing your center of gravity to add to the difficulty," says Dr. Westcott. For example, try holding a 5-pound bag of flour in one hand while your elbow is bent. Compare that with holding it with your arm extended. You will think that it got heavier. Your abs will feel the same way when your arms are extended over your head.

Get a leg—or two—up. Extending your legs straight up in the air knocks out any assistance from the thigh muscles, and you have to work harder to stabilize the pelvis.

Fight gravity. Performing abdominal exercises on an incline (head pointing down for crunches) is harder work because you're working against gravity. There's just one catch—don't hook your feet on the holders if you're using a traditional incline board. That allows your lower body muscles to help with the work.

part six

Energizers for Your Mind, Body, and Mood

6

the Hormone Connection

Most women are all too familiar with the teeth-on-edge tension that comes just before menstruation: dreaded premenstrual syndrome, or PMS.

But did you know that the subtle rise and fall of estrogen and progesterone, hormones produced by your ovaries, may orchestrate a complex ballet of your emotions and abilities at other times during the month as well? Think of estrogen and progesterone as co-workers with wildly different personalities. The demands of some projects call for the positive attitude and energetic drive of estrogen, while progesterone's calm focus is best for other tasks, according to Elizabeth Hampson, Ph.D., associate professor of psychology at the University of Western Ontario in London, Ontario, who has spent years studying hormonal fluctuations.

Dr. Hampson found that when estrogen levels are high—before ovulation and about a week before menstruation—women's fine motor skills tend to be at their best. Peaks in motor skills might help you type a report quickly and accurately, perform Bach to perfection on the piano, or run strings of numbers correctly on an adding machine.

How else can you use subtle hormone swings to your advantage?

❖ *Schedule speeches* or tough meetings with your boss about 8 to 12 days after the first day of your period, suggests Dr. Hampson. With estrogen levels high and progesterone low, your verbal fluency skills are likely to be at their prime right about then.

❖ *Wait to redecorate.* Estrogen isn't always a skill builder. In fact, Dr. Hampson found that women do best on tests measuring spatial ability during their menstrual periods, when estrogen levels are low. That's when you might want to reorganize a packed freezer, rearrange furniture, or plan the layout of next summer's flower garden.

❖ *Outwit your blues.* Progesterone may be partially to blame when your mood sours, after ovulation, during the second half of your menstrual cycle, says Elizabeth Lee Vliet, M.D., medical director and founder of HER Place women's health centers in Tucson and Dallas, in her book *Screaming to Be Heard: Hormonal Connections Women Suspect and Doctors Ignore.* If you're contemplating ending a relationship, quitting a job, or confronting a co-worker, think it through during times when you're less influenced by hormone-driven irritability, depression, and tearfulness.

Dr. Hampson notes that many things that we do in the course of a day draw on more than one skill or ability, so hormonal effects on your life may be subtle.

Escape from the Perfection Trap

35

Julia Califano always had trouble making decisions, large and small. She looked for the perfect coffee table for her apartment for five years. She cried when it was time to pick out window shades for her bedroom Both the must be other options," she pleaded with the saleswoman over and over.

Paralyzing indecision may sound funny, but it's no joke. Chronic indecisiveness is one of the hallmarks of perfectionism, a trait that psychologists often call obsessive personality and define as "the neurotic need to avoid errors or mistakes."

Contrary to what many people think, perfectionism isn't a virtue. It doesn't mean that you're perfect or even that you think you are. "Perfectionism should not be confused with the pursuit of excellence," says psychiatrist Allan Mallinger, Ph.D., associate clinical professor of psychiatry at the University of California, San Diego, School of Medicine and co-author of *Too Perfect*. "We all want to do and be our best, and no one wants to make mistakes."

But the healthy achiever is able to turn her perfection-seeking switch off. "For instance, a brain surgeon knows that she must be nearly flawless in the operating room, but not when it comes to picking out a shirt or cooking dinner for friends," Dr. Mallinger explains. "Many perfectionists feel the need to be faultless in almost everything they do."

Perfectionism: One Source of Imperfect Health

It's no surprise that women who expect a great deal of themselves—and others—tend to be more irritable than the rest of us. But did you know that perfectionists may also get sick more often? A recent study of more than 9,000 managers found that self-described perfectionists had a 75 percent higher rate of illnesses (such as migraines, heart trouble, digestive woes, and depression) than their more laid-back counterparts.

"In their quests to be flawless, perfectionists often become very dissatisfied with themselves, and that creates a lot of tension, anxiety, and stress," says Lorri Lafferty, Ph.D., clinical psychologist and chief operating officer of Human Synergistics International in Detroit, the management consulting firm that conducted the decade-long study. The catch-22 is that this fallout may result in more sick days and less productivity in the long run.

Perfectionists can change their ways to develop a healthier work style. The first two steps are accepting that it's okay not to be in control of everything and that it's fine to be merely sufficient at some tasks in your life. Give yourself plenty of time to let these two attitudes seep into your way of thinking. "Once you change your mindset, a more relaxed work style will flow from that," says Dr. Lafferty.

Unlearning perfectionism may be especially important for women for two reasons. Women often have the additional responsibility of child care, which adds to stress. And, if you expect perfection from your children, you may be raising the next generation of stressed-out perfectionists.

HEALTH FLASH

Excellence-seekers set attainable goals, while perfectionists set unrealistically high standards. "They demand a higher quality of performance than the situation requires," says Steven Hendlin, a clinical psychologist in Irvine, California.

Perfect Agony

Take Ginny Cannon, a retired teacher in Pawling, New York. For most of her life, she's been driven to be the best at everything she's done—the perfect teacher, mother, wife, homemaker, and hostess. "No matter how busy I was with work or the kids, the house had to be absolutely spotless," she says. "I had a strict routine. On Mondays, I vacuumed. On Tuesdays, I dusted. And so on."

When planning a dinner party, "I started preparing two weeks ahead, and I obsessed over every detail. The bathroom fixtures had to be sparkling, the napkins had to match the season, the menu had to be beyond compare," she says. "On the day of the party, I snapped at everyone in the family. I thought that if I could get everything perfect, I could relax. But it never worked that way. It got so bad that I hoped that people would just drop in unexpectedly so that I didn't have to put myself through all that agony."

So it goes with perfectionism. Even when these high-aiming types do meet their goals, they rarely take pleasure in the accomplishment.

When Nothing Is Good Enough

If all this sounds eerily familiar, don't be too hard on yourself: Some scientists think that perfectionism, like other personality traits, may be largely inborn. Studies by the National Institute of Aging suggest that conscientiousness, a characteristic of perfectionists, is one of the five basic building blocks of personality. (The others are agreeableness, extroversion, neuroticism, and openness.)

Of course, life experiences also play a role in honing the perfectionist personality. For instance, perfectionist parents—for instance, a mother who is compelled to redo a young daughter's attempts at making her bed—often spawn like-minded kids. "If parents are critical and hard to please, children may wind up feeling loved only when they perform perfectly," says Susan Krauss Whitbourne, a clinical psychologist at the University of Massachusetts in Amherst. This sense of not measuring up can carry on into adulthood. "Perfectionists often unconsciously believe that acknowledging their faults and weaknesses makes them unworthy of love," she adds.

Society plays its part, too. "Our culture values people who have prestigious jobs and make a great deal of money," says Hendlin. "A child learns early on that she must get good grades, go to a top college, and enter a high-paying profession to compete in a world where there's little room for failure."

Whatever forces conspire to create perfectionists, their underlying motivation remains the same. If they can avoid making mistakes or poor decisions and if they excel at everything that they do, they'll never have to face criticism, rejection, failure, or humiliation.

A Self-Defeating Outlook

Obsessive women pay a high price for their immoderation, however. Sure, these high achievers tend to accomplish many things and win approval from peers, parents, and employers. And they're usually conscientious, honest, hard-working, responsible, and highly self-motivated. But the drive for perfection can also be self-defeating. For one thing, it can take a perfectionist forever to get anything done, adding frustrating hours to an already long day.

"They need to relentlessly improve and polish every detail, no matter how inconsequential," says Dr. Mallinger. "As a result, they wind up turning out 2 units of A-plus work rather than 10 units of A-minus."

Perfectionists are also apt to be master procrastinators, both because they fear that they won't be able to meet their own high standards and because, when utter thoroughness is a must, every project looms impossibly large. Something as simple as writing a thank-you note becomes an overwhelming task to do, because the message must be perfectly composed. And so the thank-you note is delayed and delayed, until it becomes too late to send it.

Perfectionists are often reluctant to try new things, which can hold them back from what might be life-enhancing experiences. Cannon, for instance, has always avoided athletic pursuits, not because she's not interested, but because she doesn't feel that she's a natural athlete. "I don't like being a beginner," she confesses.

In many cases perfectionism also affects spouses, kids, co-workers, and employees. "Unrealistically high expectations are bad enough when applied to yourself, but when applied to other people, they can be disastrous," says Whitbourne.

Learning to Accept Imperfection

The first step toward change, say the experts, is to be aware of perfectionism's toll. "Look at what seeking perfection is costing you in terms of lost productivity, procrastination, impact on your family and co-workers, and your ability to enjoy life," says Dr. Mallinger. A cost-benefit analysis helped Cannon ease up. "I realized that keeping the house spotless was preventing me from doing things that I really enjoy, and it wasn't worth the sacrifice," she says. "Now the house isn't as neat, but I'm happier."

Awareness isn't always enough, however. You have to break your self-defeating habits. Below are five techniques for becoming a less perfect person.

Aim for average. Imagine what a B-minus worker would accomplish, and force yourself to perform to that level in the interest of getting the job done.

"You'll be amazed not only by the amount of work that you produce but also

Are You Too Perfect for Your Own Good?

Circle any of the following scenarios that sound familiar or that you can easily relate to.

1. You have just finished waxing the floor when you notice a few smudges. Instead of spot cleaning the floor, you decide to redo the entire job.
2. A paper that you've written has just been accepted by a highly respected professional journal, and your peers have been congratulating you on your success. Instead of feeling happy, however, you find yourself dwelling on the fact that it's not the most prestigious publication in the field.
3. Your child comes home from school with a score of 96 percent on a social studies test, and you can't help wondering what happened to those other four points.
4. As a result of company downsizing, you've had to take on additional responsibilities at work. Instead of being a little less thorough on every task, you run yourself ragged, putting in longer and longer hours so that you get everything done to your standard.
5. You're preparing a new dish for dinner. Halfway through, you realize that the recipe calls for fresh basil, and all you have is the dried variety. You stop what you're doing and run to the grocery store.
6. You promised yourself that you'd go to the gym during your lunch hour. Now you're running late, and you realize that you'll have only 40 minutes to exercise—not enough time for your usual workout. Still, you force yourself to do every last leg lift and stomach crunch, and subsequently miss the beginning of an important staff meeting back at the office.
7. A big report is due at work tomorrow, and you stay up late perfecting every detail. The next morning, it still doesn't read right. You continue to polish it—and you miss the deadline.

What your score means: If you circled three or more of these scenarios, chances are you have a perfectionist streak. You might benefit from taking stock of your ultrahigh standards and cutting yourself (and others) a little slack.

by its quality," says Dr. Mallinger. "It won't suffer as much as you think, and it may even improve. With fewer trivial details distracting you, your main points will carry more force and be clearer."

Give yourself clear deadlines. If you get sidetracked by details or anxious thoughts about how a project will be evaluated, slam your palm down on the desk, and say, "Move!" Then take a deep breath, refocus on your goal, and keep going.

Quash judgmental thoughts. Though your negative assessment of a friend or co-worker might occasionally be accurate, the truth is that people are imperfect, and making critical observations tends to hurt more than it helps.

Break big goals into small ones. "Realize that several small goals will add up to a major accomplishment," Whitbourne suggests.

Take risks. Tell yourself that all you can do is give it your best shot.

Taking that last bit of advice herself, Califano recently threw caution to the wind and bought custom-made nonreturnable, light-diffusing shades for her bedroom. At first, her worst fear was realized: The room was too bright in the morning. Then she discovered that this was a blessing in disguise. All that sunshine gets her going earlier, even on weekends, and that gives her more hours in the day to shop for the perfect coffee table.

36

Conquer the Fatigue Monsters

Energy is a quirky commodity. Sometimes, you get a good night's sleep, yet still you're exhausted. At other times, you feel wide awake, happy, and vital, despite a tough workday.

Wonder what is going on? The fact is, energy—whether it's physical, mental, or emotional—is a mind/body thing. How you think, and how you take care of your body, profoundly influence vitality. And some surprising techniques such as deep breathing, daily affirmations, and forgiveness can have far-reaching effects on your energy levels.

If your batteries need a charge, try these four techniques, guaranteed by experts to improve mental alertness and put some zing back into your life.

Put Affirmations to Work

Affirmations are designed to help change the often-unconscious stream of negative thoughts or emotions that go through our minds, explains Susan Jeffers, Ph.D., author of *End the Struggle and Dance with Life* and *Feel the Fear and Do It Anyway.* "Affirmations are a way to change the negative chatter that goes on in our heads all the time into something positive," she says.

And positive thinking, experts say, is more than just a pleasant interlude. Studies suggest that the more you believe in your own abilities, the better you're likely to do, says Albert Ellis, Ph.D., president of the Institute for Rational-

Love, Honor, Obey— And Fetch

"The contentment that my husband makes me feel on a really good day is the feeling that my dog gives me every day," each of several happily married women said to Karen Allen, Ph.D., a research scientist at the State University of New York in Buffalo. When she tested this claim with a study, Dr. Allen found that highly stressed women and men feel the most calm when good old Fido is nearby.

In a study of 240 happily married couples, 120 of whom owned canines and 120 of whom didn't, Dr. Allen measured the stress-busting possibilities of dogs and spouses. When study participants with high-stress, Type A personalities were given stressful tasks like doing mental arithmetic problems, making speeches, or having their hands plunged into cold water, they remained calmest when their dogs were their only attendants. Stress was highest when spouses sat in the room with them. Even being alone was less stressful than being with a spouse.

That's a good reason to entice your pooch to stay nearby when there's a stressful job to be done. "We think that this is because dogs are not evaluative," says Dr. Allen. In other words, they love you just the way you are—whether you can solve the math problem or not.

Emotive Therapy in New York City. "Affirmations may temporarily make people feel better about themselves, so they do better," he says.

From Blue to Sunny

The reason that affirmations work, says Dr. Jeffers, is that you can't think two thoughts at the same time. By putting positive thoughts in your mind, you automatically displace the negative, and that can have powerful effects.

One of Dr. Jeffers's favorite affirmations is *I let go and I trust*. "As soon as you let go—not feeling like you have to control everything, which you can't do, anyway—you have more energy," she says. "I mean, whew. You're not fighting so hard." To get the most from affirmations, here's what experts advise.

Focus on what you need and want. For affirmations to be most effective, they must be specific and focused. Pick an area of your life that you want to address, decide what you want, and formulate a concise statement that expresses the desired outcome, recommends Douglas Bloch, author of *Words That Heal*. Let's say, for instance, that you want to eat more fresh fruits and vegetables, and less fat and sugar. Your affirmation could be, "I eat only healthy foods that support my body."

Use the first person and the present tense. Affirmations are most effective when you say "I," in terms of "I want" or "I need" or "I am," according to Bloch. "When you say, 'You are healthy,' it's as though you are talking to somebody else. When you say, 'I am healthy,' you're addressing it directly to yourself and you are owning it. It's more powerful," he says.

Be positive. Which sounds better to you: "I am not poor" or "I am prosperous"? Because the subconscious usually doesn't hear the word "not," there's always the danger that an affirmation expressed negatively will send the wrong message. "You can use a negative, but only if you follow it quickly with a positive," Bloch says.

Say it aloud. "There's something about hearing your affirmations in your own voice that makes them more powerful," Dr. Jeffers says.

Repeat affirmations morning and night. Early morning and late night tend to be when people are most open to suggestion and, more destructively, when they tend to ruminate on negatives, Dr. Jeffers says. Say your affirmations when you wake up and before you fall asleep. These are almost always good times to repeat them, she says.

The Power of Deep Breathing

When you're relaxed, you breathe slowly and deeply, inhaling sumptuous streams of vital, energy-producing oxygen. When you're tense, however, you breathe lightly and rapidly, delivering less oxygen to your body's cells.

To a blood cell, stress is suffocation, says Larry J. Feldman, Ph.D., a leader of workshops on stress and burnout and author of *Feeling Good Again*. "When you're tense, your brain increases its demand for oxygen," he says. "But your shallow breaths decrease the intake of oxygen. Anxiety is the expression of each cell in the body suffocating." That's bad news on the pep and vitality front. Since each of us requires about 5,000 gallons of air every day, good breathing is important.

The good news is that by learning how to breathe correctly, you can increase your energy level. "It sounds so simple. Just take fairly deep, comfortable breaths and long exhalations, and you'll relax," says Martin Pierce, director of the Pierce Program, a yoga center in Atlanta that teaches stress reduction, and co-author of *Yoga for Life*. But even though breathing seems automatic, studies suggest that 80 percent of us don't really know how to breathe properly. "The main problem is that many people think good breathing is good inhalation," he says. "The key is breathing out completely."

Here's the full technique you'll need for breathing for stress relief and maximum energy.

Make a balloon. "Imagine that there is a balloon in your torso, somewhere below the middle of your chest," says Pierce. "Inhale and fill up the balloon in all directions—top, bottom, forward, backward. That's the ideal inhalation." Breathe in until you feel comfortably full, but not too full.

Blow it out. Exhaling is more important than inhaling, and there is an ideal way to do it. "When you exhale, pull your lower abdomen in first, then your upper abdomen," says Pierce. "Your rib cage should come in from the sides and down from the front. Make the exhalation just a little bit longer than you think it should be. Hold it for 1/2 second before you inhale again. That should be very relaxing."

Practice. The power of proper breathing is something that you have to experience for yourself. "Reading a book about how to breathe isn't the same thing as actually doing it," says Dr. Feldman. Ideas have to get out of your head and down into your body, or you won't change.

You don't need to shoehorn in 30 minutes of deep-breathing practice at the end of a time-crunched day, says Dr. Feldman. "A short exercise several times a day for 3 to 4 minutes is probably more effective in terms of tension control than one long period."

Breathe, don't fume. The next time your hair dryer blows a fuse just before you leave for work, take about 15 slow, deep breaths. You'll feel calmer, and you'll unwind all that energy-depleting tension before it has a chance to build.

Fight Fatigue with Forgiveness

The word *forgive* comes from the Greek language. It means "to let go of." And that's exactly what forgiveness is, says Dr. Jeffers. "Forgiveness is something you do for yourself, not for the other person," she says. "If anything, forgiving helps you drop the role of being the victim and take real steps to protect and assert yourself. A victim mentality brings only upset and is an incredible waste of valuable energy."

If visions of sweet revenge still tinge your thoughts, consider this: "The best revenge is being happy—and forgiveness lets you be that," Dr. Jeffers says. But it's also important to do something about your anger. Anger can mask the fear and pain that you need to address, she adds. "It's easier to be angry and to blame than to take responsibility for your life and say, 'Wait, what do I have to do to change this?'" So feel your anger, learn from it, and then let it go, Dr. Jeffers suggests.

Here are steps that can help you deal with anger and leave that grudge behind.

Have a good holler. When you feel angry with or hurt by a person or a situation, some screaming and crying may be in order. Do this alone or with a close friend, not with the perpetrator of the offense, Dr. Jeffers recommends.

"I suggest that you drive your car to an isolated place, and scream your head off to get the rage out because it is a poison in your body," she says. "Once you do that, you will feel an incredible sense of lightness." You can start your scream

A Hug a Day

In the early 1980s, researchers confirmed what grandmas have known all along: Babies who get a lot of warm physical contact thrive better and score higher on mental tests than children who aren't cuddled. Researchers also found that as adults these people have better sex lives and less illness.

But can hugging, regardless of your age, energize your life? Researchers say that hugs, like other forms of caring touch, can help banish stress, the number one energy drainer. Studies show that a calming touch can reduce stress hormones, increase the body's production of natural killer cells (which are important for immunity), reduce pain, and normalize heart rate and breathing, says Tiffany Field, Ph.D., professor of pediatrics, psychology, and psychiatry and director of the Touch Research Institute at the University of Miami School of Medicine. What better reason to be sure that you get—and give—at least one hug a day?

therapy gently by saying, "I'm angry." From there, work up to a crescendo until you feel it coming from your deepest self, Dr. Jeffers advises.

Review the details. Forget the old saying "Forgive and forget." The real process is to remember fully and forgive, says D. Patrick Miller, author of *A Little Book of Forgiveness*. "While we do eventually forget some things that we've forgiven, that kind of forgetting takes care of itself. Trying to forget is just another means of denial."

If you can, review the event that has angered you like a slow-motion movie, two or three times, until you can observe it without getting emotionally caught up in it, suggests G. Frank Lawlis, Ph.D., psychology professor at Southwestern College in Santa Fe, New Mexico, and author of *Transpersonal Medicine*. "You want to review it enough times that you begin to feel that you are observing it as an outside witness. You may still not totally understand it, but you'll have a different perspective." Ideally, ultimately, you'll feel detachment and acceptance.

Trade places. Try putting yourself mentally in the offender's place. This is crucial to the process of forgiveness, Dr. Lawlis says. "Switch places with the person who wronged you so that you can get an understanding of that person," he says. In fact, you can get an inner dialogue going that may give you some insights into what went wrong.

Acknowledge your role. Pick up a mirror, not a magnifying glass, Dr. Jeffers says. "Do this, not to blame yourself, but to understand yourself. Instead of saying, 'Why did she do it?' ask, 'Why did I react this way? What could I have possibly contributed to this? What made me choose someone who did this?'"

Let go. Hold in your mind the image of whoever is to be forgiven, then let it slowly recede, Dr. Lawlis says. Let yourself detach emotionally from the image so that it no longer controls you.

Free Your Inner Sex Goddess

Sure, you like sex. But do you lose yourself in it? Does it make the earth shake? How many times have you thought you were in for a hot date with your mate only to feel disappointed afterward? The fact is, many women don't know what they really want in bed, let alone how to ask for it. We may even feel silly discussing sex.

Even the most sexually in-tune woman can climb to dizzying heights of passion with continued self-discovery. "You can't rest on your laurels and stick to what worked in the past," cautions Ella Patterson, a professional sex educator, president of Knowledge Concepts Educational Systems in Cedar Hill, Texas, and author of the sizzling sexual-empowerment manual *Will the Real Women...Please Stand Up!* "Sex is about growing," she explains. "Passion increases the more you explore new, uncharted territories."

What's Stopping You?

There are a bunch of reasons that many of us don't allow ourselves to explore our sexuality fully. "As women, we've been culturally trained to be passive in bed because there is still a negative connotation to being assertive," says Beverly Whipple, Ph.D., associate professor of nursing at Rutgers University in New Brunswick, New Jersey; president-elect of the American Association of Sex

The Contraceptive That Can Improve Sexual Satisfaction

If you have a good relationship with your partner, then birth control pills may bring you more sexual satisfaction than other forms of contraception, according to a survey from San Francisco State University. And among users of the Pill, those who took a version that varied the hormone dose throughout the month had the most fun of all.

In the survey of 364 college-age women, those who took the triphasic pill—a contraceptive that varies the levels of the hormone progestin throughout a woman's cycle—reported more sexual interest than women who used monophasic pills with a steady hormone dose, according to Norma McCoy, Ph.D., a professor in the psychology department at San Francisco State University and the researcher who conducted the study.

Why were the triphasic pills more, well, stimulating? "I think that it's because hormones affect sexuality, and women on triphasic pills are getting more hormones," says Dr. McCoy. Women got less progestin with the triphasic pills, and progestin can depress sexual interest, she says. Other hormones that women get in triphasic pills are testosterone and estradiol. Estradiol helps increase sensitivity to stimulation, and testosterone is thought to be the sex hormone responsible for sexual interest.

But remember, the Pill won't protect you from sexually transmitted diseases such as HIV. For safer sex, your partner must wear a condom—and the two of you should talk first about your sexual histories.

Educators, Counselors, and Therapists; and co-author of *G-Spot and Other Recent Discoveries about Human Sexuality.*

It's time to embark on a path of sexual self-discovery with a brand-new attitude. Wherever you currently are on the sexual ladder, you can still discover ways to climb to new, uncharted heights. Just follow these scintillating guidelines. And remember that while these tips are geared toward your enjoyment, your honey will be the lucky co-beneficiary of your new boldness in the bedroom.

Find out what feels good. Discover something new—your body. Are you afraid of touching yourself for self-pleasuring? Many women are. "We're not encouraged to learn about our bodies, to explore and find out what is pleasurable to us," points out Dr. Whipple. Through masturbation, you can learn a lot about the areas of your body that can arouse you.

Model your birthday suit. What do you do when you've just bought a gorgeous new suit? Chances are, you rush right home and try the outfit on all over again, complete with shoes and accessories. You look in the mirror, twirling and smiling. Shouldn't you be able to wear your birthday suit with that same sassy attitude?

To help yourself build confidence, get a full-length mirror and take a good look at yourself naked, suggests Gail Wyatt, Ph.D., a professor in the psychiatry department at the University of California, Los Angeles. Don't fret over a little flab or breasts that aren't exactly the same size. Be positive. Focus on features that you admire. Do this often. The idea is to let nudity feel natural and beautiful so that you aren't preoccupied with your body during sex. Ultimately, great sex is as much about attitude as it is attractiveness.

Find a lover with a slow hand (or tutor the one you have). "Allow yourself a slow, sensuous, and relaxed attitude toward lovemaking," advises Patterson. "The best sex comes not from doing but from allowing—allowing the sexual energy between the two of you to flow." Also, men have a tendency to think of intercourse as the main event. Remind your mate that getting there is half the fun—there's plenty of time for foreplay.

And speaking of intercourse, for some reason, once the penis enters the vagina, the tendency is to go for it. The man thrusts for as long as he can, and most of us moan and groan, "More, more, more" (or some other football cheer) to bolster his ego. We might as well be yelling "more" because he isn't doing enough. Let's get real: Some women can have orgasms during sexual intercourse, but many women need clitoral stimulation at the same time. If you need to take the initiative to get your needs met (and don't we all?), then do it. For example, why not tell your honey to place his hand on your clitoris during intercourse to give you more stimulation? Or position yourself on top for better leverage.

Make sure he gets the full thrust. In-out. In-out. Ho-hum. In-out. Why is it that some men think that the only way to get our engines started is to make like a piston in a cylinder? What about sideways or in a zigzag? "The best lover I ever had did it in a circle," says Cheryl Westcott, 35, one satisfied woman.

Or how about having him just go in, and not take his penis out? Try this technique, from *The Wonderful Little Sex Book* by William Ashoka Ross, that's guaranteed to please: Without moving, lie quietly with your lover in a complete sexual embrace. His penis should remain in your vagina for as long as 20 to 30 minutes. Only if he begins to lose his erection is movement called for, and then only subtle motions—just enough for him to regain his erection.

After a while, begin to move, but only with very slow, very soft, gradual movements—no vigorous thrusting. As this goes on and on, sensations multiply and become almost unbearable in their intensity. Eventually, this becomes so intense that you feel you can hardly stand it. (Good thing you're lying down.)

Believe that you're a sensual woman—and you will be. Not all of us feel 100 percent beautiful and sexy all the time. Don't let some perceived flaw like weight keep you from doing the love thing with your man. Take more warmup time. "Kiss and pet for a while. If you allow yourself to get really turned on, your sexual energy will compensate for your feeling that you aren't the ideal size," says Patterson, who is full-figured herself. "Tell your honey that you're not feeling good about your weight and that you need his reassurance. If he lets you see that your body turns him on, it will increase your responsiveness."

Include all five senses. Touches are titillating, but what about sexual sights, smells, sounds, and even tastes? Terri Arnold, 24, swears by scented candles, fragrant bubble baths, and beautiful, silky lingerie to make her feel ultrasexy.

Valerie Anderson, 41, likes to keep those single-serve packages of honey (the kind you get at restaurants) handy in her condom drawer for life's, um, sweeter moments.

Patterson's erotic suggestion: Bring a chilled bottle of champagne to your hot tub or bath. (If your bathtub is standard size, you may prefer to take turns bathing each other.) As you and your partner bathe, sip the champagne, pour a splash into your tub, and play with the rest. Pouring small trickles down his back or on his chest while bathing can be quite refreshing. During that time, dream up the most sensuous thing you're going to do to your lover once you get him into bed, and then share it with him. Just talking and laughing add to the pleasures of a champagne bath. For auditory ecstasy, trade erotic whispers or swoon to soft, sexy music.

Call the plays. Do you have a take-charge attitude in your daily life, yet prefer to be submissive in the bedroom? "That's fine sometimes, but a relationship in which one partner always takes the initiative and the other is always submissive is unbalanced," warns Barbara J. Brown, Ph.D., a clinical psychologist in Washington, D.C. "Sex is all about interaction and sharing."

"Everybody needs to feel nurtured and desired," adds Dr. Brown, "but women are more likely than men to express to a partner the need to be held or to be submissive at times, because it's more consistent with the traditional female role."

If you're always submissive, your partner may be secretly yearning for an occasional show of initiative. Being "taken" can be highly erotic to you, so it might be to him as well.

The above ideas are just a few of the ways that you can turn up the heat in the bedroom. Let your sense of passion, romance, fantasy, and fun guide you to many more.

Discover Your Pleasure Points

Making love is the perfect time to explore sensations with your lover, but many of us put the brakes on experimentation. Touched in certain places, we get self-conscious, squirmy, or ticklish. Or even worse, we discourage our partners from touching us.

"Sometimes it is precisely those areas that we need to have touched," says Dr. Whipple. There are 36 pleasure points on the body (such as behind the knees, under the arms, and behind the ears) and a variety of touches, she explains. Touching by hand includes stroking, patting, rubbing, squeezing, pinching, and spanking. Touching by mouth includes sucking, nuzzling, licking, and nipping. "Why not try them all," she suggests, "and see what really feels good?" Try to be pleasure-oriented, as opposed to goal-oriented, during your sexual encounter. You'll be able to enjoy the here and now and not miss the joy of the experience.

Stretch Away Stress

Does tension make your neck ache? Not surprisingly, the vulnerable juncture between head and shoulders concentrates stress and strain like no other body spot does. Why? Awkward positions, like cradling a phone between your shoulder and ear or hunching over a keyboard, take their toll. So can driving a car. Plus, we naturally tend to store tension in our necks and shoulders.

If you work at a desk job, it's probably doing a number on your neck for another reason: Such jobs are notorious neck immobilizers. Necks were meant to move. When you are outdoors, your neck naturally swivels and rotates so that your senses can receive signals from all directions.

But when you're absorbed in tasks that demand intent visual focus, like staring at a computer screen, your neck is required to lock into one position.

"Static work is very hard on your neck muscles," says Joel Press, M.D., director of the Center for Spine, Sports, and Occupational Rehabilitation at the Rehabilitation Institute of Chicago.

To keep your head steady, your neck muscles must contract and hold. When your muscles contract, they produce waste products like lactic acid, much like a car produces carbon monoxide. The pumping action of exercise helps to flush away waste and bring in fresh blood for fuel. But when working muscles are immobilized, waste products have a hard time getting out and blood has a hard time getting in. This leads to cramps and aches.

Stretching: More Essential Than Ever

As American women become more sedentary, a good stretch becomes more beneficial, says John Cianca, M.D., assistant professor of physical medicine and rehabilitation at Baylor College of Medicine in Houston. Stretching can enhance circulation, help guard against injury, neutralize stress, and, if practiced just before bedtime, even help you get a better night's sleep.

And perhaps best of all, stretching wards off the stiffening effects of aging by keeping joints flexible. "Muscles act like springs," says Dr. Cianca. "If a muscle is short and tight in its resting state, then there's no place for it to go when you contract it. The longer the muscle, the more power you can generate," he says. "Muscles are also shock absorbers for the body, and the more flexible you are, the better they work."

A gentle approach to stretching is best for beginners, recommends Dr. Cianca. "Some people who embark on a stretching program try to do things that their bodies aren't capable of. It's important to keep in mind that you're not only relaxing a muscle but you're also relaxing your whole body and your mind, too." So hold stretches for just 20 to 30 seconds each, and never stretch to the point of pain, he cautions. "Try for consistency," says Dr. Cianca. "Stretching vigorously once a week won't do as much for you as stretching briefly once a day."

HEALTH FLASH

The key to warding off any neck ache is motion. Even when you are seated at your desk, you can perform a few simple stretches every ½ hour or so.

Think of them, too, as stress breaks. Allow your eyes to close, and relax as you move slowly and take deep, even breaths. And try finishing up with a minimassage. Rub your hands together to generate heat, then lay them on your neck and knead the tissue like bread dough. Breathe, and imagine your inhalations flowing right into the tense spots. On exhalations, imagine all the tension flowing out.

How to Sit

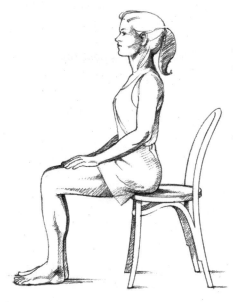

During all of the sitting stretches, keep your spine straight: Sit tall at the edge of your seat, feet flat. Stretch your torso upward, feeling your breastbone lift and your spine lengthen. Rest your hands on your thighs and relax. Breathe gently through your nose throughout the stretches.

Neck Relaxers

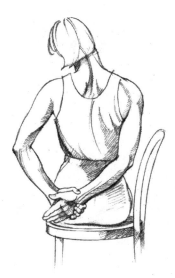

Reach your hands behind you and grasp your right wrist with your left hand. On an exhalation, slowly drop your left ear toward your left shoulder and draw your right hand to the left behind you at the same time. Maintain that position and breathe for 15 to 20 seconds, moving your chin slightly in different directions to target the spots where you feel the most tension. Don't move your head back beyond your shoulders. (Avoid full circles.) Release and pause in the center before stretching to the other side.

Head Turns

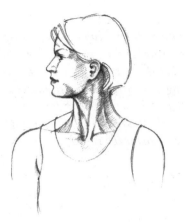

Inhale deeply, and as you exhale, slowly turn your head as far to the right as you can. Stay in this position for 10 to 15 seconds, breathing evenly and keeping your chin level. Repeat to the left.

Shoulder Rolls

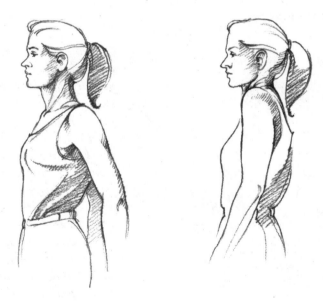

On a slow, deep inhalation, draw your shoulders up toward your ears. On an exhalation, draw your shoulders back and down in a half-circle. If you wish, pause at the top and bottom of each roll for several counts and breathe gently. Repeat for a total of three to six cycles.

Shoulder Blade Squeezes

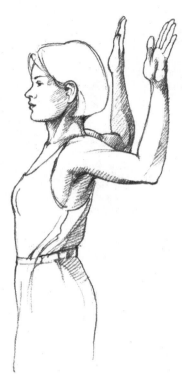

Raise your arms up to your sides with your palms facing forward. On an inhalation, draw your arms behind you, squeezing your elbows and shoulder blades toward each other. Exhale and come back to neutral. Repeat slowly 5 to 10 times.

part seven

Age-Defying Beauty Secrets

7

the Hormone Connection

Skin-Saver in a Pill?

The hormones that women take most often—birth control pills and hormone-replacement therapy (HRT)—may pay unexpected dividends for your skin. Early research shows that beyond easing night sweats and hot flashes at menopause, HRT may fight wrinkles and dry skin, too. A Belgian study found that the skin of women past menopause who took estrogen was more elastic than that of women who did not take the hormone. And at the University of California, San Francisco, School of Medicine, researchers studying 3,875 postmenopausal women discovered a significant decrease in dry skin and wrinkles among estrogenusers. The odds of wrinkling were 30 percent lower for women using estrogen, and the odds of dry skin dropped by 25 percent.

"When you're making up your list of the pluses and minuses of taking hormones, better-looking skin is definitely a plus. But it should never be the main reason to take HRT," says Karen S. Harkaway, M.D., an instructor in dermatology at the University of Pennsylvania in Philadelphia.

Estrogen may help the skin by boosting the production of collagen, the fibrous protein that gives skin its elasticity, or by slowing collagen loss that occurs with age. Other potential beauty bonuses of HRT include thicker hair and stronger nails.

Some low-dose birth control pills, meanwhile, may be as effective as antibiotics and lotions at controlling acne. When women between the ages of 15 and 46 who had moderate acne took birth control pills containing norgestimate-ethinyl estradiol for six months, 83 percent of them found that they developed significantly fewer breakouts, according to a study from the Foundation for Developmental Endocrinology in Cleveland. Women given a fake version of the Pill, as a placebo, also saw some improvement (probably because they were caring for their skin more carefully, researchers say) but still had more breakouts. The researchers note that the real Pill seemed to zap zits and that it reduced levels of testosterone, which stimulates acne.

Yet for some women, hormones have negative side effects for the skin. Two of the most common are melasma (irregular patches of darker skin pigment) and acne. If you have either problem, ask your doctor if it's possible to adjust your hormone therapy. Your skin may be reacting to the amount of estrogen or the type of progesterone that the Pill and HRT contain. You can also try over-the-counter bleaching formulas for melasma, and gentle blemish-drying lotions to fight acne.

Read This Before You Have a Facelift

Think of your skin as part plastic wrap, part gift wrap. After all, it holds your body together. It keeps out harmful environmental elements such as radiation, bacteria, viruses, and dangerous chemicals. Without it you would literally fall apart. And, it gives you personality.

Of course, none of that covering is either permanent or wrinkle-free. Smile lines around your eyes tell the world that you've been living and laughing for a while—certainly nothing to be ashamed of. Expression lines eventually crease your forehead, the skin between your eyes, and the delicate skin around your eyes. They are the result of constantly moving your face in the same patterns over a long period of time.

But of all the potential youth robbers threatening your skin, none is more destructive than the sun. A common figure cited by several doctors is that 80 percent or more of the visible aging that occurs on the skin is a result of sun exposure, a process called photoaging. Behind every wrinkle, every age spot, and every freckle, there is an afternoon spent at the beach or a picnic or a simple walk in the sunshine. More accurately, a lifetime of such moments waits until your thirties and forties to show up on your face.

Unfortunately, a lot of women don't realize that every unprotected minute spent in the sun as a child—and for most of us, there were countless, sunny hours outdoors—would show up on their faces years later, says William Cole-

C Your Way to Smoother Skin

Trusty old vitamin C is now turning up as the prime ingredient in a new generation of face creams that promise to stop the clock for aging skin. While these products are sold as cosmetics and thus have not been tested in clinical trials, researchers are discovering that vitamin C creams can shield the skin from ultraviolet (UV) light exposure and that this protection may improve signs of aging caused by sun exposure.

"Early research indicates that vitamin C serves as an antioxidant, protecting skin against damage from the sun," says Debra Price, M.D., clinical assistant professor of dermatology at the University of Miami and a dermatologist in private practice in south Florida. It may even stimulate the production of collagen, which keeps skin firm.

Dr. Price recommends a vitamin C cream called Cellex-C that was developed by a team of researchers at Duke University in Durham, North Carolina. It's available, without a prescription, through your dermatologist or by writing to Cellex-C America, 4462 Cellex-C Drive, Chestertown, MD 21690.

She says that these preparations can be useful for anyone with sun-damaged skin, discolored skin, or fine lines—though the product can cause slight skin irritation for some women.

There is no research to show how vitamin-rich creams stack up against other wrinkle fighters like a prescription tretinoin emollient cream (Renova) or over-the-counter alpha hydroxy acids, Dr. Price notes. But, she says, the most effective wrinkle warrior is you. "The best anti-aging regimen for the skin is a healthy lifestyle," she says. "That means no smoking, and wear sunscreen every single day. If you're not committed to that, then there's no point in buying these products."

HEALTH FLASH

man, M.D., clinical professor of dermatology at Tulane University School of Medicine in New Orleans. Women who have stayed out of the sun look a lot younger than those who haven't, he observes.

"Research shows that many children, by age 10, have enough sun damage to develop severe wrinkling and skin cancer later on. It's a delayed phenomenon."

Were it not for a lifetime of sun exposure, it's possible that your skin could be relatively youthful-looking up until your seventies. That is the age when intrinsic aging of skin kicks in, and studies back this up.

Outsmarting the Sun

To see the effect of the sun, doctors have looked at what happens to the outer two layers of skin, the dermis and the epidermis. The dermis is the thicker layer, which houses the sebaceous glands, or oil ducts, and the sweat glands. This layer is also filled with the collagen and elastin that make your skin tight but flexible. At the base of all that is the subcutaneous fat, which separates the dermis from the muscle and bone, insulating you from the cold.

That layer is topped off by the epidermis, a protective shield that is constantly reinforced as cells at its bottom divide and multiply, pushing the cells above them to the surface. When the very top cells get sloughed off, they're just dry and useless flakes—a miniature, invisible dust storm. These used-up cells are the materials that make up your bathtub ring and some of the dust in your house.

As sunlight exposure continues, the ridges between your dermis and epidermis keep flattening out until they completely disappear. To make things worse, the thinner the skin gets, the less tissue there is to absorb the sun's damaging ultraviolet (UV) rays and the more harmful even a small dose can be. Even reflected sunlight is damaging, and the light can be reflected off everything it touches. Sand reflects 17 percent of UV rays. Freshly fallen snow reflects more than 80 percent. This reflection can send sunlight upward to delicate areas that burn very easily, such as the top of your nose and the underside of your chin.

Photoaging doesn't just show up in the form of wrinkles. Age spots, also known as solar lentigines, are brown splotches that commonly appear on the hands and face. They're a result of the skin trying to protect itself from sun overexposure by producing an overabundance of melanin, the pigmented cells in your skin that are responsible for tanning, in uneven patches. Photoaging is also the cause of 90 percent of all skin cancer.

Save Your Face

As far as sun damage goes, what's done is done. But it's never too late to ward off crow's-feet and worry lines, says Michael Bilkis, M.D., assistant professor of dermatology at New York University School of Medicine in New York City. Here are some tactics.

Slather on sunscreen. Dermatologists sound like broken records on this point: Of everything you can do to ward off wrinkles and age spots, wearing sunscreen is the most important.

Go 15 or over. Choosing the right sunscreen can be a challenge, with sun protection factors (SPFs) ranging from 5 all the way up to 50. How can you determine how much protection you'll get from a sunscreen? It all depends on your skin type. Take the number of minutes that it takes your skin to turn red and multiply it by the SPF. If you normally burn after 20 minutes in the sun, an SPF 15 will protect you for 300 minutes, or 5 hours. (Be aware, however, that it will not be working at full strength for that length of time, so you must reapply it sooner.) Most doctors recommend an SPF of 15 or higher, according to Jonathan Weiss, M.D., assistant clinical professor of dermatology at Emory University School of Medicine in Atlanta. "I prefer one with a factor of 30 or higher."

Don't wait to renew. If you're wondering how often to put on more sunscreen, the answer is, the more frequently the better. Sunscreen gradually loses its protective power. If an SPF 15 sunscreen promises to block out 92 percent of UV rays, for instance, it's only doing that at first. After a period of time (2 hours or less), it may have diminished to an SPF of about 7. Every sunscreen has a half-life, when it's only half as effective, according to Dr. Weiss.

Up the ante to avoid beach burns. For folks who wear sunscreen every day and spend most of their days indoors, a nonwaterproof SPF 15 is adequate. Long days outside and on the beach, however, require heavy-duty protection of at least SPF 30, says Dr. Bilkis. If you spend a considerable part of your day under the sun, apply a nonwaterproof SPF 30, reapplying the sunscreen often as the day goes on.

"The lower number is for when you're not in the sun or sweating for a long time," Dr. Bilkis notes. "The other is for the beach. If you're outside sweating, you want something that will stay on your skin." A sunscreen that is truly waterproof—indicated by the label—should maintain its SPF after 80 minutes of water exposure.

Never trust a cloud. You need protection even on cloudy days, says Dr. Bilkis. Some of the ultraviolet rays aren't absorbed by the clouds; they come right through. And because you don't feel the heat, your body doesn't tell you when it's time to come inside. "The worst sunburn I ever saw was on a man who was out on his boat on a foggy day," he adds.

Make protection a daily habit. Get used to putting on a dab of sunscreen every morning, suggests Harold Brody, M.D., clinical associate professor of dermatology at Emory University School of Medicine. He recommends a combination sunscreen moisturizer with an SPF of 15, applied after you've washed and dried your face in the morning and, preferably, at least 30 minutes before you go outside. Just rub a pea-size drop on each cheek and another on your forehead. Then moisten your fingertips with water and work the sunscreen, along with the water, into your skin.

Beware: If a moisturizer simply says that it prevents aging or contains a sunscreen but it doesn't list an SPF, chances are that it won't be an effective sunscreen on its own.

Have it made with shades. Wear sunglasses every time you head outside, says Dr. Weiss. They protect the skin around your eyes to some extent and help prevent squinting, which plays a big role in expression wrinkles.

Dress for sun excess. Choose clothes that won't let those harmful rays in. Darker colors protect better than lighter ones, and tight-weave clothes are better than loose-weave, notes Dr. Weiss. "A wet white T-shirt allows rays to penetrate." One good test for a protective garment: If you can see through it only by holding it very close to your eyes, it has an SPF of at least 15.

Delay that walk. Rather than worry about sweating off your sunscreen, plan outdoor exercises like biking or jogging either before or after the sun's peak burning hours of 10:00 A.M. to 3:00 P.M. Even then, you should be smeared with sunscreen, since daily application should be a regular habit.

Keep a hat on. A hat with at least a 2-inch brim that goes all around your head offers good protection. "It should protect your ears and neck as well as your face," says Michael Martin, M.D., assistant clinical professor in the department of epidemiology and biostatistics at the University of California, San Francisco, and author of *How to Outsmart the Sun.*

More Ways to Hold Back Lines

In spite of the sun's significant influence on your skin's health, looking younger is not only about protecting your skin from UV rays. There are a lot of other strategies that can stop the boots of time from marching across your face.

Stop yo-yoing. Constantly losing and gaining weight can eventually affect the elasticity of your skin, says Melvin L. Elson, M.D., medical director of the Dermatology Center in Nashville. The cells in the subcutaneous-fat layer of the skin don't multiply—they enlarge. Excess weight pushes on the skin. "After seesawing for 40 years, the skin won't snap back anymore. Maintain a normal weight."

Quit smoking. Smoking is a major cause of wrinkling, says Dr. Elson. It's damaging in two ways. Constant facial movements result in lines, and a buildup of tar narrows the blood vessels that nourish the skin. The result is that the skin doesn't recover as well from injuries like sun damage.

Beware of anti-aging exercises. Exercises that promise to tone the muscles of your face are a bad idea, says Dr. Martin. "Any facial exercise has the effect that smiling does; it creases the skin over and over again in odd ways that you normally wouldn't use with facial expressions."

Stop smooshing your face. Sleeping on your stomach or side leads to facial creases, says Dr. Elson. One solution is to get a wrinkle pillow, available in many department stores. It holds your head in a certain position so that you can't roll back and forth.

Luscious Lips at Any Age

A lovely mouth is a thing of beauty. Its essential elements are smooth lips and fresh breath. Here's how to get, or maintain, both.

Flaking, cracking lips are completely preventable, thanks to a whole world of lip products that are a far cry from the waxy sticks and gooey potions of yesteryear. This new generation of lip-care options includes everything from aromatherapy oils to lipsticks with sunscreen to high-tech emollients in gel form. This means that there may be something out there to help you prevent or repair those flaking, chapped lips.

The ideal lip protector, says Charles Zugerman, M.D., associate professor of clinical dermatology at Northwestern University Medical School in Chicago, should perform four functions: create a moisture barrier, alleviate the tingling and itching of chapped lips, act as an antiseptic, and provide a sunscreen.

Sealing in Moisture

A waxy or oil base is key to sealing in your lips' moisture. It creates a barrier against cold winter air and drying summer winds, says Dr. Zugerman. Still, looking for a certain ingredient on a label doesn't always mean that you're going to get the best moisture barrier. There is no way of knowing how much of that ingredient is actually in the product, he says.

Taking Medication? Tell Your Dentist

Speak up before you open wide: Health conditions that seemingly have nothing to do with your teeth could make a difference in when and how you receive dental care. If you have any of the following disorders—or if you are under a doctor's care for some other reason—let your dentist know when you schedule your next appointment.

If you have a heart murmur, your doctor may prescribe antibiotics before treating you (or even cleaning your teeth), just in case you bleed during the procedure. Bacteria from your mouth can enter your bloodstream and affect your heart, says William Carpenter, D.D.S., of the University of the Pacific Dental School in San Francisco. And if you have an irregular heartbeat, certain medications—and plain old dental phobia—can cause a rapid heartbeat.

Some dental anesthetics can interact with high blood pressure medication to drive your pressure even higher. Tell your dentist about any medications that you are taking.

If you have diabetes and you must eat at specific times to regulate your blood sugar levels, let your dentist know that you need to arrange dental procedures around that schedule.

The best way to find a product that has a good moisture barrier is to test different ones. Fortunately, getting a decent level of emollience no longer has to take you back to those days of roll-on kissing potions or super-berry-flavored lip glosses. Nor do you have to settle for a product that has the consistency of car wax. Today, moisture barriers can be carnauba wax, beeswax, avocado oil, rose-hip-seed oil, or other natural ingredients.

Among those products that leave your lips nicely moist are the Body Shop's Honey Stick, which uses babassu-nut oil, beeswax, and candalilla wax; Kiehl's Baby Lip Balm, which contains rice-bran oil; and Physicians Formula Bare Radiance Protective Lip Shine, which has rose-hip-seed oil.

Taking Away the Tingle

Lips tingle when they're dry and chapped, which happens more easily as a woman ages. Oddly, the best solution for tingling lips may be more tingling. Ingredients such as camphor, menthol, and phenol are counterirritants, which means that as they add their pleasant tingle to your lips, you'll forget about the troublesome tingle that was there first.

On the more daring side is Advanced Lip Technologies' Lip Solution, which is a blue gel that tingles upon impact, then settles into a thin layer over your lips. Also pleasant is the Body Shop's ginger-spiced Thermal Lip Warmer (unfortunately, only available in two not-necessarily-flattering shades: chili and pink-spice), and Georgette Klinger's Lip Pomade in either stick or mini-compact form, which features a soothing dose of camphor mixed into a lightly whipped, creamy base.

When you're dealing with cracked, chapped lips, the fewer bacteria around, the better. Some lip products actually have antiseptic functions that keep bacteria in check, though they can't actually kill them. A well-known one is petroleum jelly. As with products that lock in moisture, there is no single ingredient to seek when you're looking for this action. Look instead for the "antiseptic" claim on the label.

Keeping the Sun Out

Most women worry about using a sunscreen on their lips only in the summer and don't bother looking for a lip product with sun protectors the rest of the year.

"That's a big mistake," points out Dr. Zugerman. During the winter, he says, this neglect is particularly threatening to skiers who are exposed to high altitudes on mountaintops and thus higher doses of damaging ultraviolet (UV) rays.

But even the lips of folks on lower ground are susceptible to sun damage. Lips lack sufficient melanin to protect them from damaging UV rays. Also, lip tissue is thinner than normal skin tissue, and the lips are in a prime position on your face to get burned. That means discomfort now and an increased risk of skin cancer later. It's no coincidence that most skin cancers occur on the lower lip, Dr. Zugerman says.

Though a sun protection factor (SPF) of 15 is recommended for most people, Dr. Zugerman says that it's smart for women who spend a lot of time outdoors to up the ante. Blistex Ultra Protection with SPF 30 isn't a bad idea. Other good, sheer sunblocks are Neutrogena's Lip Moisturizer with SPF 15, Revlon's Triple Action with SPF 19, and Almay's Demi-Sheer with SPF 15. If you want sun protection with a dash of color, Advanced Lip Technologies features lipsticks with an SPF 15.

Though most lipsticks produce some emollience and even sunblock (color alone usually provides an SPF 4), you will still want to coat your lips with an SPF-fortified balm and wait a full minute before applying your favorite shade of lipstick.

More Moisture?

Though many of these lip concoctions sound good enough to eat—or lick—by all means, don't. Most people lick their lips a lot, and while they might get moist temporarily, the saliva destroys any barrier against moisture loss that exists there, says Dr. Zugerman.

"The outer layer of skin works like a sponge," says Rodney S. W. Basler, M.D., assistant professor of internal medicine at the University of Nebraska College of Medicine and a dermatologist at the University of Nebraska Medical Center, both in Omaha. It absorbs water when you lick your lips but dries out and feels hard again quickly.

If you're looking for extra moisture from aloe or vitamin E, be aware that the jury's still out on their ability to moisturize. Meanwhile, if over-the-counter moisturizers don't work, and your lips are severely chapped or are burning, consult a physician. Cracks and chronic sores in the corners of your mouth usually are a sign of a yeast infection and require prescription medication, says Dr. Basler. In rare cases, he says, cracking may improve with oral doses of vitamins.

If you develop cold sores, the best thing to put on them is nothing; they'll heal best when kept clean and dry. Moisturize around the cold sore with your usual balm.

Whatever you do, you don't have to go overboard buying lots of different things, says Dr. Basler. Finding the right product is better than layering 10 not-so-good ones onto your lips.

Sweeten Your Breath

Smooth lips aren't the end of an attractive mouth. It's no surprise that garlic green beans at lunch can make your breath less than sweet later. But don't assume that opting for other spices is all you need to keep people close. Some seemingly innocuous factors can spoil clean breath. Here are some surprise situations to be aware of and some advice from Richard Price, D.M.D., spokesperson for the American Dental Association, about how you can keep your friendly, breathy "hello" from meeting a hasty "goodbye."

❖ Exercising. You huff and you puff as you pump through your workout. All that heavy breathing, though, can dry out your mouth, leaving you susceptible to odor-causing bacteria. Late-afternoon or evening workouts can escalate the problem, since you probably haven't brushed since morning.

❖ Feeling stressed. Anything that makes you really nervous may act like a hair dryer aimed directly inside your mouth. Stress may constrict the salivary glands, leaving you with a dry mouth.

❖ Snacking. Some people believe that there may be a link between foods heavily laden with sugar (sucrose) and a buildup of bad breath bacteria,

Spoon Out Fresh Breath

It doesn't have to be heirloom silver, just grab any teaspoon from your utensil drawer. Turn it upside down and scrape your tongue with it a few times. Voilà—a clean tongue—and fresher breath.

"Is a spoon really necessary if I already brush my tongue with a toothbrush?" you ask. In fact, yes. The relatively flat spoon doesn't trigger your gag reflex as the height of the toothbrush bristles does. So you can clean farther back on your tongue than you can with the bristled utensil, explains Richard Price, D.M.D., spokesperson for the American Dental Association.

although the evidence is sketchy, says Dr. Price. Certain foods, too, leave a pronounced aftertaste that can linger longer than you'd wish. Think of milk, peanut butter, coffee, or nacho chips breath.

❖ **Losing pounds.** Not snacking can be nearly as bad as snacking on the wrong things. Food and liquids keep saliva flowing in your mouth. (That's part of the reason that your breath is so bad when you first wake up in the morning—saliva sleeps when you do.)

Easy Steps to Good Breath

You don't have to stop losing weight or exercising to remedy bad breath. Follow these three easy steps and you can take your hand away from your mouth when you speak.

Clean up. You've heard it before—and there's a reason for that. A clean tongue, along with vigilant brushing and flossing, is the best defense against malodorous exhalations. Bad-breath-causing bacteria flock to the tongue's moist, nubbly surface.

Water your mouth. An overly dry mouth sends the same social signal as overly dry skin or hair. Blow off a major cause of temporary bad breath by increasing saliva production. Chew sugarless gum or suck on sugarless hard candies. Keep a cup of water on your desk or wherever you're working, and take a sip every time you pass by a water fountain.

Switch snacks. If you don't have access to a toothbrush and you have a close-encounter meeting in a few hours, you may want to skip the sugar. Munch on crispy vegetables like celery or carrots or on citrus fruits. These foods stimulate saliva production.

If bad breath persists despite these measures, see your dentist. You may have a more serious dental condition that requires professional attention.

The Updated

Brow

What is one of the biggest lifts that you can give your face, especially your eyes, short of plastic surgery? Many makeup artists vote for well-groomed and natural-looking eyebrows. Why pass up such an easy, inexpensive way to look more rested?

Brow care is not just about what you can do for your brows, but what your brows can do for you. The smallest brow detail, such as whether the outer edge points upward or downward, can make you look youthfully energetic or tired and old.

But don't start madly plucking away. First, heed the advice of Bobbi Brown, a makeup artist in New York City, who believes in enhancement of your natural, individual looks. Her tips, plus those from other experienced makeup artists, are ones we can all use to make the task less unpleasant and make the results more rewarding.

Basics for Beautiful Brows

"First, treat yourself to good tweezers," says Brown. "They should be sharp, balanced, and precise." There are two basic types of tweezers: the pincer-grip style and the scissors-grip style. For eyebrows the angled or slant-tip pincer-grip tweezers are the most popular.

"Tweezers are an investment that will last you a long time," says Brown. "So don't be afraid to spend a few dollars more, because it's worth it. I like the stain-

Deflating Under-Eye Puffiness

Although under-eye puffiness—what we commonly refer to as "bags"—generally develops with age, you may be able to temporarily relieve this problem or at least minimize it. Puffiness happens because, as you grow older, the muscles and tissues under your eyes weaken, and your lower lids fall into folds. Underlying fat pushes through the weakened muscles, and the baggy tissue balloons out.

Puffiness may also be a result of allergies or pregnancy. If the cause is allergies, consult an allergist or dermatologist to discuss how you can avoid what's bothering you. If it's pregnancy, well...you're not going to be pregnant forever.

Puffiness can be accentuated by too much salt in your diet and by sleeping on your face—two situations for which the remedies are obvious. If you're not pregnant or allergic, Mary Lupo, M.D., associate clinical professor of dermatology at Tulane University School of Medicine in New Orleans, recommends two additional solutions.

❖ Puffiness can be temporarily relieved by applying an eye gel. Gels are usually clear, and they are stickier than creams and contain less oil.
❖ Brew some chamomile tea, ice it, and put the ice-cold tea on gauze pads. Apply the pads to your eyes. Chamomile has a natural soothing action that can temporarily decrease puffiness. (Beware before you use this: Chamomile can contain allergy-aggravating pollen.)

If the temporary solutions don't work, surgery is a last-resort option. Depending on what needs to be done, doctors can remove a fat pocket or tighten a muscle.

HEALTH FLASH

less-steel precision ones with an angled tip by Tweezerman. Cheap tweezers can break the hair rather than pull it out."

Disinfect your tweezers with rubbing alcohol after each use and be careful not to drop them. This not only can dull the points (sharp tweezers can grab hair more easily) but can also throw the "arms" out of alignment.

Of course, the right tools don't guarantee the right aesthetic. Unless you know what you're doing, it's easy to end up with the perpetually surprised look of Phyllis Diller. If you're a do-it-yourselfer, keep in mind that a well-shaped brow should help you look naturally refreshed, not ridiculous. "Well-groomed brows can actually seem to change the shape of your face," says Denise Chaplin, makeup artist and eyebrow doyenne at Frederic Fekkai Beauty in New York City. "Your goal is to lift and soften your look." If you want to pluck years off your age, aim for a subtle arch to the brow. Don't try to give your brows a whole new shape by plucking.

To see where your eyebrows should begin, Brown suggests that you hold a ruler along the outer edge of your nose upward to your brow. That's where your brow should start. Then angle the ruler from the outer edge of your nostril to the outer edge of your eye. This gives you a guideline for how far your brow line should extend. The arch should be over your pupil.

Start tweezing at the center of each brow, at the point just above your pupil, and work out to the edge. Remove only the hairs on the bottom of your brow, nearest to your eyelid. Tweeze above your brow only if you have dark, coarse stragglers. Then clean up stray hairs that grow over the bridge of your nose. If your eyebrows are set close together, try creating a little distance between them. This will open the area around your eyes.

To make sure that your face looks balanced, try to make your eyebrows match perfectly. Allow their natural shapes to act as your guide. If you're unsure of your judgment, go to a professional. She can give you the clean, natural brow that you want. Then all you have to do is pluck unwanted hairs as they start to grow in.

Techniques and Tips

Plucking doesn't have to be a pain. Try these techniques to sideline irritation.

Shower, then tweeze. Tweeze your brows after a shower. That's when your pores are open, and plucking may hurt less. If you take a nighttime shower, do the plucking then since you won't be applying makeup afterward. To prevent slipping, tweeze on dry skin, says Chaplin.

Keep it germ-free. "Pluck your eyebrows after you've washed away any makeup," says Chaplin. Apply an astringent to the area to keep it germ-free. "This is both sanitary and practical as it allows you to see stragglers that might otherwise be hidden by makeup."

Brush, brush, brush. Brush your brows in the direction of hair growth and in the shape you want so that you can see where you need to tweeze. Then, pluck them in the direction of hair growth, too. Not only is this a bit more comfortable, but you also increase the chance of removing the entire hair, rather than breaking off just a portion.

Ease the pain. "To take the sting out of the process, you can numb the area with Anbesol," says Brown. "Then hold a hot facecloth over your brow to open the hair follicle a bit before plucking. Some people find that using a finger to stretch the surrounding skin also helps. Try not to pluck right before your period; your skin may be more sensitive at this time."

Don't race. "Take your time, and make sure that you're pulling out the right hair, because every hair counts," Chaplin says. "Pluck out only a single hair at a time. If you pull two hairs and they're not from the right area, you can create a hole in your brow."

Afterward, cool down. After tweezing, rinse your brows, first with water, then astringent. If there is slight swelling, cool, wet teabags placed on the area can be soothing and help reduce the puffiness. Give your brows a rest from makeup immediately afterward, as your skin may be a little sensitive. "Hang in there. The good news is that the more you tweeze, the less painful it becomes," says Chaplin.

Get a good mirror. If you're farsighted, invest in a magnifying mirror. That way, you can avoid trying to pluck with your glasses on.

Keep It Natural

You can ruin the best-shaped brow with eyebrow pencil that's too dark. "For a natural look choose a color that matches your hair color," says Brown. "For example, someone with brown hair should choose a rich brown eyebrow color. Women with lighter brown hair should choose a taupe or sable, while blondes look most natural with a light cocoa shade."

It's not just a case of color but also of technique. If you can use a brow pencil and get a natural color, great. But if it creates a harsh look, try one of the powder eyebrow colors that are applied dry but with a brush. "Women's eyebrows become more sparse with age. Brushed-on powders give a softer line," says Brown. They're especially helpful if you have a few gray hairs. "Never pluck gray hairs—that will leave a bald spot. Instead, brush over them with the powder brow shadow."

Whether you opt for a brow pencil or brush for your application, always apply color in short, diagonal strokes in the same direction that you're going to train your brows. Try using a brow gel as a finishing touch. All you have to do is comb one of these gels (the clear is the most mistake-proof) through your eyebrows in an up-and-out direction, and the hairs will stay that way all day. Clear mascara will work in a pinch. Not bad for a 30-second investment of time.

What if you've already plucked your brows into an unflattering, overplucked shape? If brows have been reduced to a thin line, let the brow hair grow back naturally. Only tweeze the hairs that grow below the browbone or over the bridge of your nose. "It takes about two weeks for hairs to start growing back," says Chaplin. "They don't all grow back at once." If you're happy with your eyebrow shape, maintain the brow's natural curve by tweezing new hairs as they grow in.

Credits

"Love, Lust, and Your Hormones" on page 14 was adapted from "Love, Lust and Hormones" by Emma Segal, originally published in *New Woman*, February 1997. Copyright © 1997 by *New Woman*. Reprinted with permission.

"Prelude to the Change" on page 23 was adapted from "Welcome to Peri-menopause: Life in Hormonal Hell" by Rita Baron-Faust, originally published in *American Health*, January/February 1997. Reprinted with permission from *American Health for Women*. Copyright © 1997 Rita Baron-Faust.

"The Pill's Surprising Health Benefits" on page 29 was adapted from "The Pill" by Teresa Carr, originally published in *American Health*, September 1996. Reprinted with permission from *American Health for Women*. Copyright © 1996 Teresa Carr.

"Estrogen and Cancer: What Every Woman Needs to Know" on page 41 was adapted from "Long-Term Hormone Therapy: Issues of Risk and Safety," which appeared in *The Hormone Replacement Handbook* by Paula Brisco and Karla Morales. Copyright © 1996 by People's Medical Society. Reprinted with permission.

"Beyond Estrogen: New Hormones on the Horizon (Melatonin: Too Good to Be True)" on page 51 was adapted from "The Bottom Line on Melatonin," originally published in *The Johns Hopkins Medical Letter Health After 50*, August 1996. Adapted with permission from *The Johns Hopkins Medical Letter Health After 50*, copyright © MedLetter Associates 1996.

"Beyond Estrogen: New Hormones on the Horizon (Estrogens of the Future)" on page 53 was excerpted from "Designer Estrogens" in the September 1996 issue of the *Harvard Women's Health Watch*, copyright © 1996, President and Fellows of Harvard College. Reprinted with permission.

"Beyond Estrogen: New Hormones on the Horizon (DHEA: Not Ready for Prime Time)" on page 53 was adapted from "DHEA: Not Ready for Prime Time," by David Schardt and Stephen Schmidt, originally published in *Nutrition Action Healthletter*, March 1997. Copyright © 1997 by the Center for Science in the Public Interest in Washington, D.C. Reprinted with permission.

"Beyond Estrogen: New Hormones on the Horizon (Prometrium: Not (Yet) Available in the United States)" on page 54 was excerpted from "Prometrium: Where Is It?" in the October 1996 issue of the *Harvard Women's Health Watch*, copyright © 1996, President and Fellows of Harvard College. Reprinted with permission.

"Beyond Estrogen: New Hormones on the Horizon (Testosterone: The "Male" Hormone That Women Need, Too)" on page 54 was excerpted from "Testosterone and HRT" in the June 1996 issue of the *Harvard Women's Health Watch*, copyright © 1996, President and Fellows of Harvard College. Reprinted with permission.

"Are You Turning Into Your Mother?" on page 59 was adapted from "To See Your Future, Look Into Your Past" by Steven Finch, originally published in *Health*, October 1996. Reprinted from *Health*, copyright © 1996.

"Relief from Fibroids—With or without Surgery" on page 110 was adapted from "Politically Incorrect Surgery" by Rita Rubin, originally published in *Health*, November/December 1996. Reprinted from *Health*, copyright © 1996.

"Escape from the Perfection Trap" on page 257 was adapted from "The Perils of Perfectionism" by Julia Califano, originally published in *American Health*, June 1996. Reprinted with permission from *American Health for Women*. Copyright © 1996 Julia Califano.

Index

Arthritis
    body mass index risk for, 219
    relief, <u>154</u>
Aspartame, as migraine trigger, 144
Asthma, 3, 5–6
Astroglide, for vaginal dryness, 50
Atherosclerosis, magnesium as protection
        from, 194
Athletic shoes. *See* Sneakers
Atypical hyperplasia, 72
Autoimmune disease, 122, <u>124</u>
AutoPap QC, 100
Avocado oil, as lip barrier, 287

B

Baby lip balm, 287
Back stretch, <u>229</u>
"Bags," under eyes, <u>292</u>
Beans, as source of fiber, 179
Bed rest, extra calcium after, <u>205</u>
Beef(Not), soy product, <u>208</u>, 210
Beeswax, as lip barrier, 287
Behavioral therapy, for panic attacks, 9
Belladonna, as sore throat treatment,
        151–52
Benzoyl peroxide, for acne, 4
Beta VLDL particle, 76
Biceps curls, *238*
Bingeing
    night, 180
    vs. snacking, 182
Biological clock, resetting, <u>168</u>
Biopsies
    breast, 69
        alternative to, 134–35
    endometrial, alternative to, 27
Birth control pills. *See* Oral contraceptives
Birth defects, vitamin A overload and, 193
Black cohosh (*Cimicifuga racemosa*)
    for cramps, 22
    for hot flashes, 49
Blackheads, 3–4
Bleeding, abnormal menstrual, 25, <u>27</u>
    oral contraceptives and, 27
    menstrual, relief from, 22
Blisters, foot, 160, 161
Blood test(s), 135, 136
    AIDS, 127
    cholesterol, 129
    diabetes, 136
    estrogen level, <u>24</u>
    fecal occult, 134
    thyroid-stimulating hormone, <u>122</u>, 123,
        126
    triglyceride level, 76, 129

Blood clots, risks of
    using with oral contraceptives, 31
    with estrogen replacement therapy, 40
Blood pressure. *See* Hypertension
Blues, outwitting, <u>256</u>
BMI. *See* Body mass index
Body changes, at menopause, <u>214</u>
Body image, 218
Body shapers, 234–45
    toning, self-esteem and, 232
Body Mass Index (BMI), 180, 218–19, <u>219</u>
Body Shop lip products, 287, 288
Bone(s)
    brittle, hormones and, 3
    density
    effect of estrogen on, <u>138</u>
        increased with oral contraceptives, 33
        test, estrogen replacement therapy, 37
    scan, 133
    tissue, impact of estrogen, <u>2</u>, 138
Bonemeal, calcium supplement, 201, 205
Borage oil, arthritis relief from, <u>154</u>
Bowel scintiscan, as diagnostic test, 135
BRCA1 gene, <u>63</u>
Breast(s)
    biopsy, 69
        alternative to, 134–35
    cancer, 44, 67, 131
        BMI risk for, 219
        estrogen, relation to, 44
        genetic predisposition to, 61, <u>63</u>
        and hormone replacement therapy,
            44–45
        oral contraceptives and, <u>30</u>, 33
        risk factors of, <u>30</u>, 45, 71
        sigmoidoscopy and, 134
        soy products and, 210
        testing for, <u>60</u>, 134–35
        walking as preventative, <u>227</u>
    dense, 69
    self-examination, 131, 132
Breath, bad, 289–90
Breathing, as stress-relief technique,
        265–66
Brow gel, shaping with, 294
Bunions, foot, 158, 160, 161

C

Caffeine
    as diuretic, 187
    impact on premenstrual syndrome, 21
    lumpy breasts and, <u>72</u>
    as migraine trigger, 144
    in over-the-counter medicine, 170
    withdrawal, headaches from, 8, 21

Dermis, 283
DEXA test, 133
DHEA. *See* Dehydroepiandrosterone
Diabetes, <u>287</u>
  body mass index risk for, 218
  dehydration and, 185, 189
  genetic predisposition for, 61, <u>63</u>
  heart disease risk in, 75
  high risk groups, <u>63</u>
  hypertension and, 107
  magnesium protection, 194
  test, 136
  prevention, <u>63</u>
  waist/hip ratio, as risk indicator, 220
Dicalcium phosphate, 201
Diet, 175, 218
  cancer prevention, 81–86
  changes, at menopause, <u>174</u>
  disease prevention and, <u>63</u>
  fruits and vegetables, 84–86
  high-fiber, <u>174</u>, 178–79
  pain tolerance with, 144
  lumpy breasts and, <u>72</u>
  migraine prevention with, <u>140</u>
  portion sizes, 178
Dieting. *See* Weight loss
  skin damage from, 285
Digital rectal exam, 133
Dilation and curettage (D and C)
  hyperplasia, 43
  perimenopausal, 25–26, <u>27</u>
Dimetapp, 170
Diuretics, dehydration and, 185
Dolomite, calcium supplement, 201, 205
Domeboro, for phlebitis, 10
Dong quai (*Angelica sinensis*), for
  menopausal symptoms, <u>47</u>
Droloxifene, 53
Dry skin, impact of hormone replacement
  therapy on, <u>280</u>
Dual energy x-ray absorptiometry
  (DEXA) test, 133
Dual photon absorptiometry test, 133
Dumbbells, 233, 236–39, 244
DV, <u>176</u>, 181

E

Eating habits, 180–81, 183, 217
Echinacea, 147, 150
Ectopic pregnancy, 32
Elder flower (*Sambucus canadensis*), for hot
  flashes, 49
Electrocardiogram, test for heart disease,
  <u>128</u>, 129

Electrosurgical vaporization, for fibroid
  tumors, <u>116</u>
Ellagic acid, 82
Endometrial ablation, for fibroid tumors,
  116–17
Endometrial biopsy (aspiration)
  for hyperplasia, 43, 44
  perimenopausal, <u>24</u>, 25–26, <u>27</u>
Endometrial cancer
  hormone replacement therapy, 41–44
  oral contraceptives and, 31–32
  sigmoidoscopy and, 134
  test for, 131
Endometrial hyperplasia, 42–43
Endometrial tissue sample, 131
Endometriosis, and oral contraceptives, 33
Endometrium, overgrowth of, 25
Energy, recharging techniques, 263–67
Epidermis, 283
ERT, 35, 40
Essential oils, as nasal congestion remedy,
  149
Estrace (Rx), 39
Estraderm patch (Rx), 39
Estradiol, 35, <u>52</u>, <u>58</u>
  impact on acne, <u>280</u>
  in triphasic birth control pills, <u>269</u>
Estratest (Rx), 55
Estrogen(s), <u>2</u>, <u>24</u>, 35, 37, 38–40, 138, <u>256</u>
  acne and, <u>280</u>
  during adolescence, 14–15
  during adulthood, 16–17
  analogs, 53
  asthma and, 5–6
  breast cancer and, 44
  bone loss and, 9, 138
  calcium and, 88
  cardiovascular risk of, <u>36</u>
  cholesterol and, 77, <u>138</u>
  gum disease and, 7
  headaches and, 8
  insomnia and, <u>4</u>
  in males, 15, 17
  memory and, <u>138</u>
  in oral contraceptives, 30–31
  patches, 35, 38–40
  during perimenopause, 25
  skin problems and , <u>280</u>
  snoring caused by, 11
  teeth and gum condition and, <u>2</u>
  in triphasic birth control pills, <u>269</u>
  wrinkles and, <u>280</u>
Estrogen-replacement therapy (ERT), 35,
  40. *See also* Estrogen(s); Hormone
  replacement therapy
Eucalyptus, as decongestant, 149, 151

G

Gallbladder disease, risk of, with estrogen replacement therapy, 40
Gamma linolenic acid, arthritis relief from, 154
Garlic, 83, 147–48
Genetic testing, 60
Georgette Klinger's Lip Pomade, 288
Gingivitis, 7–8
Glucose check, 136
Gn-RH agonists, for fibroid tumors, 117
Gonorrhea, 32
Gum disease, 7–8
Gynecologist, for Pap tests, 97
Gyne-Lotrimin, for yeast infections, 13

H

Hair, impact of hormone replacement therapy on, 280
Hammertoes, 158, 160
HDL. See High-density lipoprotein
Headaches, 8, 143. See also Migraine headache
　food triggers, 143, 144
　perimenopausal symptom, 26
Head turns, 276
Heart
　dehydration and, 186–87
　estrogen benefit for, 138
　murmur, 287
　palpitations, as perimenopausal symptom, 26
Heart attack symptoms, 74
Heartbeat, irregular, 287
Heart disease
　African-American risk of, 63
　anger and, 78
　body mass index and risk for, 219
　calcium benefit, 201
　depression and , 79
　estrogen and, 2, 36, 138
　genetic predisposition to, 63
　hormones and, 3
　iron excess and, 193
　loneliness and, 79
　perfectionism and, 258
　prevention, 39–40
　　folate, as prevention, 192
　　folic acid, as prevention, 194
　risk factors, 75–77, 78–79, 80
　stress and, 12
　vitamin E benefit, 198
　waist/hip ratio, 220

Heel, 159
　cup, 161
　pain, acupuncture for, 142
Heel raises, 240
Heel-to-toe walking, 227–29, 229
Hemochromatosis, iron overload and, 193
Herbal teas, rice cooking with, 225
HER Place, 2
Herbs, medicinal
　black cohosh, 22, 49
　calendula, 50
　chamomile, 292
　chickweed, 49
　crampbark, 22
　dong quai, 47
　echinacea, 147, 150
　elder flower, 49
　feverfew, 8
　garlic, 83, 147–48
　lady's mantle, 22
　motherwort, 21–22, 49
　raspberry leaves, 21
　rose-hip-seed-oil, 287
　St.-John's-wort, 50
　slippery elm, 50
　violet, 49
High blood pressure. See Hypertension
High-density lipoprotein (HDL), 36, 36, 39, 129, 195, 233
Hip
　exercise, 93, 242
　flexion, 248
　fractures, complications from, 132
　heel-to-toe walking and, 228, 230
　overweight and, 219–20
Hodgkin's disease, breast cancer risk, 71
Ho-ku, acupuncture, 142
Horizontal chest presses, 243
Hormone replacement therapy (HRT)
　breast cancer and, 33, 44–45
　dry skin and, 280
　endometrial cancer and, 41–44
　endometrial tissue sample, 131
　estrogen testing during, 24
　heart disease prevention with, 77
　for hot flashes, 207
　mammograms and, 42
　during perimenopause, 27–28
　during postmenopause, 31–32
　testosterone in, 52
　side effects, 41
　wrinkles and, 280
Hot flashes, 26, 38, 49, 207
HRT. See Hormone replacement therapy
Hugging, as an energizer, 267
Huntington's disease, genetic testing for, 60

Hyperplasia
   atypical, 72
   endometrial, 43, 44
   test for, 44
Hypertension, 106–9. *See also* High blood
      pressure
   genetic predisposition for, 61, <u>63</u>
   home monitoring, 104–5, 109
   magnesium and, 194
   physical fitness and, <u>103</u>
   testing for, 128, 129
   undetected, 102, 104
   waist/hip ratio, risk test for, 220
   "white-coat," 104
Hypertension Network, 106
Hyperthyroidism, 121, 122, <u>124</u>
Hypothalamus
   and estrogen, <u>2</u>, 48–49
   impact on thirst mechanism, 186
Hypothyroidism, 119
   risk factors for, 123, <u>124–25</u>
   symptoms of, 120–21
Hysterectomy, 112–13, 114, 118
   fibroid tumors and, 110, 114, 112
   sexual responsiveness and, 115–18
Hysterectomy Education and Referral
      Service (HERS), 115

I

Ibuprofen, for menstrual symptoms,
      <u>19</u>
Idoxifene, 53
Indecision, chronic, 257
Infertility, 32, 33
Insomnia, 164, 166
   hormonal change and, <u>4</u>
   perimenopausal symptom, 26
Intercourse. *See* Sexual intercourse
International Soundex Reunion Registry,
      <u>64</u>
Iron, as supplement, 193
   and calcium, 206
   in combined supplements, 192–93
   foods rich in, 21, <u>174</u>
   replacement for menstrual bleeding, 21,
      193
Irritable bowel syndrome (IBS), test form,
      135
Isoflavones, 208, <u>208</u>, 209, 210, <u>211</u>

J

Junk-food diet, avoiding, 182
Just Veggies, 85

K

Kidney disease, 194–95
Kidney stones
   calcium risk and, 206
   vitamin C overload, 198
Kiehl's Baby Lip Balm, 287
K-Y Jelly, for vaginal dryness, 50

L

Labels, <u>195</u>, 204, 288
Laboratory, for Pap test, 98–99
Lachesis
   cold relief from, 148
   sore throat treatment, 152
Lactaid milk, advantages of, 89
Lady's mantle (*Alchemilla vulgaris*)
      tincture, 22
Laparoscopic myomectomy, <u>116</u>
Lateral shoulder raises, *235*
LDL. *See* Low-density lipoprotein
L-Dopa, for sleep, 172
Lead content, calcium and, 205
Levothyroxine sodium (Rx), <u>122</u>
Light therapy, sleep disorders and, <u>168</u>
Limbic system, and estrogen, 2
Lip care, 286–87
Lip sores, as yeast infection symptom,
      289
Lithium, as risk factor for
      hypothyroidism, <u>124–25</u>
Loneliness, effects of, <u>79</u>
Low-blood sugar rebound effect, 20
Low-density lipoprotein (LDL), <u>36</u>, 39,
      <u>63</u>, <u>120</u>, 125, 129, <u>233</u>
Lp(a) cholesterol, <u>36</u>
Lumpectomy, effectiveness of, 69
Lumpy breasts, <u>72</u>, 132
Lunges, *241*
Lungs, effect of estrogen withdrawal, 5
Lupron (Rx), for fibroid tumors, 114
Lycopne (phytochemical), 82
Lying side stretches, *245*

M

"Macho hormone," 15
Magnesium, as supplement, 194–95, 202
Mammography, 67–69, 132
   getting the best, <u>70</u>
   hormone replacement therapy and, <u>42</u>
   false-negative rate, 132
   screening guidelines, 71–72

Ogen (Rx), 39
Oil glands, 3
Omega-3 fatty acids, _19_
Oral contraceptives, 27–33, _32_, 34, _280_
   mini-pill and, 31
   safety of, _30_
   "Second generation" pills, 31, 34
   sexual satisfaction with, _269_
   side effects of, 31, _280_
   "Third generation" pills, 31
   triphasic, _269_
   yeast infections and, 13
Ortho-Est (Rx), 39
Osteoarthritis, 153–57
Osteoporosis, 8–9, 39, 86, 210
   magnesium, as protection against,
      194
   oral contraceptives, as protection
      against, 33
Ovarian cancer
   genetic predisposition, 61
   oral contraceptives and, 31–32
   sigmoidoscopy and, 134
   testing for, 131
Overhead presses, _237_
Over-the-counter drugs, caffeine in,
   170
Overweight
   body area and, 219
   heart disease risk, 80
   hypertension risk factor, 108
   osteoarthritis and, 153–55
Oxalate, and kidney stones, 206
Oxytocin, 14–15
Oyster shell, calcium supplement, 201, 205

P

Pain, management, 139, 140
   acupuncture for, 142
Panic attacks, 9–10
Panty hose, for varicose veins, 12
Papnet, 100
Pap test, 96–101, 130
   estrogen level, _24_
   false negative, 95
   preparation for, _98_
   sampling errors, 97
Pelvic exam, 130
Pelvic inflammatory disease (PID), 32
PEPI, 54
Perfectionism, 257, 259, 260
   goal setting, 258
   modifying, _258_, 260–62
   personality quiz, _261_
   sickness and, _258_

Perimenopause, 24–25
   vs. premenstrual syndrome, 26–27
   decreased libido in, 21, 26
   depression rates, 27
   diet for, 28
Periodontitis, 7
Personality, basic building blocks of,
   259
Petroleum jelly, as lip barrier, 288
Phenol, for tingling lip, 287–88
Pheromones, 16
Phlebitis, 3, 10
Photoaging, 281, 283
Physical examination, estrogen
      replacement therapy, 37
Physician's Formula Bar Radiance
      Protective Lip Shine, 278
Phytochemicals, 82
Phytoestrogens, 46–47
PID, 32
Pill, the. _See_ Oral contraceptives
Pimples, formation of, 3–4
Pirbuterol (Rx), 6
Plantar fasciitis, 160
Plaque, dental, 7, 8
Pleasure points, 272
PMS. _See_ Premenstrual syndrome
Postmenopausal Estrogen/Progestin
      Intervention (PEPI), 54
Postmetabolic syndrome, 76
Postpartum thyroid problems, 125–26
Posture, heel-to-toe walking and, 228,
   229–30
Potbelly, aging and, _247_
Pregnancy
   gum disease during, 7
   and hormones, 3
   phlebitis during, 10
   under-eye puffiness, _292_
   unintended, rates of, 29
   varicose veins during, 12
Premarin (Rx), 38, 39, 55
Premenstrual syndrome (PMS), 18, 19
   insomnia and, _4_
   symptom relief, _19_, 20–22
Procrastinators, perfectionists as, 260
Progesterone, 11, _256_
   gum disease and, 7
   insomnia and, _4_
   panic attacks and, 9
   during perimenopause, 25
   premenstrual syndrome and, 19
Progestin
   and diminished sexual interest, _269_
   in oral contraceptives, 30–31
   side effects of, 43
Progressive relaxation, 9-10

Prometrium, in hormone replacement
therapy, 54
Prostaglandins, as cause of cramps, 19
Proventil (Rx), 6, 170
Prozac (Rx), 19
Pullovers, *244*
Push-ups, *234*

Q

Quantitative computed tomography test,
133
Quibron (Rx), 170

R

Racewalking, 227–29, 229
Radiation therapy, as hypothyroidism risk,
124
Raloxifene, 53
Raspberry leaves (*Rubus idaeus*), for
cramps, 21
Red wine
antioxidants in, 223
as migraine trigger, 143
Rehydration, 187–88, 190
Relaxation techniques, for panic attacks, 9
Renova (Rx), 282
Replens, 50
Resistance training, for osteoporosis
prevention, 93–94
Reverse crunch, *253*
Revlon's Triple Action lip protection, 288
Risk taking, perfectionism and, 262
Ritalin (Rx), 170
Rose-hip-seed oil, as lip barrier, 287
Rotating delivery of excitation off
resonance (RODEO), 134–35
Runner's knee, acupuncture for, 142
Running shoes. *See* Sneakers

S

St.-John's-wort, for vaginal dryness, 50
Salicylic acid, with acne, 4
Saline infusion sonohysterography (SIS),
26, 27
Salt
hypertension risk factor, 108
pills, avoiding, 189
under-eye puffiness and, 292
Scents, sleep-inducing, 167, 169
"Second generation" pill, 31, 34

Self-talk, for panic attacks, 9
Serotonin, migraine pain and, 140
17-beta estradiol, 2
Sexual empowerment, 268
Sexual incompatibility, 15
Sexual intercourse, 15, 270–71
Sexuality, exploring, 268–69
Sexually transmitted diseases (STDs) and
oral contraceptives, 33
Sexually transmitted infections, as cause
of pelvic inflammatory disease, 32
Shoes, selecting, 162–63
Shoulder blade squeezes, *277*
Shoulder raises, *235*
Shoulder rolls, 229, *276*
Shoulders, tension in, 273
Side stretch, 229
Sigmoidoscopy, 63, 134
Single-arm rows, *236*
Single energy x-ray absorptiometry test,
133
Sinuses, clogged, relief from, 151
SIS, 26, 27
Skin, 187, 281, 283
aging, 282
hormones and, 280
Sleep, 169–72, 171
activities to induce, 167–68
apnea, 164
disorders, 164
estrogen for enhancing, 138
food to induce, 166–67
inadequate, 164–65
problems, relaxation techniques for,
142–43
recovery techniques, 165
Slippery elm powder, for vaginal dryness,
50
Smoking
breast cancer and, 45
cholesterol and, 120
heart disease and, 80
hormone replacement therapy and, 42
hot flashes and, 28
hypertension risk, 108
insomnia and, 171
oral contraceptives and, 31
osteoporosis and, 90
skin damage from, 282, 285
Snacks
bad breath and, 289–90
vs. bingeing, 182
fruit, 224
Sneakers, foot problems and, 161, 163
Snoring, 10–11
disturbance of, 171–72
low estrogen and, 11

Sodium. *See* Salt
Sore throat, causes of, 151
Soy, 210
  cheese, 48
  foods rich in, <u>174</u>
  isoflavones lacking in, <u>211</u>
  menopausal symptom relief, 46–47, 207–11
  milk, 47, 48, <u>208</u>
  protein, 47
Soybeans, roasted, 208
Soy butter, roasted, <u>208</u>, 211
Spatial abilities, low estrogen and, <u>256</u>
SPF, 283–84, 288
Sphygmomanometer, 128
Spices
  as nasal congestion remedy, 148
  as weight loss aid, 224
Spina bifida, preventing, <u>192</u>
Spine toner, 94
Sports drink, advantages of, 190
Squats, *235*
Steam, for nasal congestion, 148–49
Steroid use, bone scans and, 133
Strawberries, free radicals in, 82–83
Strep throat, treatment for, 151
Stress, 11–12
  bad breath and, 289
  dogs, to calm, <u>264</u>
  panic attacks and, 9
  relief
    breathing technique for, 265–66
    stretching, *275–77*
  spouses and, <u>264</u>
Stress-management, for premenstrual syndrome relief, 20
Stretching, <u>274</u>, *275–77*
Stroke
  high blood pressure and, <u>63</u>, 102
  oral contraceptives and, <u>30</u>
  risk of, <u>30</u>
Sudafed, 170
Sun
  skin damage and, 281, <u>282</u>
  protection
    face, 284–85
    lip, 288
Sun protection factor (SPF), 283–84, 288
Sunscreen
  choosing, 283–84
  lip protection with, 286, 288
Supermilk, <u>90</u>
Supplement labels, information on, <u>195</u>
Sweating, hydrating before, 188–89
Syndrome X, 76
Synthetic supplements, label information, <u>195</u>

T

Take Care High Protein Beverage Powder, <u>208</u>, 211
Tamoxifen (Rx), 131
Tartar, gum disease, 7, 82
Teeth, care of, 7–8, 142, <u>287</u>
Tempeh soy product, 208, <u>208</u>
Testosterone, 15, 16–17
  acne and, <u>280</u>
  in females, 15, 16–17, 54–55, 138
  in hormone replacement therapy, <u>52</u>, 54–55
  in triphasic birth control pills, <u>269</u>
Tetracycline (Rx), 206
Textured soy protein (TSP), 210
Theophylline (Rx), 170
"Third generation" pill, 31
Thirst mechanism, sensitivity of, 186
ThyroChek, thyroid-stimulating hormone home test, 126
Thyroid
  reproductive problems and, 121, 124–25
  screening, for problems, 123–24
  surgery, risk factors, <u>124</u>
Thyroid Foundation of America, 121, <u>122</u>
Thyroid-stimulating hormone (TSH), 122
  home test, <u>122</u>, 123, 126
Thyroxine, thyroid hormone, 119, 121–22, <u>122</u>
Time-released supplements, label information, <u>195</u>
Tingling, lip, 286, 287–88
Toe taps, <u>229</u>
Tofu soy product, <u>208</u>, 208, 210
Tongue, cleaning, <u>290</u>, 290
Toremifene, 53
Touch, <u>267</u>
  sexual, 272
Toxicity level for
  calcium, 205
  chromium, 196
  copper, 195
  folic acid, 194
  vitamin A, 193
Transient insomnia, <u>4</u>
Transvaginal ultrasound, 131
Tretinoin (Rx), <u>282</u>
Triceps kickbacks, *239*
Triglyceride level, 40, 76, 129
Triphasic birth control pill, <u>269</u>
Tryptophan, for pain tolerance, 143–44
TSH, 122
TSP, 210
Tubal pregnancy, 32

Turkey, increased pain tolerance from eating, 143-44
Tweezers, for brow maintenance, 291, 292
Tylenol, caffeine in, 170
Tyramine, food rich in, 144

U

Ulcer, testing for, 135–36
Ultrafast computed tomography, 136
Ultrasound, as D and C alternative, 24
United States Pharmacopeia (USP), 195, 204
United States Preventive Services Task Force, 123
United States Public Health Service, 194
Urine, well-hydrated, 188
Urogenital atrophy, 35
Uterine cancer, 25. *See also* Endometrial cancer

V

Vagina, 13
  dryness, 15, 37-38, 50
  hysterectomy, for fibroid tumors, 117
Vaginal ring, 35, 37–38
Valerian (*Valeriana officinalis*), for menstrual pain, 22
Varicose veins, 3, 12
  compression hose, 12
Vasomotor symptoms, 35
Vegetable juices, as cough relief, 149–50
Vegetarian diet
  calcium for, 89
  iron intake and, 21
Ventolin (Rx), 170
Violet (*Viola odorata*), for hot flashes, 49
"Viropause," symptoms of, 17
Vitamin A, as supplement, 176, 193
Vitamin B$_6$, as supplement, 194
Vitamin C, as supplement, 197–98
  cold relief from, 147
  creams, 282
  foods rich in, 156, 176, 198
  osteoarthritis and, 156–57
  osteoporosis prevention, 92
  skin protection of, 282
Vitamin D, as supplement, 193–94
  calcium absorption and, 180
  in combined supplements, 193–94, 202
  osteoarthritis and, 157
  supermilk and, 90

Vitamin E, as supplement, 198, 174
Vitex (*Vitex agnus-castus*), irregular period treatment, 22

W

Waist/hip ratio, as heart disease risk determinant, 77, 220
Waist-strengthener exercise, 94
Walking, for premenstrual syndrome relief, 20
Water, 185, 187, 188
Weight, 180, 216–17
  gain
    aging and, 247
    at menopause, 214
  loss, 215, 217
    bad breath and, 290
    deprivation, avoiding during, 222
    cooking for, 224–25
    goals for, 220–21
    plate redesign and, 223–24
  maintenance, 220
Wet dreams, 15
Wheat bran, avoiding calcium with, 206
"White-coat hypertension," 104
Whiteheads, 3–4
Whole grains, weight loss and, 225
WOMAC pain score, 155
Worry diary, as sleep-inducing activity, 167
Wrinkle pillow, 285
Wrinkles, impact of hormone replacement therapy on, 280
Wrist strengtheners, 94

X

Xanax (Rx), 19

Y

Yeast infections, 13, 289
Yoga
  for premenstrual syndrome relief, 20
  for sinus relief, 151

Z

Zinc, 195
  calcium absorption and, 206
  cold relief from, 146–47
  in combined supplements, 195, 196, 202
  use with copper, 196